⟨ **W9-DIO-692**

---

brought to you as a service by

MSD
MERCK
SHARP &
DOHME

LEADER
IN INNOVATIVE
ANTIBIOTICS

---

the maker of
MEFOXIN® IV/IM
(Cefoxitin Sodium | MSD)
and
PRIMAXIN®
(Imipenem-Cilastatin Sodium | MSD)

Please see enclosed Prescribing Information for MEFOXIN and PRIMAXIN.

Current Therapy Series

CURRENT THERAPY

OF TRAUMA - 2

DONALD D. TRUNKEY, M.D.

Chief of Surgery
San Francisco General Hospital
Professor and Vice-Chairman of Surgery
University of California
San Francisco, California

FRANK R. LEWIS, M.D.

Assistant Chief of Surgery
San Francisco General Hospital
Professor of Surgery
University of California
San Francisco, California

1986

B.C. DECKER INC • Toronto • Philadelphia

Publisher

B.C. Decker Inc.
3228 South Service Road
Burlington, Ontario   L7N 3H8

B.C. Decker Inc.
P.O. Box 30246
Phildelphia, Pennsylvania   19103

Sales and Distribution

United States and Possessions	**The C.V. Mosby Company** 11830 Westline Industrial Drive Saint Louis, Missouri 63146
Canada	**The C.V. Mosby Company, Ltd.** 5240 Finch Avenue East, Unit No. 1 Scarborough, Ontario M1S 4P2
United Kingdom, Europe and the Middle East	**Blackwell Scientific Publications, Ltd.** Osney Mead, Oxford OX2 OEL, England
Australia	**Holt-Saunders Pty. Limited** 9 Waltham Street Artarmon, N.S.W. 2064 Australia
Japan	**Igaku-Shoin Ltd.** Tokyo International P.O. Box 5063 1-28-36 Hongo, Bunkyo-ku, Tokyo 113, Japan
Asia	**Holt-Saunders Asia Limited** 10/F, Inter-Continental Plaza Tsim Sha Tsui East Kowloon, Hong Kong

Current Therapy of Trauma - 2   ISBN 0-941158-82-9

© 1986 by B.C. Decker Incorporated under the International Copyright Union. All rights reservedd.
No part of this publication may be reused or republished in any form without written permission of
the publisher.

Library of Congress catalog card number: 85-072317

10   9   8   7   6   5   4   3   2

CONTRIBUTORS

HENRY M. BARTKOWSKI, M.D., Ph.D.

> Assistant Professor of Neurosurgery, University of California School of
> Medicine; Assistant Chief of Neurosurgery, San Francisco
> General Hospital; San Francisco, California
> *The Head*

GREGORY L. BORAH, M.D., D.M.D.

> Assistant Professor of Surgery, Division of Plastic Surgery,
> University of Massachusetts Medical School, Worcester, Massachusetts
> *Maxillofacial Trauma*

JURIS BUNKIS, M.D.

> Assistant Clinical Professor of Surgery, University of California
> School of Medicine, San Francisco, California
> *Wounds*
> *Maxillofacial Trauma*
> *Burns*

C. JAMES CARRICO, M.D.

> Professor and Chairman, Department of Surgery, University of
> Washington School of Medicine; Attending Surgeon, University of
> Washington Affiliated Hospitals, Seattle, Washington
> *The Spleen*

HOWARD R. CHAMPION, F.R.C.S.(Edin), F.A.C.S.

> Clinical Associate Professor and Chief, Division of Surgery for Trauma,
> Department of Surgery, Uniformed Services University of the Health
> Sciences, F. Edward Hébert School of Medicine, Bethesda, Maryland;
> Chief, Trauma Service and Director, Surgical Critical Care Services,
> Department of Surgery, Washington Hospital Center, Washington, D.C.
> *Triage of Trauma Victims*

RICHARD A. CRASS, M.D.

> Associate Professor of Surgery, University of California School of
> Medicine; Chief, Gastrointestinal Surgery Service, San Francisco
> General Hospital, San Francisco, California
> *Duodenum, Small Intestine, and Colon*

E. PATCHEN DELLINGER, M.D.

Associate Professor of Surgery, University of Washington School of Medicine; Attending Surgeon, Harborview Medical Center and University Hospital, Seattle, Washington
Antibiotic Use

MARTIN L. FACKLER, M.D., F.A.C.S.

Director, Wound Ballistics Laboratory, Letterman Army Institute of Research; Staff General Surgeon, Letterman Army Medical Center, Presidio of San Francisco, California
Wound Ballistics

HENRY BARRIE FAIRLEY, M.B., M.S.

Professor and Chairman, Department of Anesthesia, Stanford University School of Medicine, Stanford, California
Anesthesia

MICHAEL P. FEDERLE, M.D.

Professor of Radiology, University of California School of Medicine; Chief of Radiology, San Francisco General Hospital, San Francisco, California
Special Diagnostic Testing

DAVID V. FELICIANO, M.D., F.A.C.S.

Associate Professor of Surgery, Baylor College of Medicine; Staff Surgeon and S.I.C.U. Director, Ben Taub General Hospital, Houston, Texas
The Heart
The Esophagus

CHARLES F. FREY, M.D.

Professor and Vice Chairman, Department of Surgery, University of California School of Medicine, Davis, California; Attending Surgeon, University of California, Davis, School of Medicine and Veterans Administration Medical Center (Martinez), Sacramento, California
Pancreas and Duodenum

THOMAS A. GENNARELLI, M.D.

Associate Professor of Neurosurgery, University of Pennsylvania School of Medicine, Philadelphia, Pennsylvania
Triage of Head-Injured Patients

RUSSELL D. HANDS, M.D.

> Resident, Surgery, University of California School of Medicine,
> Davis, California

Pneumatic Antishock Garment

JAMES W. HOLCROFT, M.D.

> Professor, Department of Surgery, University of California School of
> Medicine, Davis, California

Pneumatic Antishock Garment

FRANK R. LEWIS Jr., M.D.

> Professor of Surgery, University of California School of Medicine;
> Assistant Chief of Surgery, San Francisco General Hospital,
> San Francisco, California

Prehospital Care: An Overview
Prehospital Fluid Resuscitation
Primary Assessment
Chest Wall
Hemopneumothorax
Special Problems

ROBERT E. MARKISON, M.D., F.A.C.S.

> Assistant Professor of Surgery, University of California School of
> Medicine; Chief of Hand Surgery, San Francisco General Hospital,
> San Francisco, California

The Extremities

KENNETH L. MATTOX, M.D.

> Professor of Surgery, Baylor College of Medicine; Chief of Surgery,
> Ben Taub General Hospital, Houston, Texas

The Esophagus
The Heart

JACK W. McANINCH, M.D.

> Associate Professor and Vice Chairman, Department of Urology,
> University of California School of Medicine; Chief of Urology,
> San Francisco General Hospital, San Francisco, California

Genitourinary Tract

NORMAN E. McSWAIN Jr., M.D., F.A.C.S.

> Professor, Department of Surgery, Tulane University School
> of Medicine, New Orleans, Louisiana

Victim Extrication

LAWRENCE H. PITTS, M:D.

> Associate Professor and Vice-Chairman, Department of Neurosurgery,
> University of California School of Medicine; Chief of Neurosurgery,
> San Francisco General Hospital, San Francisco, California

Peripheral Nerve
The Head

H. DAVID ROOT, M.D., Ph.D.

> Professor of Surgery and Assistant Chairman, University of Texas
> Medical School; Attending Staff and Emergency Center Director,
> Medical Center Hospital; Attending Staff, Audie L. Murphy Memorial
> Veterans Hospital, San Antonio, Texas

Diagnostic Peritoneal Lavage

RONALD E. ROSENTHAL, M.D., F.A.C.S.

> Associate Professor of Clinical Orthopaedic Surgery, State University
> of New York Health Sciences Center; Chief, Division of Trauma,
> Department of Orthopaedics, Long Island Jewish Medical Center;
> Chief of Orthopaedics, Queens Hospital Center, Stony Brook, New York

Splinting

WILLIAM J. SACCO, Ph.D.

> Associate Professor, Department of Neurosurgery, University of Virginia
> School of Medicine, Charlottesville, Virginia

Triage of Trauma Victims

RONALD D. STEWART, M.D., F.A.C.E.P.

> Associate Professor of Surgery and Assistant Professor of Anesthesiolo-
> gy/Critical Care Medicine, University of Pittsburgh School of Medicine;
> Medical Director, Emergency Medical Services Department, City of
> Pittsburgh, Pennsylvania

Airway Management

GERALD O. STRAUCH, M.D.

> Professor of Surgery, University of Connecticut School of Medicine,
> Farmington, Connecticut; Clinical Professor of Surgery, Uniformed
> Services University of the Health Sciences, F. Edward Hébert School of
> Medicine, Bethesda, Maryland; Chief of Surgery, New Britain General
> Hospital, New Britain, Connecticut

The Uterus

ERWIN R. THAL, M.D., F.A.C.S.

> Professor, Department of Surgery, University of Texas Southwestern
> Medical School, Dallas, Texas

The Neck

PETER G. TRAFTON, M.D., F.A.C.S.

> Associate Professor of Orthopaedic Surgery, Brown University Program
> in Medicine; Surgeon-in-Charge, Division of Orthopaedic Trauma,
> Rhode Island Hospital, Providence, Rhode Island

Fractures

DONALD D. TRUNKEY, M.D.

> Professor of Surgery, University of California School of Medicine;
> Chief of Surgery, San Francisco General Hospital, San Francisco,
> California

Secondary Assessment
Special Diagnostic Testing
Treatment Priorities
Force in Blunt Trauma
Torso Trauma: An Overview
Air Embolism
The Great Vessels
The Pelvis

FRANKLIN C. WAGNER Jr., M.D.

> Professor and Chairman, Department of Neurologic Surgery, University
> of California School of Medicine, Davis, California; Chief, Department
> of Neurologic Surgery, University of California, Davis, Medical Center,
> Sacramento, California

Spine and Spinal Cord

ROBERT L. WALTON, M.D.

> Professor and Chairman, Division of Plastic Surgery, University of
> Massachusetts Medical School, Worcester, Massachusetts

Wounds
Maxillofacial Trauma
Burns

RICHARD E. WARD, M.D.

Associate Professor of Surgery, University of California School of Medicine, Davis, California; Director, Transplant Program; and Vascular Lab, University of California, Davis, Medical Center, Sacramento, California

The Diaphragm

JOHN A. WEIGELT, M.D., F.A.C.S.

Associate Professor of Surgery, Department of Surgery; Director, Critical Care and Trauma Surgery Fellowship, University of Texas Southwestern Medical School; Medical Director, Surgical Intensive Care Unit, Parkland Memorial Hospital, Dallas, Texas

The Liver

RICHARD B. WEISKOPF, M.D.

Associate Professor of Anesthesia, University of California School of Medicine; San Francisco General Hospital, San Francisco, California

Anesthesia

ROBERT F. WILSON, M.D., F.A.C.S.

Professor of Surgery, Wayne State University School of Medicine; Director of Thoracic and Cardiovascular Surgery, Chief of Surgery, Detroit Receiving Hospital, Detroit, Michigan

Larynx, Trachea, Bronchi, and Lungs

PREFACE

Since the appearance of the first volume of *Current Therapy of Trauma* there have been very few changes in health care delivery to diminish the effect of trauma as a health and social issue. It is still the number one cause of death in those under 40 years of age. A white male aged 15 years has a risk of 1 in 110 of dying from a motor vehicle related injury by the time he is 30 years old. A black male aged 20 years has a 1 in 50 risk of dying from homicide by the time he is 35 years old. One in every eight hospital beds is occupied by a trauma patient. Only 1 in 10 critically injured Americans has access to a rehabilitation program. Although these statistics point out the social consequences of trauma, this book is primarily directed to the acute treatment of the trauma patient.

The present volume has been expanded substantially in scope and in authorship. The purpose is to broaden the trauma management concepts and at the same time provide opinions that might differ somewhat from our own at San Francisco General Hospital. Consistent with our original volume we have continued to provide what we consider the best treatment and have avoided alternative treatments, particularly if they are controversial. In all instances we have presented a treatment modality that will offer the best and most consistent results both in an academic and community practice.

In contrast to our first volume we have introduced a number of illustrations and tables. We have avoided references and extensive bibliography since the purpose of the book is to provide a quick reference to current treatment rather than an extensive review of the literature or alternative methods. The intent of the volume remains to present a simple, direct means of describing what we consider optimal management of the trauma patient.

We gratefully acknowledge the cooperation and forebearance of the publisher in bringing this book to fruition. We particularly wish to thank our new coauthors and our original contributors who are colleagues and members of the "Trauma Team". Finally, we must give particular thanks to the many surgical residents who have worked with us through the years. Not only did they provide most of the direct care involved in managing the severely injured patient at our institutions, they also led us to improved therapy through their questioning and skepticism of established practices.

Donald D. Trunkey
Frank R. Lewis
December, 1985

CONTENTS

TRAUMA TO THE EXTREMITIES

SPECIAL TYPES OF INJURY

PREHOSPITAL TRAUMA CARE

PREHOSPITAL CARE: AN OVERVIEW

FRANK R. LEWIS Jr., M.D.

Prehospital care services for the trauma victim have evolved largely as an extension of paramedic skills used to treat the cardiac arrest victim, though the role of these services in reducing prehospital trauma deaths or later morbidity has yet to be validated. In the case of cardiac arrest, the patient loses physiologic function relatively instantaneously, and definitive care for the arrest can be provided in the field. In the case of trauma, physiologic function is lost more gradually, and definitive care can be provided only in the hospital. As a result, the time taken in the field to provide any particular advanced life support (ALS) intervention must be critically weighed against the time it will take. If the intervention is not essential to the maintaining of life, it should not be done because time is more important. In the case of cardiac arrest, this is not true because the patient who is nonperfusing must be resuscitated on the spot to have any chance of survival.

The major causes of death in the prehospital period are severe CNS injury, exsanguination, and respiratory compromise due to either airway obstruction or mechanical disruption of ventilation. If one is to reduce the number of deaths in the prehospital period, it must be by more effective treatment of these problems. Patients with severe head injury who die in the field are, for the most part, non-salvageable even if treated. Those who have lesser degrees of injury and are treatable do not usually develop symptomatic intracranial mass lesions or cerebral edema until some minutes after their initial injury. The exception to this generality are patients who lose consciousness immediately with their injury and fail to control their airway. Such patients may suffocate, or may vomit and aspirate. It has been well shown that head injury patients are commonly hypoxic as a result of these circumstances. For the potentially salvageable head injury patients, therefore, the most effective therapy consists of controlling and protecting the airway and ventilating the patient. This can best be accomplished by endotracheal intubation and positive pressure ventilation. If endotracheal intubation has not been taught to the paramedics in a given locale, use of the esophageal obturator

1

airway may allow some degree of protection and ventilation, but it is decidedly inferior in effectiveness. The net benefit that can be expected from prehospital intubation of the CNS victim who would otherwise die is unknown, but is estimated to be at least 20 percent.

Other treatments, to reduce intracranial pressure, are hyperventilation and intravenous administration of mannitol. In long transport time systems, such therapy may be beneficial, but in the usual urban environment, they have little place, as cerebral edema is rarely a problem in less than 30 to 60 minutes. Mannitol, in particular, should be avoided as it would only exacerbate the hypovolemia that might be present in such a victim.

Exsanguination is the second most common cause of prehospital mortality, typically accounting for one-third of the total. Two modalities are potentially useful: intravenous fluid replacement and application of the pneumatic antishock garment (PASG). The arguments pro and con regarding intravenous fluid have been presented in another chapter in this section and will not be recapitulated in full here. Suffice it to say that intravenous infusions are useful only when prehospital time exceeds 30 minutes, when the bleeding rate is greater than 15 ml per minute, and when intravenous fluids are given at approximately the same rate as the bleeding is occurring.

The PASG, which is the subject of great controversy at present, has been used for at least 10 years and has achieved the status of essential tool in prehospital care. However, the critical evaluation of its usage currently fails to show any objective demonstration of its overall effectiveness, and it has been well shown to produce multiple complications. As a result, recent studies have sought to compare actual PASG usage in the field with nonusage, to see if effectiveness can be shown. Although the PASG clearly raises blood pressure in the hypovolemic patient, there is no indication that it has any impact on overall survival. Two studies have now been completed (Lewis FR, J Trauma 1982; 24:882 and Mattox et al. J Trauma 1986; 26: [in press]), and both fail to show any evidence of benefit. In one study, it was shown to contribute to a few minutes of delay in the field; in the other no delay could be shown. Its efficacy in rural prehospital trauma care has yet to be shown.

Other studies have also shown that the mechanism of action of the PASG is principally that of increasing the peripheral resistance of the lower half of the body and redirecting available blood flow to the upper trunk and head. The degree of autotransfusion that is produced is relatively minimal, approximately 200 ml. Disadvantages are (1) the ischemia that is produced beneath the garment, (2) the lack of access that results, particularly to the abdomen, (3) the restriction of motion of the lower thorax when the abdominal portion of the garment is inflated, and (4) the profound hypotension that results when the garment is deflated rapidly. It appears at the present time that use of the PASG is of no value in the urban system, whereby the patient can be delivered rapidly to definitive care, although it may have definite value in the rural setting, where transport times are longer. It is most valuable, in all cases, when the bleeding site lies beneath the garment and can benefit from the partial tamponade, as when there is a pelvic or femoral fracture.

The final cause of death is respiratory compromise owing to either direct airway problems or mechanical thoracic disruption. The major treatment for both is endotracheal intubation with positive pressure ventilation. As with head injury, the esophageal obturator airway can be substituted if paramedics are untrained in endotracheal intubation, but it must be viewed as distinctly secondary in effectiveness, and it does not produce absolute airway protection from vomiting and aspiration. Among its numerous other hazards are rupture of the esophagus or stomach and inadvertent placement in the trachea with airway occlusion and suffocation.

The benefits to be derived from endotracheal intubation, both for airway problems and for CNS injuries, would seem to mandate its inclusion in ALS skills training whenever possible. Among the various ALS skills available, its potential for salvage far exceeds that of all the others combined. Ironically it is the only one that is not routinely taught. Stewart has clearly shown that it can be taught effectively and can be practiced by paramedics with 80 to 90 percent success in placement. Since its complications would be expected to be less than for the esophageal obturator airway, there seems little reason not to proceed with its implementation generally.

The other modality that has been advocated by some for the patient with ventilatory compromise due to pneumothorax is placement of an intrapleural cannula (needle or McSwain dart) in the field. This is mentioned only to condemn it, because in my opinion, the diagnosis of pneumothorax in the field would be erroneous most of the time, and placement of the aforementioned devices would cause more pneumothoraces than they would treat. Most patients tolerate simple pneumothorax well, and it is not life-threatening. When the pneumothorax is open, the proper treatment is to effectively close it with an occlusive dressing; this usually relieves the respiratory distress produced by the open pleural communication. True tension pneumothoraces are rare in patients who are not being ventilated with positive pressure, and as a result the need for pleural decompression to save life in the field is exceedingly rare.

The final paramedic skills that are most useful in the traumatized patient are those related to fracture stabilization and protection of the spine. When fractures are obviously present with gross extremity deformity, the extremity should be gently brought into alignment while maintaining axial traction. Splinting should then be achieved with either a pneumatic splint, if available, or, if not, with whatever devices are present. For fractures of the femur, a Thomas splint with traction applied to the ankle is best.

Spinal protection should also be sought for any patient who has head injury or obvious head trauma. The cervical spine is particularly vulnerable and should be protected, unless other threats to life are present which demand more immediate treatment. It should be recognized that there are situations in which exsanguination or airway problems can cause death unless the patient is extricated, treated, and delivered to definitive care. In such situations, treatment should focus on the greatest immediate threat to the patient. It should also be recognized that most patients who suffer cervical spine cord transections do so at the moment of injury, when the forces causing displacement are greatest. The true incidence of unstable fracture without immediate cord damage is probably in the range of 10 to 20 percent, and so the hazard should be recognized. However, to allow patients to exsanguinate or suffocate because of fear of mvoing them or extending their head, is an absurdity that has been known to occur because of the overemphasis on spine protection. In stable patients, every precaution should be taken; in unstable ones whose life is threatened, the greatest threat to the patient should be treated.

TRIAGE OF TRAUMA VICTIMS

HOWARD R. CHAMPION, F.R.C.S.(Edin), F.A.C.S.
WILLIAM J. SACCO, Ph.D.

Triage refers to the classification of injured patients. The triage process was first applied by Baron Dominique Jean Larrey, Napoleon's chief medical officer. Larrey's goal was to perform surgery as soon as possible after injury. He developed the principle of sorting patients for treatment based on medical need. According to his plan, those who were dangerously wounded were treated first; the less severely injured would wait until the gravely wounded were treated.

Triage of mass casualties still involves the urgent prioritization of trauma patients, initially at the site of an accident, and later, on arrival at the emergency room. However, the triage process is more commonly applied in the daily operation of an emergency medical service (EMS) system to define a threshold of injury severity which separates the severely injured from the lesser injured.

The development of a two-tiered system for the treatment of trauma victims has resulted in this new application of the triage process. In many parts of the United States and other developed countries, the victim of major trauma can be directed into one of two systems of care:

1. Transport to the local community hospital for routine emergency department evaluation and outpatient or inhospital care. This system is appropriate for over 90 percent of patients seen in an emergency department and admitted following injury.
2. Rapid transport to a trauma center, bypassing facilities that do not have this appellation. This system concentrates technology, personnel resources, and substantial expertise into the early care of the 5 to 10 percent of patients who are at risk of dying from their injuries. It is costly, but effective.

The difference between the two systems of care is substantial. The triage decision, therefore, determines the level, pace, intensity, and cost of care, and, in certain subsets of patients, the ultimate outcome in terms of life or death.

The triage decision is based on an evaluation of the patient and a judgment of the apparent, actual, or possible severity of injury as determined by the prehospital personnel at the accident scene. It is generally held that any patient with more than a 10 percent chance of dying should be treated in a trauma center. This equates with a physiologic Trauma Score of less than 13 or an (anatomic) Injury Severity Score of more than 15. The Injury Severity Score ranges from 0 to 75 and represents the effects of multiple injuries in different body areas as scored by the Abbreviated Injury Scale (AIS).

Only a fraction of those injured each year have injuries severe enough to warrant trauma center care. For example, there are about 15.3 million automobile accidents each year involving 3.6 million injured patients. Most of these injuries are minor and many do not require hospitalization; however, in this patient population there are 160,000 severe injuries and over 25 percent of this latter population (45,000 persons per year) die. Thus, the prehospital personnel evaluating the patient at the scene of an automobile accident must identify those who need trauma center care—about 1 percent of all those involved in automobile accidents or less than 5 percent of all those injured. Likewise, there are 3.7 million hospital admissions each year for injury, but only 250,000 hospital admissions for major trauma, i.e., only about 7 percent of all hospital admissions for injury require admission to a trauma center.

Clearly, the odds are not good that patients needing trauma center care in the prehospital phase can be easily and rapidly selected in the process of triage. Further complicating the identification and sorting process is the fact that the physical evidence of lethal intra-torsal injury may not be detectable and the physiologic state of the patient immediately following injury may not have deteriorated enough to alert the health care team to the presence of significant injury.

This chapter discusses the factors that assist in prehospital and interhospital triage of patients and focuses on information that is available at the scene of the accident to indicate whether the injury is severe enough to merit trauma center care.

FIELD TRIAGE

Evaluation of the severity and nature of injuries at the scene of an accident requires an assessment of the anatomic damage that resulted from the injuring forces, as well as an evaluation of the physiologic status of the patient. Precise determination of anatomic damage is not possible at the scene of an accident. Therefore, one must seek surrogates for this level of diagnostic precision—information to indicate how substantial a force has been applied to the body. The components of evaluation that permit a reasonable assessment of injury severity will be discussed under the headings: (1) physiologic status of the patient, (2) anatomy of injury or forces applied to the body, and (3) other factors.

Physiologic Factors

There have been many attempts to use vital signs and level of consciousness information in a manner that facilitates triage decisions. The most widely applied such scheme has been the Trauma Score which, although well tested and validated, has been found by some to be too time-consuming for field application. The CRAMS score was devised as a simplification of the Trauma Score; however, the CRAMS score added another variable, physical examination of the abdomen, to be assessed in the field. Unfortunately, such examination is of dubious accuracy when performed by ambulance personnel in the field.

Physiologic assessment can be simplified for field triage. The assessments of respiratory rate (RR), systolic blood pressure (SBP), and Glasgow Coma Scale (GCS) are sufficient to characterize respiratory, circulatory, and neurologic physiologic distress. Patients with GCS less than 13 or SBP less than 90 or RR less than 10 or greater than 29 should be triaged to a trauma center. Most such patients would have more than a 10 percent chance of death. All patients, including those with normal physiology, initially should be reevaluated during transport and at hospital admission for deterioration and for other evidence of potentially significant injury. The prehospital or admission values of GCS, SBP, and RR can be incorporated into an abbreviated Trauma Score, which has a high correlation with mortality and retains the capacity of the original Trauma Score for process audit and quality assurance.

No physiologic scoring system suffices for prehospital triage of trauma victims. Patients with abnormal physiology following injury need to be in a trauma center. Many with normal physiology have lethal injuries, but have yet to experience physiologic defects. Use of physiologic assessment as a primary triage tool abets rapid identification of those at risk of dying from their injury and their prompt and rapid transport to a trauma center. This leaves a population of individuals with an initially normal physiologic status, some of whom have to be triaged to a trauma center to rule out or treat significant injury.

Irrespective of the components of physiologic assessment, provided they represent the cardiovascular, respiratory and central nervous system in a valid and structured manner as described above, they identify patients needing trauma center care with a positive accuracy of above 80 percent, a specificity of about 90 percent, and a sensitivity of above 40 percent. These are then augmented by decision rules which are intended to identify the other at-risk patients with normal physiologic status.

Anatomic Diagnosis

Actual anatomic diagnostic information can be somewhat sparse at the scene of an injury. Patients with penetrating wounds that may involve vital organs or major vascular structures are usually triaged to a trauma center irrespective of physiologic status, particularly in the case of projectile or ballistic injuries. Thus, patients with penetrating wounds to the head and neck, chest, abdomen, and groin are certainly candidates for a trauma center evaluation. Some systems exclude trauma center triage of nonballistic chest injuries lateral to the nipple line, since these injuries usually result in a simple pneumo- or hemothorax, which can be easily treated in most emergency departments.

Blunt torsal trauma is extremely difficult to accurately diagnose at the scene. Yet it is here that delayed or inappropriate therapy can often result in preventable deaths from exsanguination or increased morbidity from hypoxia and hypercarbia. Thus, prehospital personnel should give considerable attention to identifying information available at the accident scene which portends a risk of significant blunt anatomic injury to the chest and abdomen. Research has shown that patients with two or more proximal long bone fractures have twice the risk of thoracic or abdominal trauma than those with just one such bone injury.

The change in velocity that occurs when a person hits an object (or vice versa), the "Delta V" (or ΔV), has been correlated with injury severity. Significant injuries are rare at Delta Vs of less than 12 miles per hour (mph) and more common toward 20 mph. Patients whose Delta Vs are greater than 20 mph should be evaluated in trauma centers; those with Delta Vs above 30 mph have a high risk of significant trauma. The obvious problem with using Delta Vs is that they are difficult to identify at the scene of an accident. However, there is information available at the scene of the automobile accident that gives an indication of high velocity changes. This includes (1) death of another passenger in the same car, (2) significant (greater than 1 foot) intrusion of the car into the passenger compartment, (3) rearward displacement of the front axle, and (4) passenger ejection.

Factors which should be evaluated as a part of an anatomic assessment of injury are shown in the two-step triage decision rule given in Figure 1.

It should be stressed that, unlike the physiologic scores, these indicators of potential anatomic damage have not been precisely correlated with injury severity or risk of death. Nevertheless, they serve as a checklist to raise the index of suspicion and to prompt continuous close patient monitoring and detailed evaluation in patients whose physiologic status following injury is initially normal.

Other Factors in Evaluation

The mortality associated with a given severity of injury increases substantially among victims over age 55. It is generally held, therefore, that patients below the age of 5 and over the age of 55 who have a moderately severe injury should be triaged to a trauma center for evaluation. Likewise, the presence of significant cardiovascular respiratory disease should modify the threshold of severity meriting trauma center care.

ERRORS IN TRIAGE

The aforementioned components provide the basis for prehospital triage. Formulations of these components into triage decisions can reduce mistriage decisions. False-positive triage decisions incorrectly classify patients as needing trauma system care; false-negative decisions incorrectly classify patients as not needing trauma center care. Although any triage rule produces incorrect triages, concerted efforts should be made to minimize these. Unfortunately, false-negative and false-positive mistriages are interdependent. The medically desirable low false-negative triage rate is achieved at the expense of a higher, politically sensitive, false-positive triage rate. In some parts of the country, the needs of the patient prevail over institutional and physician differences.

Strong medical control in prehospital triage is desirable. Inclusion of well-trained physicians into this process may help to minimize incorrect triage decisions.

INTERHOSPITAL PATIENT TRIAGE

Interhospital patient triage sometimes occurs after admission of the patient to the receiving hospital when it becomes clear that the hospital is unable to provide promptly the level of care required by the patient. In these situations, the decision is prompted either by deterioration of the patient's condition or by an initial examination by the physician which reveals anatomic diagnoses that clearly require the focus and depth of care available in a trauma center. Interhospital triage criteria are listed in Table 1.

DISASTER TRIAGE

The factors cited as important for prehospital triage are also those used for mass casualty triage in military or civilian environments. Application of prehospital factors to disaster triage is not identical, however, because under disaster circumstances the life-saving resources may be insufficient to sustain the lives of all those in need.

Modern disaster triage often operates under a different premise from that used by Larrey, whereby medical treatment was secured first for those with the gravest injuries. Priority is given to patients who will derive the most medical benefit from treatment. That is, injured victims who will probably live even *without* treatment as well as those who probably will die even *with* treatment are of lower priority. Highest priority is given to those victims who will probably live *only* if they are treated. This triage principle is based on the need to maximize scarce medical resources by minimizing the possibility that use of these resources would be wasted on those for whom it would make no difference in ultimate survival or death.

Disaster triage, then, must identify those patients whose probability of survival can be increased significantly by medical care. A physiologic indicator of severity that is correlated with probability of survival is, thus, an appropriate adjunctive disaster triage tool. Table 2 shows the suggested relationship between the familiar disaster triage tag classifications and the Trauma Score. Some scien-

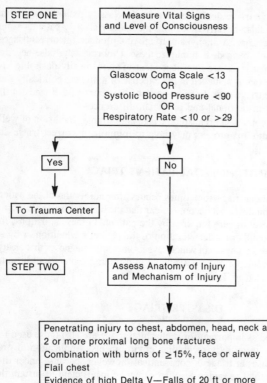

STEP ONE

Measure Vital Signs
and Level of Consciousness

Glasgow Coma Scale <13
OR
Systolic Blood Pressure <90
OR
Respiratory Rate <10 or >29

Yes

No

To Trauma Center

STEP TWO

Assess Anatomy of Injury
and Mechanism of Injury

Penetrating injury to chest, abdomen, head, neck and groin
2 or more proximal long bone fractures
Combination with burns of ≥15%, face or airway
Flail chest
Evidence of high Delta V—Falls of 20 ft or more
—Auto Delta V
20 mph or more without
restraints *25 mph* or
more with restraints
—Rearward displacement of
front axle
—Rearward displacement of
front of car by 20 inches
—Passenger compartment
intrusion of 15 inches on
patient side of car;
20 inches on opposite
side of car
—Ejection of patient
Roll over
Death of same car occupant
Pedestrian hit at 20 mph or more

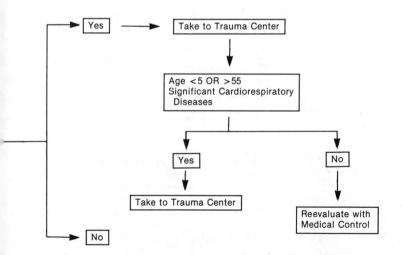

Figure 1 Triage algorithm.

TABLE 1 Interhospital Triage Criteria: Indication (any one) for Prompt Transfer to Trauma Hospital

Trauma

    Central Nervous System
        Head injury, with
            Requirement for CT scan
            Severe obtundation (GCS <10)
            Lateralizing signs
            Deteriorating level of consciousness
            Penetrating injury
            Depressed skull fracture
        Spinal cord injury
    Chest
        Wide superior mediastinum on upright chest film
    Abdomen/Pelvis
        Disruption of pelvic ring in two or more places
    Combination injuries
        Severe face injury and head injury
        Chest injury and head injury
        Abdominal or pelvic injury and head injury
        Thoracic injury and abdominal injury
    Secondary deterioration
        Respiratory failure or sepsis in combination with later onset (>24 hours) of deterioration of cardiac, hepatic, renal, or central nervous system function

Burns

    Greater than 20% total body surface
    Involving the respiratory system
    Involving the face, head, feet, hands, or perineum

TABLE 2 Relationship Between Disaster Triage Tag and Trauma Score

Tag Definition	Priority	Trauma Score
Immediate	1st	4–10
Secondary	2nd	11–12
Delayed	3rd	15–16
Deceased	4th	3 or less

tific basis to the process of mass casualty triage will minimize unschooled subjectivity under extremely difficult conditions and provide some basis for auditing the process. Again, disaster triage decisions should be made under the general direction of a physician trained in the triage process (Table 2).

VICTIM EXTRICATION

NORMAN E. McSWAIN Jr., M.D., F.A.C.S.

The extrication of a patient who is trapped in any situation requires the use of specialized tools, training, and experience. Although the most common of such situations is the automobile accident, which will be discussed in detail here, the principles and steps are the same for any extrication; only the methods differ. The details of such specialized forms of extrication as mountain extrication, aerial extrication, sea extrication, and snow extrication will not be discussed here. The reader is referred to the National Association of Search and Rescue for that information.

Automobile extrication is not removal of the patient from the automobile, but removal of the automobile from the patient. This is accomplished after first gaining access to the patient and providing initial basic medical care. The automobile parts restraining the patient are removed (disentanglement). The patient is immobilized so that removal can be accomplished without causing further harm. Extrication is required when the patient cannot or should not remove himself from his precarious situation under his own power; this description is not necessarily limited to a trapped patient. The patient cannot remove himself when he is unconscious or has severe injuries; nor can a patient remove himself if trapped because of deformation of the automobile. The patient should not remove himself when he is in danger of causing further harm to himself by the active use of his muscles. Some bending of the metal is necessary to free the trapped patient. The unconscious patient or the severely injured patient requires stabilization before removal, so that further harm is not produced during the removal process.

Extrication can be accomplished by either of two methods: (1) deliberate slower method when the initial assessment reveals that the patient's condition is stable and time is available for adequate immobilization of fractures and (2)

TABLE 1 Steps in Extrication and Initial Patient Care

Scene Survey
Access Patient
Primary Survey and Initiation of Resuscitation
Disentaglement
Stabilization of the Patient
Removal of the Patient
Reassessment and Restabilization
Transportation
Continued Reassessment and Management

a rapid removal without use of stabilizing devices if the patient's clinical condition is deteriorating and time does not permit adequate fracture immobilization and careful removal.

There are basically eight steps in extrication. Initial access to the patient must be gained. Once the patient has been reached, initial assessment and resuscitation is begun while the auto is removed from around the patient. When stabilization devices, such as backboards, can be gotten to the patient, these are applied and the patient is carefully removed from the car. After removal, the patient is reassessed, and management of critical conditions is begun as rapid transport is started (Table 1).

ACCESS

Access to the patient should be rapidly achieved by the flexibility and agility of the emergency medical technician (EMT). The best and easiest approach to the patient is through the doors of the car. Even though the door on the side of the injured patient is blocked or deformed so as to prevent access, the other doors of the car, particularly on the uninvolved side, frequently provide easy access to the patient. It is an obvious waste of time to utilize extrication tools to remove a door when easy access is provided simply by going around to the other side. Although this sounds extremely obvious and straightforward, many neophyte EMTs are overzealous and do not examine this possibility. In this modern age of prehospital care, physicians are infrequent visitors on the scene and are far more often guilty of this oversight than other members of the health-care team. The Medical Director of an EMS system should be in the field much of the time during a difficult extrication and should be experienced in the extrication process. Physicians who do not have an understanding of this process should admit it, step back, and allow EMTs experienced in extrication to do their job quickly and efficiently.

The windshield of almost all cars driven in the United States is laminated with a piece of plastic between two pieces of glass. The windshield shatters, but does not break. Because there is no penetration, this provides face protection for the occupants. However, these safety features make removal of the front windshield one of the slowest and most difficult ways to gain access to the patient (Fig. 1). Patient access via side or rear windows is usually the preferred approach, whereas patient removal is more often done through the removed doors or the roof. The agile EMT can quickly get through a small hole through which the patient cannot be easily removed (Fig. 2). The side and rear windows, because they are heat-treated but not laminated, shatter readily when struck with a sharp-pointed object, such as a fire axe. At one of the four corners, the EMT breaks the window into a multitude of small fragments that can be easily pushed in, allowing free and easy access to the patient (Figs. 3 and 4). A simple, readily available tool to shatter the glass is a spring-loaded center punch which is carried by most EMTs in their belt pouch (Fig. 5).

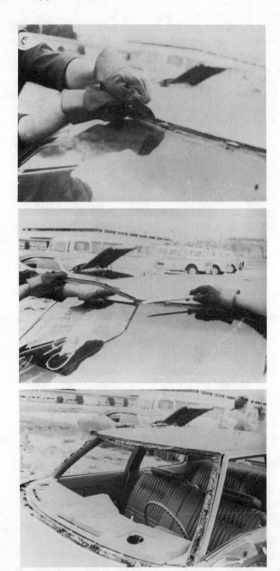

Figure 1 Removal of the windshield is a slow process. The windshield should not be used as the primary entry point unless preferred points of entry are blocked.

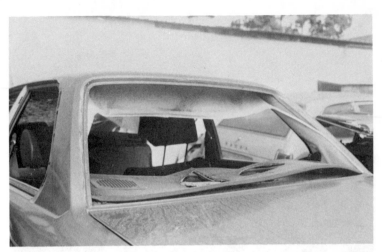

Figure 2 Access to the patient can be through a small opening, such as the rear window.

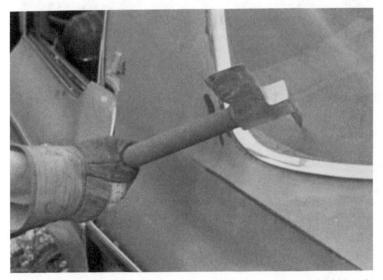

Figure 3 Fire axe or other sharp-pointed object easily shatters windows other than the windshield.

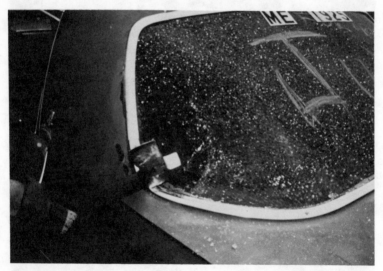

Figure 4 Hit at the corner, the window shatters. The shattered window can be easily punched in to provide rapid access.

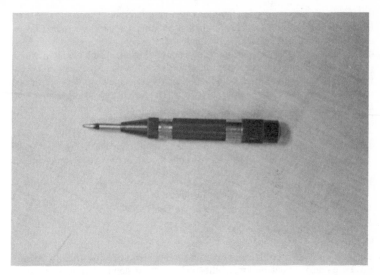

Figure 5 A simple tool to shatter windows is the spring-loaded punch, which is carried by most well-equipped EMTs.

Assessment and Resuscitation

As soon as adequate access to the patient is available, the EMT crawls to the patient, accomplishes a primary survey, establishes an airway, begins ventilation if necessary, and administers oxygen to achieve a high FiO_2 unless there is an extreme danger of fire. When the danger of fire exists, a bystander, police officer, or other EMT (if available) should have a dry-powder fire extinguisher aimed directly at the patient and the extricating EMT, whose chance of rapid exit from the auto is reduced. No attempt should be made by nontrained personnel to put out a fire with a small (5 to 25 lb dry-powder) fire extinguisher. Although this can easily be accomplished by someone with sufficient training, someone without sufficient training simply wastes time and does not protect the patient and the EMT.

After initial assessment is accomplished and resuscitation is begun (which may include initiation of intravenous therapy), the EMT carries out a secondary survey with two goals in mind: (1) to identify the injuries of the patient and (2) to determine whether any body parts of the patient are trapped and will further complicate the extrication. Further description of initial assessment and resuscitation, because it does not differ from that accomplished in the hospital or in the field with a nontrapped patient, can be found in other chapters in this text. However, this resuscitation differs from that performed in the Emergency Department in that the EMT must be welltrained and experienced to accomplish resuscitative maneuvers (e.g., starting intravenous infusions, establishing airways, placing endotracheal tubes) under the adverse conditions of the prehospital environment. Techniques differ from those used for the same procedure performed inside the hospital. For example, body position, use of the laryngoscope, and ET tube insertion are different when the patient is elevated on a roller in the Emergency Department than when he is supine in the street.

The EMT must have the judgment to distinguish between techniques that are lifesaving and should be accomplished in the prehospital period and those that are not and thus should be delayed until the patient arrives in the hospital.

Disentanglement

In a difficult extrication, there may be so much deformation of the automobile that easy access to the patient cannot be accomplished. In general, the first step is to provide a large enough portal of entry (and of exit) to allow enough EMTs to reach the patient for stabilization. The next step is to enlarge the space surrounding the patient so that backboards and other fracture-stabilizing devices can be applied in preparation for removal. A portal of exit through which to remove the patient is then created.

The first area to be investigated for the portal of exit is the doors; the second, the roof; the third, the front windshield; and the fourth, the entire roof, which is removed by cutting the two or three supporting pillars on each side.

There are basically four types of equipment used in extrication. Although there are many variations in the way that these equipment pieces are powered, they function by one of four methods: pulling, ripping, cutting, or spreading.

Spreading devices pry apart jammed or bent doors, or spread separate bent pieces of metal (Fig. 6). Pulling devices can be used to pull the seat or the steering wheel off the patient (Fig. 7). Snipping tools cut through large supporting structures, such as the "A" or "B" pillars to allow removal of the entire roof (Fig. 8). Cutting tools cut sheet metal auto parts to create holes for removal of the patient (Fig. 9).

Stabilization

While disentanglement is proceeding, the EMT who is with the patient is maintaining the airway, starting intravenous infusions, ventilating as necessary, initiating fluid replacement, and completing the secondary survey.

Rapid immobilization may then be carried out as soon as appropriate, and

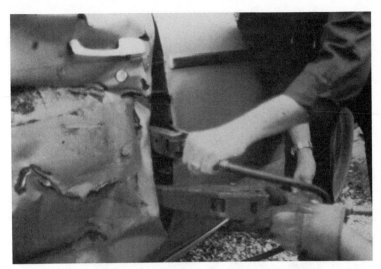

Figure 6 Spreading devices and the rescue tools move tightly bent or attached pieces of metal.

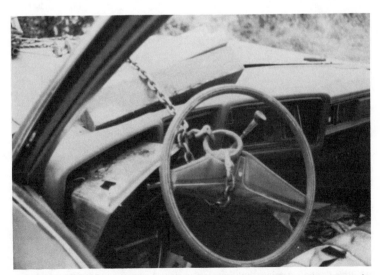

Figure 7 Pulling devices move steering wheels or seats to allow patient removal.

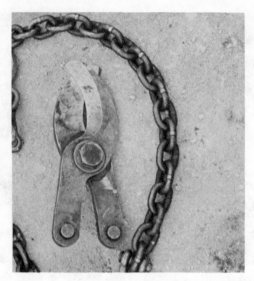

Figure 8 Snipping tools can be used to cut through large supporting pillars.

equipment can be gotten to the patient (Fig. 10). Although the hands may be used for immobilization of the patient's fractures (maintaining in-line stability or traction) during removal, this method is not so efficient as the rigid devices used proximal and distal to possible fractures in preventing undue fracture motion during complicated removal sequences.

The short backboard is the most frequently used device for spinal immobilization (Fig. 11). There are many such devices on the market that work well. The rescuer (and his Medical Director) should choose the device that most effectively stabilizes the joint above and the joint below the fracture. Thus, at least three points of the patient's body must be stabilized: the head, the thorax, and the pelvis. Failure to stabilize any of these three points constitutes failure to immobilize the entire spine, and therefore a risk of aggravating the patient's inju-

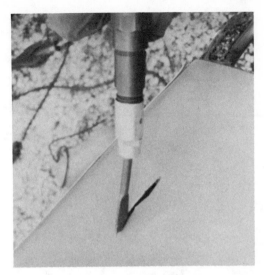

Figure 9 Cutting tools open metal sheets to form doors.

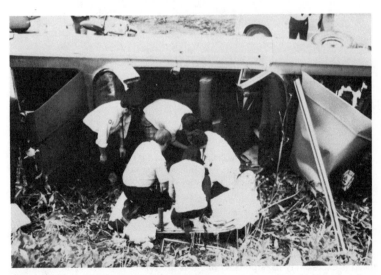

Figure 10 Immobilization on a long backboard and management of individual fractures is the ideal method of patient removal.

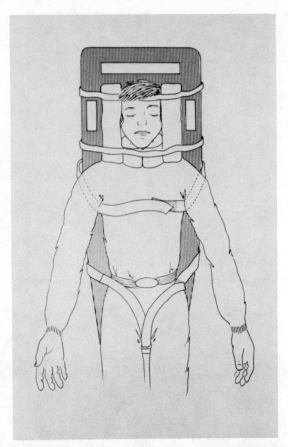

Figure 11 The short backboard is the correct device for removal from the seat. To provide proper stabilization of the entire back (lumbar spine is the most frequent spinal fracture in automotive trauma) the backboard used must immobilize the head, the trunk, and the pelvis.

ries exists. The Committee on Trauma of the American College of Surgeons has reaffirmed that use of the chin as one of the immobilization points for the head is excessively hazardous. If the jaws are forced together tightly by a chin restraint to hold the head and neck in a neutral position, the possibility of aspiration, should the patient vomit, is such a major hazard that backboards incorporating such immobilization techniques should be abandoned. Head immobilization is best accomplished by supports on either side of the patient's head to prevent rotary movement and straps to prevent anterior-posterior movement. The cervical collar has been identified in numerous articles as totally inadequate for purposes of extrication; although it should never be used alone, it is extremely useful in combination with a good backboard.

The vertebrae most commonly injured in automotive trauma are T_{12}, L_1, and L_2. These are not adequately stabilized unless the pelvis is included in the stabilization. Stabilization devices that do not provide such immobilization are inadequate.

REMOVAL

Once the patient has been immobilized on the short backboard, the entire body of the patient can be turned and allowed to slide onto a long backboard. The patient can then be lifted through a hole cut in the roof, manipulated over the seat and out the back window, through the windshield, or through the door. When time, space, and conditions permit, other stabilization devices such as pneumatic, traction, or rigid splints should be applied to possible fractures before extrication.

Reassessment

After extrication, reassessment should be rapid and continued in the ambulance enroute to the hospital.

Rapid Patient Removal

In some situations, the patient is not trapped in the car because of car damage, but because severe injuries prevent his emerging. Such injuries, as well as other conditions such as fire, cardiac arrest, and rapid deteriorating vital signs, make rapid removal imperative. Rapid removal techniques require that rescuers be well trained and experienced.

To illustrate: Assume that the patient is unconscious, severely hypotensive, and in the front seat without deformation to the automobile so that easy access to the patient exists. *EMT No. 1* gains access to the patient through the rear doors and provides in-line stabilization of the C-spine (Fig. 12). *EMT No. 2* rolls a gurney, on which is placed a long backboard, to the door. He slides the long backboard under the patient's hips (Fig. 13). *EMT No. 3* enters the car through the opposite door. *EMTs 2 and 3* rotate the patient 45 degrees against the "B"

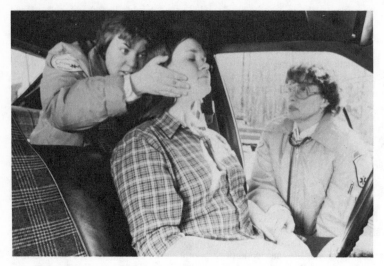

Figure 12 In-line stabilization is the initial step for rapid patient removal.

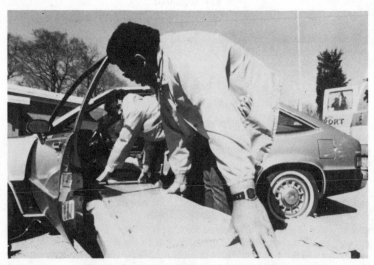

Figure 13 Long backboard moved into position.

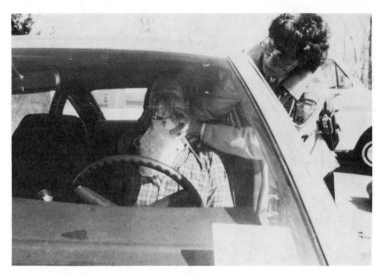

Figure 14   In-line spinal stability transferred outside the car.

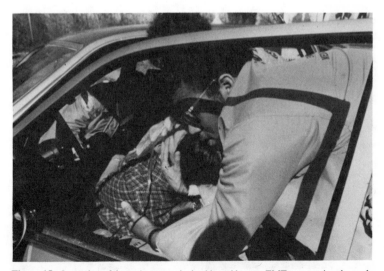

Figure 15   Lowering of the patient onto the backboard by two EMTs supporting the neck, head, and back.

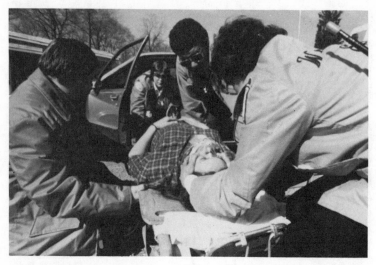

Figure 16 Movement of the patient as a unit on the backboard.

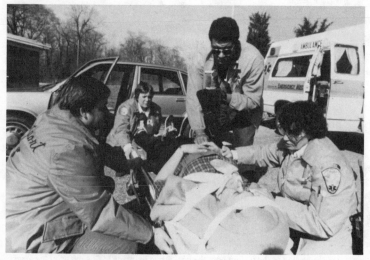

Figure 17 Stabilization of the patient to the backboard.

pillar. *EMTs 1 and 2* exchange control of the in-line stability of the cervical spine (Fig. 14). While *EMT No. 3* manages the legs and lower extremities, *EMT No. 1* then exits the car to provide stabilization of the patient's shoulders and torso. As the patient is lowered to the supine position of the backboard (Fig. 15), *EMT No. 3* is assisting by lifting the patient's hips and legs from inside the car, while *EMTs 1 and 2* move the patient onto the backboard (Fig. 16). After the patient has been moved onto the backboard and strapped to it, the patient is removed from the automobile (Fig. 17). This can be easily accomplished by well-trained and practiced EMTs in 30 to 90 seconds, as has been demonstrated and taught by the Prehospital Trauma Life Support Course (PHTLS), developed by the National Association of EMTs in cooperation with The Committee of Trauma of the American College of Surgeons.

At the scene, the bottom-line of patient care is quick assessment of the patient, rapid identification and management of the patient's needs, removal of the patient from the precarious environment as quickly as possible, provision of continued respiratory management, stabilization of fractures, and initiation of shock resuscitation during the extrication maneuvers. As soon as practicable, the patient is placed in the ambulance where other resuscitative measures, such as initiation of intravenous therapy, are carried out enroute to the hospital. When the patient is trapped, intravenous therapy should be started in the car while disentanglement is in progress. Except for the actual maneuvers necessary to bend or cut the car in order to accomplish patient removal, only under unusual circumstances should more than 10 minutes be required on the scene before transportation to the hospital. These techniques, which have been developed by the National Association of Emergency Medical Technicians in cooperation with the American College of Surgeons, are taught by the Prehospital Trauma Life Support Course.

AIRWAY MANAGEMENT

RONALD D. STEWART, M.D., F.A.C.E.P.

In the management of the trauma patient in the field, few challenges are as great as that of airway control, often under the most uncontrolled and adverse conditions. Witness the paramedic who must intubate a patient trapped under the rubble of a collapsed building, or one who has to provide positive pressure ventilation while transporting a deteriorating patient down the narrow staircase of a tenement. Combine with this the problem of avoiding undue movement of the head and neck in those at risk of cervical spine injury, and the dilemma of field airway control becomes even more evident.

Despite the controversy of "swoop 'n scoop" and the debate over the effect on outcomes of time-on-scene, few would dispute the essential nature of adequate airway control in the trauma patient. Whether it be through the simple yet important act of applying supplemental oxygen by face mask to the patient or more complex procedures such as endotracheal intubation, the airway must be attended to immediately. Assessment of the airway cannot be delayed, and securing a patent airway cannot be postponed until the ambulance arrives at the hospital. More than 15 years have passed since Frey estimated that many of the patients who die at the scene of road crashes die because of airway obstruction, and without proper roadside care, this would perhaps be true today.

The difficulty of ensuring appropriate airway care to the patient is complicated by the surroundings in which field teams must work. The basic task of adequate bag-mask ventilation, for example, is made almost impossible in the back of a fast-moving ambulance. Helicopters are notorious for their confined space and their ambient noise levels, both of which so restrict the activities of rescue teams.

To provide proper airway care to the trauma patient in the prehospital setting, the essentials of skill and experience must be combined with preparation and innovation. Our discussion will center around the basic skills needed to maintain the airway in the trauma patient, as well as a presentation of several innovations that might make for easier and safer airway maintenance in prehospital care.

EQUIPMENT

It is essential that field teams be prepared and *organized* well in advance of the need to use their skills and equipment in the care of the injured. Ready access to properly maintained equipment is essential to successful airway control because time is the crucial element in the care of the trauma patient. Proper maintenance includes the daily rechecking of equipment as well as the establishment of protocols for disinfection and cleaning.

All equipment necessary for immediate control of the airway should be contained in a lightweight, portable bag or case. Such a kit should include the following:

1. A "D" or "E" cylinder of oxygen, preferably aluminum.
2. Oxygen tubing, cannulae, and masks for administering supplemental oxygen to awake patients.
3. Oro- and nasopharyngeal airways.
4. A portable battery or manually operated suction device.
5. A demand valve (oxygen-powered resuscitator).
6. A ventilating bag-valve-mask device.
7. Equipment for endotracheal intubation. This should be further contained in a portable "apron" or "kit," which can be carried into "tight" spaces or situations.

Inclusion of a suction device is imperative, particularly for the trauma patient, in whom blood and other secretions can often lead to disastrous consequences. The airway kit used in our system is of a modular design in a durable nylon case and contains a new lightweight battery-operated suction, an aluminum "D" oxygen cylinder, and all equipment needed for endotracheal intubation (Fig. 1). This has allowed us ready access to the equipment needed to quickly manage the airway of almost any patient.

SUPPLEMENTAL OXYGEN

All seriously injured patients should be supplied with supplemental oxygen, especially if history and physical findings are consistent with chronic obstructive lung disease. A simple face mask at 6 to 8 L per minute or a nonrebreathing mask at 10 L per minute should be sufficient to prevent hypoxia in patients who are able to control their own airways.

Although it is generally understood that supplemental oxygen at a rate of at least 15 L per minute must be added to a bag-mask device, it is not equally appreciated that an oxygen reservoir must be attached to ensure delivery of a high oxygen percentage (FDO_2) from the ventilating port of the resuscitator bag. In at least six cases personally observed in the field, errors in tubing connections or equipment malfunction caused the patient to be ventilated with air (FDO_2 of 21). To alleviate the problem, it is now our practice to connect the demand valve (which delivers 100% oxygen at flow rates up to 110 L per minute) to the reservoir port of the resuscitator bag (Laerdal) (Fig. 2).

We have performed a comparative study of the various techniques of supplementing oxygen to the ventilating bag and have found that connecting the

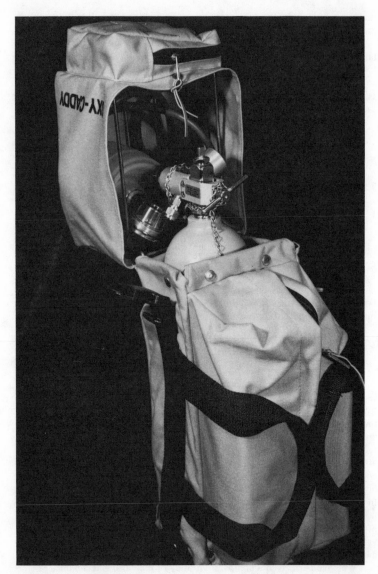

Figure 1 A lightweight kit contains all essentials for immediate field airway control: oxygen, suction, ventilating devices, and equipment for intubation.

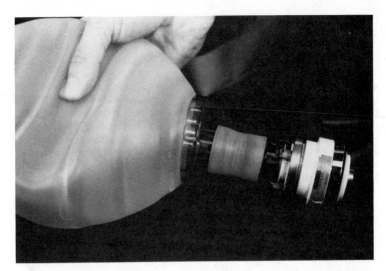

Figure 2 Connecting a demand valve ensures that 100 percent oxygen is supplied to the bag and avoids the problems posed by bag or tube reservoirs.

demand valve in this way allows 100 percent oxygen to be delivered from the ventilating port of the bag. The bag is quickly filled with 100 percent oxygen, and there is an audible "hiss" when the demand valve is triggered. Should the oxygen tank empty, the bag does not refill, and the person caring for the airway is immediately aware of the problem. When corrugated tube reservoirs are used, there is nothing to alert the clinician should something interfere with supplemental oxygen flow into the ventilating bag. Connecting the demand valve to the reservoir port of the ventilating bag eliminates these problems as well as the variables that affect the concentration of oxygen inside the bag. These include the flow rate of oxygen from the oxygen source into the ventilating bag, the possible malfunction of the reseroivr, and the "filling time" of the bag when released. We have found this demand valve to be superior to either reservoir bags or corrugated tubing.

POSITIVE PRESSURE VENTILATION

One of the most difficult tasks facing the field team is the provision of adequate positive pressure ventilation in patients who need it. Ventilation is often required in the most adverse surroundings and in the most challenging of patients. Although endotracheal intubation could be considered the solution to the problem, it is necessary to oxygenate the patient prior to placing the tube, and in such cases bag-mask devices are frequently used.

Positive pressure demand-valve resuscitators are available for use in patients, but they carry with them serious disadvantages including very high flow rates, which can lead to gastric insufflation and very high airway pressures if the devices are improperly used. Demand-valve resuscitators should not be used with endotracheal tubes because they can generate high intrapulmonary pressures. I prefer to avoid these problems and rely on careful use of the bag-valve-mask with supplemental oxygen. There are several advantages to this practice, among which is the ability to feel compliance of the lungs once the endotracheal tube is inserted. Several cases of tension pneumothorax and some cases of right mainstem bronchus intubation have been identified by field teams who detected a *change* in the ease with which patients were ventilated with the bag-mask device.

Adequate ventilation with ventilating bags appears to be a function of mask seal. Most traditionally designed face masks seem to be incapable of providing adequate seals, and our center has been instrumental in the design of a new mask, which appears to lessen the problem of mask leak (Fig. 3). In our recent mannikin studies, we found this mask to significantly reduce mask leak and to deliver better volumes. Our clinical field trials have been equally promising.

BASIC MANEUVERS

The performance of any maneuver to maintain a patent airway in the trauma patient assumes an ability to judge when the maneuver is indicated. Clinical judgment and skill in assessing the airway of a patient are therefore essential to all personnel. Even fundamental interventions that are easily performed require judgment, particularly in the case of trauma patients who have associated injuries that may worsen with movement or in instances of inept attempts at airway control.

Although not emphasized in most texts and teaching, positioning of the patient with a potential or actual airway compromise is an essential element of proper care. Although most emergency medical services (EMS) practitioners are careful to consider the possibility of injury to the cervical spine in most unconscious trauma patients, few equally emphasize measures that help to ensure adequate airway control.

The tongue is still the most common cause of upper airway obstruction even in the trauma patient, and simple measures such as the jaw thrust or chin lift are important first steps to open the airway while minimizing movement of the cervical spine. Patients who are unconscious and whose protective airway reflexes are depressed should be placed in a position that reduces the likelihood of airway obstruction and aspiration. When no adjunctive airway equipment, such as suction, is available, patients should be placed in the right or left lateral position with the upper hip and knee flexed and a pillow, blanket, or coat placed under the chest or abdomen to prevent the patient from rolling to the prone posi-

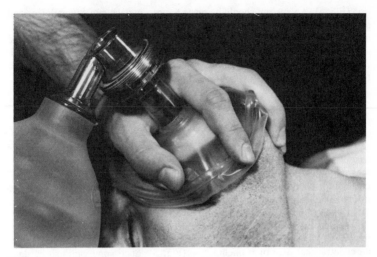

Figure 3 The SEALEASY balloon mask provides a more secure and effective seal, obliterating dead space beneath the mask and allowing easier ventilation, particularly when the patient is being moved.

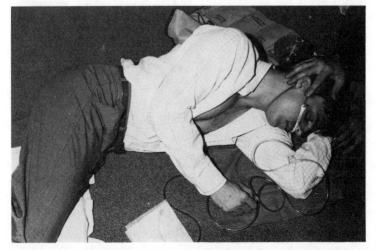

Figure 4 The lateral "COMA" position, allowing the tongue to fall forward and airway secretions to drain.

tion (Fig. 4). An attempt should be made to prevent neck movement during and after positioning, someone being assigned the task of ensuring a patent airway and limiting movement. When equipment is available, patients can be strapped solidly to a backboard and suction used to remove secretions and prevent aspiration. In the absence of suction, the lateral (coma) position is preferred in patients who are unconscious from any cause.

ADJUNCTS

Adjuncts helpful in airway management include oropharyngeal and nasopharyngeal airways, the latter of which are not used perhaps as often as they might be. Both these devices hold the tongue forward and provide an open channel for air exchange. Although these are simple to use and usually easy to insert, the choice of the correct size is important, and gentle placement is crucial to guard against dental and oral or nasal soft tissue trauma.

A recent redesign of the original Guedel airway (the Williams airway) removes the lingual surface and enlarges the central opening to allow passage of an endotracheal tube or bronchoscope (Fig. 5). Suctioning can also be done through this opening. The device can be used as a guide for blind endotracheal intubation using a curved or directional-tip endotracheal tube, a fiberoptic laryngoscope, or a lighted stylet.

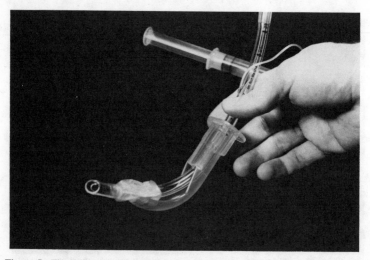

Figure 5 The Williams' Airway Intubator, facilitating suction, guided intubation, and fiberoptic laryngoscopy/bronchoscopy.

Soft nasopharyngeal airways can be especially useful in patients who have trismus or whose upper airway reflexes are not completely depressed because these are better tolerated than oropharyngeal devices. Care must be taken on insertion; the airway must be well lubricated so that the bevel can slide along the floor of the nasal cavity or against the septum to avoid getting caught on the lateral turbinates. In most cases of facial trauma, especially suspected nasal fracture, these airways should not be used.

ESOPHAGEAL AIRWAY

The introduction of the esophageal obturator airway (EOA) in the early 1970s brought hope that prehospital care personnel would now have an effective ventilating device offering the advantages of easy insertion and requiring less training to use than did endotracheal intubation. Early clinical experience with the EOA appeared to fulfill expectations, and use of the device became widespread in EMS systems.

Controversy concerning the safety and effectiveness of the device soon arose, and recent evidence in the literature has tended to dampen our original enthusiasm. Not only has endotracheal intubation been shown to be safe and effective in the hands of well-trained and medically monitored paramedical personnel, but some doubt has been cast on the ability of the EOA to maintain a patent airway with acceptable risks.

The major concern about the EOA is that it does not provide an adequate airway under field conditions. Reported complications have included esophageal lacerations in patients undergoing prolonged external chest compression. Ventilation with the device requires an adequate mask seal, and this is difficult to maintain with the present mask design. Simultaneous decompression of the stomach is possible with the esophageal gastric tube airway (EGTA), which permits the passage of a nasogastric (NG) tube through the obturator.

Recent redesign of the EGTA allows for a better mask seal by increasing the size of the inflatable cuff and may improve ventilation with the device. Suction of the oropharynx can be carried out through a small port built into the face mask.

Such improvements may make the device itself more effective, but will not lead many to accept the EOA as a substitute for endotracheal intubation. In fact, it has never been proposed as such by the physicians who developed it, although most studies have elected to compare the two methods of airway control. We have decided to teach endotracheal intubation to our prehospital care personnel and do not use the EOA except when personnel have failed to successfully pass an endotracheal tube. We are convinced that the use of the EOA and the recognition of inadequate ventilation or complications require almost as much training and skill maintenance as does endotracheal intubation.

A recent variation in the EOA, the pharyngeotracheal lumen airway (PTL airway), employs a two-tube, two-cuff system that seals the oropharynx when the cuffs are inflated. Following blind insertion and cuff inflation, the longer tube can function as an endotracheal tube or an esophageal obturator, depending on whether it enters the trachea or the esophagus. Ventilation can be carried out through the longer tube if it is in the trachea, or through the shorter pharyngeal tube if the longer tube is blocking the esophagus. Several encouraging preliminary studies have been reported comparing the PTL airway with endotracheal intubation, but much remains to be done in the form of controlled clinical trials before it can be recommended as a method of ventilating comatose trauma patients.

ENDOTRACHEAL INTUBATION

The challenge of airway maintenance in a field setting can be one of the most difficult in the care of the trauma patient. Not only can rescuers face the problem of anatomic disruption in the patient, but they are often required to carry out airway control maneuvers in some of the most adverse environments. Poor lighting, patient positioning, ambient noise, the necessity of moving the patient, and the weather may combine to make even the simplest of airway maintenance procedures prohibitively difficult. The field setting also reduces the ability of personnel to identify problems in airway control, such as inadequate ventilation, the development of tension pneumothorax, or a misplaced endotracheal tube. Auscultation is notoriously unreliable at the scene of an accident or major trauma event.

We are convinced that paramedical personnel can safely and effectively manage the airway by using endotracheal intubation in unconscious patients. However, this applies only to systems in which medical personnel work closely with physician team members who are responsible for training and ensuring skill maintenance; a program of adequate quality assurance and monitoring of personnel performance and patient outcomes must be in place. In addition, protocols for endotracheal intubation must include specific guidelines to ensure against unrecognized complications, particularly esophageal placement (Table 1).

Few will argue that endotracheal intubation is the definitive method of airway control in comatose patients. This is particularly true of trauma patients, in whom chest wall or lung injury may make difficult adequate air exchange, or in whom controlled hyperventilation may be indicated for rapid lowering of carbon dioxide and hence intracranial pressure.

Not only are field teams presented with the challenge of intubation under adverse conditions, but they are also required to perform the task in patients who may have neck injuries made worse by movement. Although the percentage of trauma patients sustaining injury to the cervical spine and the risk of creating or worsening cord damage is relatively small, the consequences are so catastrophic that each patient should be managed in the field as if a vertebral

**TABLE 1   Field Protocol for Confirmation of Tube Placement
(Pittsburgh EMS)**

1. Feel lung compliance—bag should be firm, no air leak.
2. Watch for breath condensation on tube.
3. Auscultate the following 6 sites:
   a. Right/left apical areas
   b. Right/left mid-axillary lines
   c. *Epigastrium*
   d. Sternal notch—tracheal sounds should be readily heard here
4. Feel the chest wall for movement.
5. Palpate pilot balloon*

* Triner L. A simple maneuver to verify proper positioning of an endotracheal tube. (Letter)
  Anesthesiology 1982; 57:548-549.

injury existed. Gentle in-line traction on the head with the placement of immobilization devices and the liberal use of the short board (in whatever form) helps to reduce the risk to the patient. There is some experimental evidence that standard airway control maneuvers can move the cervical spine at a fracture site. Whether this motion is clinically significant or not, we must do as much as possible to minimize such movement.

TECHNIQUES OF FIELD INTUBATION

Direct-vision laryngoscopy is most commonly used to place an endotracheal tube and many suggest that this can be done without excessive movement of the head and neck. It has the distinct advantage of affording a view of the upper airway, but blood or vomitus in the oropharynx may render it difficult if not impossible. To protect the neck of the patient, an assistant is required to hold the head firmly in a neutral position. Posterior pressure on the laryngeal prominence displaces the cords posteriorward and may make visualization easier. We as well advise our personnel to apply cricoid pressure (the Sellick maneuver) to prevent regurgitation with possible aspiration, since many patients have food in the stomach. As has already been mentioned, a strict protocol to verify correct tube placement is essential. This protocol must be applied immediately after placement of the tube and each time the patient is moved, e.g., from the floor to the stretcher or after being placed in the ambulance.

Digital (tactile) intubation, the original method of placing an endotracheal tube, fell into disuse with the invention of the laryngoscope. For several years we have conducted clinical trials of the method, first in cadavers and then in field and emergency department patients. The endotracheal tube may be used with or without a stylet. If the stylet is used, the tube is formed into an open ''J'' and the tip and balloon are well lubricated. The index and middle fingers of the gloved left hand are first slid down along the tongue, pulling it forward (Fig. 6). The epiglottis is palpated and the endotracheal tube is guided along the middle finger, using the index finger to keep the tip of the tube against the middle finger and from slipping laterally. The tip is then guided into place against the epiglottis anteriorly and the middle and index fingers posteriorly. The fingers lift forward on the tube and epiglottis as the tube is slipped distally through the glottic opening. As the cords are passed and some resistance is felt, the stylet (if one is used) is withdrawn slightly to reduce the rigidity of the distal tube and lessen the likelihood of damage to the tracheal wall.

The intubation procedure can be completed in the usual way and proper placement confirmed. The identification of correct placement of endotracheal tubes is doubly important in the case of those techniques in which placement of the tube is not done under direct vision. This technique has been reported as successful in several field trials.

The transillumination method for placement of endotracheal tubes was first suggested in the fifties and later was refined by investigators at home and abroad. For the last 3 years we have carried out studies of this method in the laboratory and operating room as well as in the field and emergency department. Our experience has led to a redesign and improvement of the lighted stylet as a device for guiding the endotracheal tube into place through the transillumination of the tissues of the neck.

Orotracheal intubation with a lighted stylet is a particularly attractive alter-

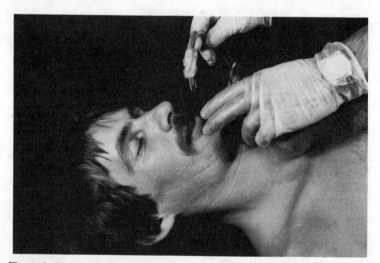

Figure 6 Digital (tactile) intubation can be useful in patients who are without airway reflexes and whose head and neck ought not to be moved.

native to the conventional laryngoscopic technique in trauma patients since the head can be kept in the neutral position with little or no movement required. The procedure is simple. The intubator kneels or stands at the left (or right) shoulder, facing the patient. Following lubrication, the lighted stylet (STAT-TUBE, Concept Corporation, Clearwater, FL) is inserted into a transparent endotracheal tube 25 cm in length, and then bent to a right, or slightly more acute, angle. After proper oxygenation and preparation of equipment, and with suction at the ready, the patient's tongue is drawn forward or the tongue and jaw are lifted. The tube with the stylet in place is then slid along the tongue and is used to lift the epiglottis and bring the tip of the tube through the glottic opening (Fig. 7A).

The position of the tip of the tube can be readily discerned through transillumination of the soft tissues of the neck; placement of the tip in the right or left pyriform fossa can be recognized as a glow lateral to the midline, whereas correct placement at or below the cords is seen as an intense glow illuminating the laryngeal prominence (Fig. 7B). Should the tube be in the esophagus, no light is seen, or a very faint glow may be visible. The transilluminated light can be more readily seen in low ambient lighting, although successful intubations have been done in bright sunlight (with some shielding of the neck) and bright overcast.

When the light is seen midline in the correct position, the tube/stylet is advanced slightly to ensure passage through the cords, and the stylet is then held firmly and steady while the tube is slipped off and into the trachea. The intubation can be completed in the usual way, with care being taken to confirm correct placement (see Table 1).

The advantages of endotracheal intubation in the trauma patient using the lighted stylet are several. First, it does not require special positioning or movement of the head and neck, and the patient may therefore be placed at less risk than with more conventional techniques of orotracheal intubation. We have performed lighted stylet intubations in patients with cervical immobilization devices in place, including C-collars and halos. Second, the technique is easier to perform in confined spaces, such as helicopters, or in the often crowded environment of the field. It is most easily accomplished from the side of the patient, and uncomfortable crouching or lying flat is not required of the rescuer.

However, the technique is essentially a ''guided'' one and direct visualization of tube placement is not possible. Care should be exercised in pulling the tongue forward, since the frenulum can be lacerated, a complication that caused us to modify the initial maneuver to pulling forward on the tongue and jaw as one.

Nasotracheal intubation is a valuable method of endotracheal tube placement in some patients but we have rarely used it in the field setting. Among its disadvantages is the fact that placement in many cases must be guided by the sound and feel of the patient's breathing, something that is not easily done in the environment of the field.

Whatever the method of endotracheal intubation used in prehospital care,

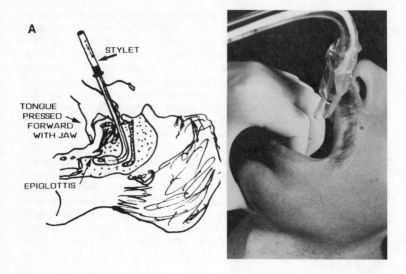

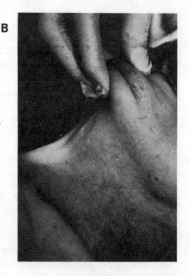

Figure 7 *A*, The lighted stylet ''hooks'' up the epiglottis and can be advanced when the laryngeal prominence is illuminated. *B*, Transillumination of the soft tissue of the neck and the lighted stylet permits easy identification of correct placement and guided passage of the endotracheal tube.

it is crucial that correct placement be ensured and the position of the tube frequently reconfirmed. This is particularly true in the instances in which blind or guided methods are used to intubate. In order to reduce the risk of the catastrophe of unrecognized esophageal placement, we have devised a protocol (see Table 1) that is to be carried out immediately following placement of the tube and every time the patient is moved (e.g., to the stretcher, into the ambulance). We consider this to be one of the most important aspects of the procedure of endotracheal intubation, particularly in the rather adverse environment of the field. In our recent study of 779 patients intubated in the field, three incidents of esophageal placement were unrecognized by the intubator (but recognized by a preceptor). In each case the protocol was not followed in its entirety. We particularly emphasize the importance of epigastric auscultation which, when combined with clearly audible breath sounds and chest wall movement, appears to be the most reliable sign of correct intratracheal placement of the tube.

TRANSLARYNGEAL JET VENTILATION

Fortunately, most problems of airway control in the trauma patient can be solved with relatively simple techniques and adjuncts. A small percentage of patients, owing either to anatomic disruption of the face or inability to pass an endotracheal tube, require access to the trachea below the level of the cords.

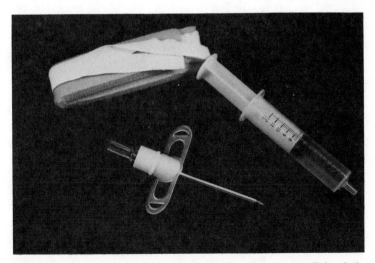

Figure 8 A 13-gauge cannula with attached manually triggered jet ventilating device, delivering 100 percent oxygen at 40 to 50 psi.

In these rare instances, I favor translaryngeal jet ventilating using a 13-gauge curved cannula with side holes, connected to a manually triggered oxygen insufflator (Fig. 8). When used with high-frequency jet ventilation, this technique provides adequate oxygenation and control of $PaCO_2$. When used with a manually triggered system at rates of 20 to 30 per minute, the 13-gauge cannula should be adequate for at least 45 to 60 minutes until high-frequency ventilation is established, endotracheal intubation is accomplished, or cricothyroidotomy is performed. With these adjuncts available, I do not advocate field cricothyroidotomy, but if these were not on hand, our resident or faculty physician on the scene would not hesitate, for the purpose of temporary ventilation, to perform cricothyroidotomy and insert a 5- or 6-mm endotracheal tube through the incision.

PREHOSPITAL FLUID RESUSCITATION

FRANK R. LEWIS Jr., M.D.

The use of intravenous (IV) fluid replacement for trauma victims in the pre-hospital period would seem to be noncontroversial; complications of IV catheter placement and fluid administration are few and costs are minimal. Unfortunately, it is difficult to start an intravenous line in a moving ambulance; as a result, paramedics usually delay transport until the IV catheter is placed. The time taken to accomplish this is poorly documented in the literature, and would no doubt vary greatly according to the skills and experience of the paramedic as well as the patient's degree of hypovolemia. Nevertheless, such documentation as does exist suggests that the average time is at least 10 to 12 minutes. (McSwain et al. Ann Emer Med 1980; 9:341; Gervin and Fisher. J Trauma 1982; 22:443; and Smith et al. J Trauma 1983; 23:317.)

There seems to be a clear tradeoff between the benefits of the IV infusion versus the extra time taken to deliver the patient to definitive care when an IV is started. If the time from scene to definitive care is less than 15 to 20 minutes, then no matter what the rate of bleeding, it will be nearly impossible to make up for the 10 minutes delay in starting the line. On the other hand, if delivery of the patient is expected to take 60 minutes, the 10-minute delay is fully war-ranted. To totally evaluate the problem, one would also need to consider the failure rate in starting an IV line in the field, which has been reported at 10 to 40 percent; again, the data are not comprehensive enough to verify this number.

Because of the multiple factors involved, we undertook to model this problem on a computer and have recently reported the results. (Lewis. J Trauma 1986; 26:[in press].) It appears from this work that when bleeding rates are either very slow (< 15 ml per minute) or very fast (> 100 ml per minute), use of an IV line is of no benefit. In the former situation the patient does not become signifi-cantly hypotensive for at least 2 hours, and in the latter he exsanguinates within 30 minutes, before he can reach definitive care in most systems. Within these limits, IV replacement is potentially beneficial, provided two other conditions are fulfilled: (1) The total prehospital time must be at least 30 minutes, and usually greater than 45 minutes, and (2) the IV replacement rate must equal the rate of bleeding, which means it must be in the range of 25 to 100 ml per minute. Available evidence seems to show that these conditions are rarely fulfilled, and suggests that prehospital systems should be monitoring IV usage more closely to see that it is omitted in a short transit time system and that, when fluids are given, they are given in appropriate amounts.

When IV fluids are administered to a trauma victim, the need for large volumes mandates a large-bore IV cannula, a 14- or 16-gauge cannula. The type with a plastic catheter mounted over the steel needle is best because it optimizes the size of the catheter that is inserted. With the type that allows the plastic catheter to be passed through the needle, the catheter that is ultimately placed in the vein has a much smaller internal diameter and in general should not be used. The catheter should be placed in an upper extremity vein if at all possible, and no attempt should be made to do internal jugular or subclavian punctures because of the danger of producing a pneumothorax. If no other venous access can be secured, the common femoral vein just below the inguinal ligament can be punctured. Because of the danger that the femoral artery rather than the vein may be cannulated in this location when patients are profoundly hypotensive, vasoactive drugs such as epinephrine should never be infused through such a line, as loss of the extremity can result from intra-arterial infusion. For IV infusion in an emergency, however, when arterial pressure is near zero, the artery works as well as the vein for infusion of balanced salt solution.

After placement of the line, it is essential to verify accurate intravascular placement by (1) lowering the bottle of infusate and noting that there is a prompt backflow of blood, (2) observing that the infusion is dripping freely, and (3) checking the site of placement to ascertain that there is no infiltration.

After placement, verification, and securing of the cannula, some form of pressure infusion is used if needed to maintain an adequate rate of fluid flow. As already noted, in the hypotensive patient with moderate-to-major blood loss, it is essential to give fluids at a rate approximating the rate of bleeding; this cannot be done with gravity infusion. At a minimum, manual pumping of the fluids should be utilized. However, it is more effective to use an inflatable pneumatic device that can be placed around the plastic bag of fluid and blown up to approximately 300 torr pressure. As this is done, the patient's blood pressure should be monitored at 5-minute intervals and the infusion rate turned down as soon as blood pressure is maintained above 90 to 100 torr.

The fluid that is used should be a balanced salt solution such as Ringer's lactate or one of the proprietary formulas that approximate human plasma in ionic composition. Normal saline should not be used since large volumes of it may cause hyperchloremic acidosis; however, it is well tolerated in volumes up to 4 or 5 liters.

PNEUMATIC ANTISHOCK GARMENT

RUSSELL D. HANDS, M.D.
JAMES W. HOLCROFT, M.D.

Use of the pneumatic antishock garment (PASG) remains controversial. Although its use is widespread and recommended, much remains to be learned about the mechanism of its effect, safety, and indications for use. In this chapter, we will outline the history of its use, the proposed physiology, indications for use, contraindications, complications, and clinical trials.

The antishock garment, also known as Military Anti-shock Trousers, MAST suit, G suit, circumferential pneumatic compression device, and external counterpressure suit, is comprised of inflatable overalls with three compartments. There are two leg compartments and one for the abdomen. These may be inflated independently. The PASG is equipped with pop-off valves, which prevent pressures from increasing to more than about 100 mm Hg. The patient is placed on the open garment and is enveloped within it; the suit is then secured with Velcro straps and inflated with a foot pump.

An inflatable rubber suit was used as early as 1903 by Crile to treat orthostatic hypotension. He later described its use in hemorrhagic shock to 1909. Those suits were complicated by troublesome air leakage and fell into disuse. The ideal of external compression was re-introduced in World War II to prevent blackouts experienced by pilots during rapid ascents. Since then, its modern medical use has been founded on many reports of external compression to treat multiple different causes of intra-abdominal bleeding. Interest in prehospital use of the garment was sparked by a report in 1971 by Cutler and Daggett on their experience in Vietnam with lower extremity and perineal blast injuries. Civilian prehospital garment use became more ubiquitous after the report by Kaplan and Civetta in 1973. They noted substantial blood pressure increases after PASG application. Since then, these easy-to-use, rapidly placed suits have become part of prehospital care throughout the United States.

PHYSIOLOGY

It is generally accepted that the blood pressure can increase after an external compression device is applied. The exact mechanism of blood pressure augmentation by PASG has been the subject of much debate. The commonly held mechanism for years was that of "autotransfusion." The idea is that suit inflation displaces lower extremity and abdominal venous blood, which in turn causes an increase in blood pressure. A figure of 750 to 1,000 ml of blood often has been quoted. Measured "autotransfusion" volumes are probably much smaller than this.

The report by Gaffney demonstrated no sustained autotransfusion effect with simple leg raising, suggesting that available leg venous volume is small. He noted an initial increase in stroke volume and cardiac output (by 8% to 10%), which disappeared in 7 minutes.

Lee, in 1983, reported the use of an in-line electromagnetic flow probe in dogs subjected to hemorrhagic shock and concluded that inflation of a pneumatic antishock garment resulted in the autotransfusion of only 4 ml per kilogram. Using radioactive microspheres, Bivens et al determined the amount of blood displaced by inflation of the antishock trousers at presssures of 40 and 100 mm Hg. This was repeated after these healthy volunteers had had approximately one liter of venous blood withdrawn. They found that less than 5 percent of the total blood volume was displaced by the antishock trousers. Goldsmith and his group compared transfusion of 750 ml of saline with PASG inflation to approximately 70 mm Hg. The central venous pressure increased (to the same level) with both maneuvers. However, the blood pressure responded only to PASG application in these healthy volunteers. Thus "autotransfusion" is not the major factor responsible for the pressure effect.

Possibly, the increase in blood pressure seen with PASG application is due to increased cardiac output. Gaffney and Thal applied pneumatic antishock garments to 10 healthy adults at pressures of 40 and 100 mm Hg in the supine and 60 percent head-up tilt position. In the supine position, the cardiac output decreased by 30 percent with PASG application. In the head-up tilt, where presumably venous pooling occurred in the legs, application of the PASG increased stroke volume 14 percent.

The effect of the garment on venous return, which must equal cardiac output in the steady state, was evaluated in baboons by Holcroft et al and reported recently. Normovolemic and hypovolemic baboons were assessed with full garment pressures. Inflation of the pneumatic antishock garment did little to augment venous return. It was noted that the driving pressure for venous return increased markedly, presumably secondary to compression of small venules under the garment. However, venous resistance was also increased. The overall effect on venous return and, therefore, cardiac output was minimal. Inferior venacavograms showed progressive narrowing of the inferior vena cava with increased garment pressures. Increases were seen in central arterial pressures only because systemic vascular resistance increased. Burchard et al recently applied the garment to postoperative cardiac surgery patients at low pressures. Although some increases of central venous pressure and of left atrial pressure were noted, there was no increase in cardiac index. Bellamy et al confirmed the autotransfusion estimate of 3 ml per kilogram using the radiomicrosphere technique. In the same paper, they assessed cardiac output and aortic pressure before and after hemorrhage of 30 percent of blood volume. Although there was no increase in prehemorrhage cardiac output, posthemorrhage cardiac output increased markedly in their swine model. They noted a minimal increase in peripheral vascular resistance. The apparently short equilibration time after hemorrhage may make the cardiac output data difficult to interpret.

It is increasingly apparent that PASG elevates blood pressure by increasing peripheral vascular resistance rather than by an "autotransfusion" enhancing cardiac output. This was demonstrated by Niemann and his group in an elegant study on dogs at various suit pressures. They found no significant difference in inferior vena cava flow during and immediately following antishock garment inflation. Cardiac output was not significantly different from control values at each inflation pressure. However, there was a significant increase in aortic pressure and right atrial pressure. They found that the peripheral vascular resistance was significantly increased at all inflation pressures. Gaffney and Thal felt that PASG acts as a "local nonpharmacologic vasoconstrictor" when they demonstrated that blood pressure increases were caused by increasing peripheral vascular resistance by 48 percent.

It is reasonable that the increase in peripheral vascular resistance is due to direct compression of the vessels of the lower half of the body. Wangesteen et al demonstrated in 1968 that the direct compression of the arterial vasculature decreased flow in accordance with Poiseuille's law. This law related flow as directly proportional to the fourth power of the radius of the vessel. Therefore, a small decrease in the radius of the artery would cause a substantial decrease in its flow and a concomitant increase in peripheral vascular resistance. It is this increase in resistance within the garment, which encompasses the lower rib cage distally to the ankles, that sacrifices blood flow to the lower half of the body to increase blood pressure and flow in the upper half of the body. In fact, increased blood flow was seen in the cardiac and cerebral circulation in Bellamy's study. Gaffney and Thal demonstrated increased forearm flow with PASG trouser application.

The increase in peripheral vascular resistance could be a pharmacologic or generalized response to PASG application. However, when forearm vascular resistance (noncompressed tissue) was measured by Gaffney and Thal, it did not increase, suggesting that the contribution to peripheral vascular resistance is one of direct compression under the suit.

What of the claims of augmented hemostasis with pneumatic antishock garment application? There have been numerous reports in the literture of increased blood pressure and presumed cessation of bleeding in such conditions as ruptured aortic abdominal aneurysm, bleeding from percutaneous renal biopsy, retroperitoneal hematomas, bleeding from pelvic fractures, bleeding from disseminated intravascular coagulation, intractable intra-abdominal bleeding, and lower body mutilation from blast type injuries. According to the law of LaPlace, circumferential wall tension is equal to the transmural pressure times the radius of the vessel. An increase in external pressure would thereby decrease the transmural pressure and therefore decrease the wall tension. This would decrease the amount of flow through the vessel laceration. As already noted, decreased flow in the vessel would result from the compression-induced decrease in vessel radius. Studies by Wangensteen and Ludewig substantiated this when they made incisions in the aortas and inferior vena cava of dogs. Control dogs bled rapidly from the surgical longitudinal incisions. With external compression in place, however, the dogs survived much longer, even when anticoagulated. The fact that the external compression affected pressure within the vessels was substantiated. Pressure transducers passed from subdiaphragmatic inferior vena cava (outside the suit) to the leg demonstrated an abrupt jump in intravenous pressure of the veins within the suit. Approximately 50 percent of the external compression pressure can be measured intravenously.

USES OF PASG

It has been recommended that pneumatic antishock garments be used on any patient with a systolic blood pressure less than 80 mm Hg or with a systolic blood pressure less than 100 mm Hg if other signs of intravascular depletion are present such as tachycardia, pale clammy skin, or peripheral vasoconstriction. Their use has been recommended in all kinds of shock except that of cardiac origin. Interestingly, although the number of patients was small, Mahoney found, in a controlled, prospective, randomized study of nontrauma cardiac arrest patients, the pulseless patients with idioventricular rhythms did significantly better with PASG application. It has been recommended that causes of hypotension other than hemorrhagic shock may be treated, such as sepsis, shock secondary to extracellular volume contraction, or shock secondary to a drug such as alpha-blockers or vasodilators.

Hypotension caused by cardiac tamponade and tension pneumothorax should be treated by decompression and chest tube placement respectively. Palafox et al noted that PASG application, including the abdominal portion, accentuated hypotension caused by cardiac tamponade and tension pneumothorax in their canine experimental model. This was presumably caused by increased intrathoracic pressures when the abdominal portion was inflated, which caused an increase in CVP and a decrease in venous return and cardiac index.

The PASG may be used for fracture stabilization. The suit, inflated to a pressure of 30 to 40 mm Hg, should satisfactorily function as an air splint to the pelvis, femur, and lower extremities.

As already mentioned, PASG has been advocated for hemostasis. This should be effective for bleeding sources within the garment. There have been questions raised regarding possible PASG-induced augmentation to bleeding above the diaphragm. The pulmonary artery has an increased diameter with PASG application which would promote bleeding from a vessel injury. This will require further evaluation.

DISADVANTAGES

Cardiogenic shock has been described as a possible contraindication, given the mechanism of increased afterload. Other contraindictions include pulmonary edema, pregnancy, an impaled object in the abdomen, evisceration, esophageal varices, and possibly traumatic quadriplegia (to be discussed). Tension pneumothorax and cardiac tamponade have been discussed in other chapters.

The garment could harm patients. Time is necessary to apply and inflate the garment. Much more time is required in deflating it. McSwain has advocated a deflation protocol that takes 20 to 30 minutes to accomplish completely. This could delay evaluation of the patient by emergency room personnel. Its presumed mechanism of diversion of blood flow from the lower body to the upper body may be harmful. Presumably, it decreases blood flow to the liver, stomach, spleen, pancreas, intestines, and kidneys. Renal blood flow has been shown to be significantly increased in hypovolemic baboons and dogs. Since normal homeostasis involves decreased blood flow to splanchnic organs during hemorrhagic shock, a further decrease in flow could conceivably cause irreversible tissue damage. Ransom and McSwain noted severe metabolic acidosis followed by hyperkalemia in dogs with trouser pressure greater than arterial pressure. Furthermore, central pH dropped dramatically after trouser deflation. Wangensteen demonstrated a substantial acidosis after suit deflation. Thus, although the only controlled study on suit pressures found no benefit for the majority of patients at low pressure inflation, high pressure may cause deleterious pH and potassium levels. Furthermore, Burchard found a significant increase in lactate levels in the postcardiac surgery patient even when low pressures up to 20 mm Hg were assessed. Very slow release of suit pressure has been emphasized. Patients who arrive in the emergency department with PASG cannot have 60 percent of their body examined. Time consuming suit removal delays assessment and treatment of injuries within the suit. Also, the saphenous veins at the ankle—reliable access sites for high-volume fluid resuscitation—become inaccessible in patients wearing pneumatic antishock garments.

SUIT PRESSURE

Further controversy surrounds optimal suit pressures. Recommendations have included inflation of the suit until an adequate hemodynamic response is achieved (i.e., a minimum blood pressure of 100 to 110 mm Hg systolic) or until the pneumatic trousers indent with firm pressure, or the Velcro straps begin to slip, or the pop-off valve releases. The latter occurs at approximately 104 mm Hg. In Wayne's prospective study, 70 percent of the patients did not respond to inflation pressures of 20 to 30 mm Hg. For those patients, inflation was continued to 60 to 80 mm Hg, i.e., when the Velcro began to slip. Approximately 30 percent of those patients improved their blood pressure at the higher pressures. He also noted that the patients that seemed to respond to the lower pressures had only mild shock. This seems to lend further credence to the theory that impedance to lower body flow is the mechanism of augmentation of blood pressure, and that is why low pressure inflation was not effective in a majority of patients.

Bellamy found an equivalent response at all inflation pressures. Gaffney found that the blood pressure increase was only 8 mm Hg at 40 mm Hg suit inflation pressures, whereas there was a 21 mm Hg increase in blood pressure at full suit inflation (100 mm Hg). His ten healthy volunteers all noted abdominal discomfort and pain beneath the suit at 100 mm Hg inflation pressure. Niemann et al could not demonstrate a change in interior vena cava flow and cardiac output with PASG from the control dogs at any pressure. They did note that garment inflation significantly increased peripheral vascular resistance and that aortic pressure and peripheral vascular resistance correlated significantly. Therefore, given that the blood pressure response seems to be derived mainly from an increase in peripheral vascular resistance, higher suit pressure is necessary for the best possible blood pressure response. However, the higher suit pressures are more dangerous for the patient.

Although there has been some discussion regarding the sequence of suit inflation, Hanke and Bivins recently demonstrated no difference between simultaneous and sequential inflation of the suit. Using radioisotope scans on 10 healthy male volunteers at pressures of 10, 40, and 100 mm Hg, they confirmed that approximately 200 ml of blood is displaced and that only occurred at pressures of 40 and 100 mm Hg. They suggested low pressure inflation first to see whether clinical response occurs. If the patient does not respond, they then suggest full pressure inflation. They believe that all suits should be equipped with gauges so that the pressures can be documented in all patients.

Sanders and Meislin have shown that intrasuit pressure increases almost threefold as the altitude changes from 2,500 to 9,500 feet. They have also shown that each increase of 1 degree centigrade in temperature increases the intrasuit pressure approximately 1 mm Hg.

SUIT DEFLATION

The deflating of PASG can lead to sudden hypotension. This can be dramatic and irreversible, even with reinflation of the suit, presumably because of the sudden decrease in peripheral resistance that was caused by suit deflation, as well as peripheral vasodilatation under the suit due to acidosis. It has been recommended that satisfactory intravenous volume be replaced prior to suit removal. Furthermore, if surgery is anticipated immediately, it has been suggested that suit deflation should be deferred until after the induction of anesthesia. Of course, this would require an operation to be performed on a patient who has not had his lower body examined.

McSwain outlines a technique for careful deflation in which blood pressure is monitored during gradual deflation of the abdominal portion and then the leg portion. For each 5 mm Hg drop in systolic blood pressure, he recommends that deflation be stopped and additional IV fluid be administered. He suggests that 20 or 30 minutes may be required for this deflation procedure.

COMPLICATIONS OF PASG USE

Numerous complications have been attributed to PASG use, namely skin necrosis beneath the garment, compartment syndrome, intracranial pressure increases, alterations of respiratory function, and possible renal alterations.

Wayne and MacDonald assessed 821 patients and found no evidence of compartment syndrome. However, they did note ischemic skin changes in 33 patients or 4 percent. It would make sense that prolonged application of pneumatic antishock garments at high pressures would lead to ischemic changes beneath the garment. Chisholm and Clark used the Wick catheter method on healthy volunteers and found that approximately 90 percent of the externally applied pressure was transmitted to the muscle compartments. All subjects developed intramuscular pressures greater than 50 mm Hg at 60 mm Hg suit inflation. Hypotensive patients could have compartment pressures well exceeding arterial pressure. The garment may increase the incidence of deep venous thrombosis. There are reports of compartment syndrome resulting in amputation in trauma patients without lower extremity trauma. In short-term urban uses, this would probably be of little consequence. However, if long transport times are anticipated, or if the garment is used for hemostasis for several hours, low pressures would be prudent.

Experimental evidence indicates that pneumatic antishock garments probably have little detrimental effect on intracranial pressure. Palafox induced experimental intracranial lesions in hemorrhagic dogs and found that intracranial pressures were increased with PASG application. If the function of the suit is to increase upper body perfusion at the expense of lower body perfusion, cerebral perfusion pressures may be augmented with the use of the PASG.

The increase in intra-abdominal pressure caused by the abdominal portion of the PASG probably limits inspiration. Burchard noted a statistically significant increase in peak respiratory pressures of the mechanically ventilated patients he studied even though the suit pressure was only a maximum of 20 mm Hg. Espinoza noted that many patients would complain of dyspnea on inflation of the G suit. In healthy volunteers, he found an 18 percent reduction in vital capacity. The G suit encompassed the upper abdomen as well; however, modern suits could cause decreased respiratory excursions by the same mechanisms. McCabe found a 5 percent reduction in vital capacity in healthy volunteers using shock trousers. Increased intra-abdominal pressure could lead to emesis and possibly aspiration. Shenasky and Gillinwater showed a statistically significant increase in respiratory acidosis and CO_2 retention with suit inflation. This was reversible with deflation. Gilbert demonstrated marked Pco_2 elevation with PASG in traumatic quadriplegia. Lee et al found that Pco_2 was elevated significantly with the antishock trouser inflation as well. Therefore, PASG probably causes some degree of resistance to respiratory effort and should be monitored carefully in patients with spinal cord injuries and depressed consciousness.

Controlled clinical evaluation of the pneumatic antishock garment effect on renal function is lacking. A decreased renal plasma flow in the baboon has been demonstrated. External counterpressure caused significant decreases in renal blood flow, glomerular filtration rate, and urine output in dogs. More studies are warranted.

CONTROLLED CLINICAL STUDIES

Two controlled clinical studies evaluated the effect of standard prehospital care as compared to the addition of PASG application. MacKersie, Christensen, and Lewis recently assessed over 200 patients retrospectively in San Francisco. They evaluated trauma scores, which take into account respiratory function, blood pressure, and the Glasgow coma scale as well as blood pressure index. The patients were well matched regarding injury, average time in field, and transport time. The success rate for intravenous line placement was similar in both groups, approximately 85 percent. PASG did not appear to enhance the intravenous line placement success rate. In this study of short urban transit time, there was no demonstrable beneficial effect of PASG on trauma score, blood pressure index, or mortality. There was no apparent advantage to field use of PASG in fully arrested patients. PASG did not delay transport. There was no advantage of using PASG in addition to conventional in-field treatment.

A prospective, randomized assessment of PASG in trauma patients was reported recently by Bickel et al. They evaluated the trauma score of the patient in the field as compared to the trauma score as determined by the evaluating physician in the emergency room. Both groups, control and PASG-treated groups, were well matched for types of injuries and response time. Treatment differed only in whether or not PASG was used. Each group received approximately 650 ml intravenous fluid during transport. They used full 105 mm Hg PASG inflation to allow maximal effect. Although there was a small increase in the trauma score from the field to the emergency room in both groups, there was no statistical difference between the control group and the group treated with PASG. Mortality was not assessed. Thus, the only prospective study of PASG use on trauma patients has shown no benefit to patients.

SUGGESTED READING

Bellamy RF, Leonides R, DeGuzman R, Pedersen DC. Immediate hemodynamic consequences of MAST inflation in normo- and hypovolemic anesthetized swine. J Trauma 1984; 24:889–895.

Bickel WH, Pepe PE, Wyatt CH, Dedo WR, Appelbaum DJ, Black C, Mattox KL. Effect of antishock trousers in trauma score: A prospective analysis in the urban setting. Ann Emerg Med 1985; 14:208–222.

Cutler BS, Daggett WM. Application of G-suit to control hemorrhage and massive trauma. Ann Surg 1971; 173:511–514.

Holcroft JW, Link DP, Lantz BMT, Green JS, Weber CJ. Venous return in the antishock garment in hypovolemic baboons. J Trauma 1984; 24:928–937.

Mackersie RC, Christensen JM, Lewis FR. The pre-hospital use of counterpressure: Does MAST make a difference? J Trauma 1984; 24:882–888.

SPLINTING

RONALD E. ROSENTHAL, M.D., F.A.C.S.

The goal of splinting is immobilization of the injured part, and this immobilization can be accomplished in many ways, with many different devices. A properly applied splint can accomplish a great deal in the early management of the injured patient: it helps to alleviate pain; decreases tissue injury, bleeding, and contamination in an open wound; and simplifies transportation. It also helps to realign fractured extremities and minimizes the risk of further injury to skin and deeper structures.

A well-padded splint must be applied carefully. This can be a time-consuming process that usually requires more than one person to accomplish; it should not be rushed. Extremity injuries in themselves are rarely life-threatening, and there is usually time for adequate evaluation of the patient in the field and application of the necessary splints. However, a severely injured patient with unobtainable vital signs may be brought into the emergency department without any splints at all if the emergency service medical back-up team feels it is important to transport him rapidly.

With the exception of the patient with unobtainable vital signs, facing imminent death from intra-abdominal exsanguination, splinting of all obvious and suspected extremity injuries should be part of the emergency care and transportation of the injured patient.

GENERAL PRINCIPLES OF IMMOBILIZATION

Splinting should be carried out as soon as a suspected extremity injury is identified, the airway is protected, and obvious bleeding is controlled. Ideally, splints are applied as part of the prehospital care. All obvious and suspected injuries to the extremities and/or spine should be splinted. It should be assumed that a wound on a fractured extremity is an open fracture. Any tender, discolored, swollen, or deformed area should be treated as a fracture or dislocation. Any extensive extremity or spinal injury—sprain, laceration, contusion, avulsion— even if it does not appear to include an obvious fracture or dislocation, should be splinted.

The splint must include the joints proximal and distal to a fracture and the bones proximal and distal to a dislocation. A splint should not be applied until the suspected injury has been exposed and examined closely. Except in unusual circumstances, the clothing must be removed for this purpose. Beware of the occult open fracture. Most open fractures are obvious because of associated bleeding, but this is not the case with the occult open fracture; instead, the examiner must look for a wound, for tenting of the skin, or for obvious discoloration.

All wounds should be covered with sterile dressings. I prefer a dry, fine-mesh gauze-base dressing. Some local protocols call for use of an antiseptic such as Betadine on the wound. I do not believe that soaking the wound in the field is helpful, although obvious clumps of foreign matter should be removed.

If a bone end is visible, it should be covered with a dressing, and the extremity should be aligned so that it will fit into a splint. If the bone then disappears into the tissue, this should be noted so that definitive treatment of the wound includes a more extensive debridement. If the bone end does not go back into the wound, one should not make a direct attempt to replace it, but the dressing should be reinforced and the splint applied. Virtually all open fractures require surgical debridement in the operating room, and the sooner this is accomplished, the less the likelihood of sepsis, the greatest enemy of fracture healing. An open fracture of any bone constitutes a true surgical emergency.

The neurovascular status of the extremity distal to the injury is determined and documented. A nerve injury should be identified before splinting and the neurovascular status of the extremity rechecked after splinting. If a previously unnoted nerve deficit is detected after splinting, the splint and dressings are removed and the extremity replaced to its original position. Vascular injuries occur with nerve injuries, and the presence of adequate capillary filling in the fingers or toes does not, in itself, ensure an intact vascular tree. Injuries about the knee and elbow should be suspected of involving the vascular tree, particularly if there is a peripheral nerve deficit. Major dislocations about the knee or elbow are also true surgical emergencies.

The extremity should be handled as little as possible. When a splint is manipulated or a dressing is applied to an obviously fractured extremity, gentle but firm manual traction is applied on the long axis of the extremity. The splint should be left in place until definitive treatment can be carried out or until it is determined to be unnecessary. The splint should be padded, and particular attention should be paid the bony prominences to avoid undue compression. The malleoli, epicondyles, styloid processes, and greater trochanter are the sites most susceptible to pressure problems. The splint must allow inspection of the hand or foot. If a vascular injury is suspected, provision should be made for palpating pulses and/or using Doppler ultrasound. The splint must not be so tight that it constricts the blood vessels. Cast padding, such as Webril, is inelastic and can be as constricting as roller gauze. I prefer not to use any circumferential dressing about a splint except elastic bandages and elastic gauze such as Kling or Kerlex.

An attempt should be made to align a grossly deformed fracture of a long bone so that it can fit into a splint. This can usually be done without causing much pain if the extremity is handled gently and traction is maintained in the long axis of the extremity. However, if there is obvious resistance, the extremity should be splinted without repositioning. Also, clinically apparent dislocations with obvious deformity about the joint should be splinted without attempting to realign. This often precludes the use of standard splints. Pillows, folded towels, and boards can help to minimize further trauma and discomfort in these cases.

Major dislocations about the ankle may be an exception to that rule. The skin is often tented over the deformity, and the neurovascular bundle of the foot is compromised. In that circumstance, an experienced paramedic may be able to reduce the dislocation with gentle, direct traction on the foot, in line with the deformity. In many cases the dislocation is easily reduced. I believe that this is one of the few instances in which joint manipulation can be carried out in the field, prior to obtaining roentgenograms. Obvious dislocation about the shoulder, hip, fingers, or toes should not be manipulated before radiologic documentation of the dislocation and/or fracture is obtained. Unreduced dislocations are difficult to splint and are painful, but they are not in themselves life-threatening and should be thoroughly evaluated before treatment is begun.

All unconscious or unresponsive patients are assumed to have sustained a spinal injury. All patients with suspected injuries to the spine should be splinted with a back board and a collar until such injury is ruled out. The patient with obvious or suspected spinal injury requires careful handling. Most fractures of the spine are reasonably stable in extension, but not in flexion or rotation. The face and head must be kept forward and not allowed to flop from side to side. Turn the patient supine using three people to roll him like a log onto a back board, and keep him there. A Philadelphia-type collar should be placed around the patient's neck. If the patient has neurologic deficit implicating a spinal cord or nerve root injury, it is assumed that an unstable vertebral fracture or dislocation has occurred. The patient with a spinal injury must not be allowed to leave the ambulance or the emergency facility with a neurologic deficit that was inapparent at first.

Specific Types of Splints

Any lightweight, radiolucent material that will fit around the extremity can be used for a splint. The splint should hold the adjacent joints in a neutral position. Flat boards, such as intravenous arm boards, make poor extremity splints. Whatever the splinting material, it should be well padded and comfortable once in place.

The aluminum or gutter splint is probably the one most widely used. It is inexpensive, simple to use, easily carried in the ambulance, and available in a variety of sizes. It is important that the splint be large enough and well padded with ABD or similar pads. The extremity is fitted into it, and both are wrapped with an elastic wrap. This is a good splint for injuries of the hand, foot, wrist, ankle, forearm, or leg. It is *not* a satisfactory splint for injuries proximal to the knee or elbow, for dislocations, or for severe, deforming injuries.

The pneumatic or air splint is popular because it takes up little room, is easy to apply, is lightweight, and allows inspection of the skin. However, this splint has some serious potential consequences. It should be inflated only by mouth, never with a pump. It is completely impervious to water or perspiration and can cause skin maceration. It can deflate itself by cracking or leaking. If a patient is to be transported by air with a pneumatic splint in place, the pressure should be released slightly. Air splints lack the flexibility of the gutter splint and cannot be used for injuries proximal to the knee or elbow.

The traction splint has been used to splint fractures of the femur since Hugh Owen Thomas described its use in 1860. Several kinds are commercially available, but all work on the same principle. The extremity is cradled on a series of bands between two metal rungs. A padded ring, designed to fit over the upper thigh at the groin, is used for countertraction, while traction is applied by a bandage or tie around the foot, which is attached to the end of the splint. This splint, in my experience, is the most difficult to apply and the one most often incorrectly applied. At least two people are needed to apply a traction splint. The patient must be supine while one person holds the extremity flexed slightly at the hip and abducted sufficiently to slide the splint into the groin, then stabilizes the extremity while the traction hitch is applied. This splint does not apply strong traction, but produces enough traction to help stabilize and align a fracture. The patient should be placed on a spine board before the traction splint is applied so that he or she can be moved more easily with the splint. If there is a palpable pedal pulse before a traction splint is applied, it should be present after the splint is applied. The Thomas splint cannot be used on a patient with a pelvic fracture. In contrast to most splints, the traction splint is often uncomfortable, particularly in the groin. Do not keep the patient with a femoral shaft fracture in a traction splint longer than is absolutely necessary.

The pneumatic antishock garment (PASG) has been suggested as a splint for the patient with pelvic and femoral fractures, as well as for those with massive intra-abdominal bleeding. It would seem that, in a hemodynamically unstable patient, a PASG has advantages over a conventional traction splint since it is lighter, less bulky, and easier to apply. However, there are no data indicating its effectiveness as a femoral splint, while there are data suggesting its danger in cases of fracture below the knee. The pressures generated inside an inflated PASG can cause ischemia in a previously compromised extremity. I believe that the PASG should be used primarily in patients who are hemodynamically unstable from intra-abdominal or intrapelvic hemorrhage. The PASG may help stabilize a pelvic fracture. If the victim has a femoral fracture as well, the PASG can stabilize the femur sufficiently to allow the necessary procedures to restore hemodynamic stability. If a PASG must be used on a patient with an extremity fracture, bear in mind that the extremity may be compromised by its use; therefore, the PASG should be removed as soon as possible. A standard traction splint cannot be properly applied over or under a PASG.

The plaster splint is among the easiest to use. Plaster should be available in every emergency department, although it is not commonly used in the field. Plaster is inexpensive and can be custom-fitted to the extremity. A well-applied plaster splint may, in some fractures, serve as early treatment and need not be changed for days. A plaster splint should be compact and need not be excessively heavy. I prefer plaster splints for the emergency treatment of most injuries distal to the knee or elbow.

There are many different ways of making a sugar-tong (upper extremity) or stirrup (lower extremity) splint, but all involve the same basic principles. The splint must be able to accommodate swelling; therefore, the elastic cannot be too tight, and a circumferential dressing should not be used unless it can expand. If cast padding is rolled around the extremity before the splint is applied, it should be either very loose or, preferably, cut before the splint is applied. The plaster should never touch the skin directly, but should be covered with padding on both sides. If the elastic bandage is applied directly over the wet plaster it will stick to the plaster and lose its ability to stretch. Avoid making dents in the plaster with your hands. As with all splints, continuous monitoring is necessary.

Regardless of the type of splint used, the patient should not be moved until he is "packaged." It is difficult if not impossible to apply any kind of splint in a moving ambulance. Occasionally, the splint has to be removed in the hospital for special radiologic studies, but as a rule it remains in place until definitive treatment begins. In the interim, the extremity should be monitored for signs of vascular compromise, neurologic dysfunction, or swelling. The wrapping around the splint may have to be loosened, the extremity repositioned, or a different splint applied. Increasing pain in a splinted extremity is a danger sign and demands immediate attention. The correctly splinted extremity should be comfortable.

EMERGENCY ROOM CARE

PRIMARY ASSESSMENT

FRANK R. LEWIS Jr., M.D.

The majority of trauma patients who present in an emergency department do not have life-threatening injuries. Such patients may be assessed by working through the orderly sequence of diagnostic criteria that physicians are traditionally trained to use. However, when dealing with the 5 to 10 percent of patients who do have major injuries, a different approach must be adopted, and treatment and diagnostic maneuvers are interspersed as required in order to treat immediately life-threatening conditions. It is essential that the emergency physician or surgeon who initially manages such patients have an organized plan. This plan should enable assessment of the most urgent problems first, while, at the same time, it allows a comprehensive evaluation of the patient. In this way no injuries will be missed. The primary priorities in this sequence are evaluation of the airway and pulmonary function, evaluation of blood volume and cardiac function, and evaluation of neurologic function.

AIRWAY AND PULMONARY FUNCTION

Airway obstruction is generally recognized as the most rapidly fatal problem seen in the emergency setting; however, not as well recognized are injuries to the lung or chest wall which can impair ventilation almost as severely as an obstructed airway. Such injuries are an open pneumothorax (sucking chest wound), a tension pneumothorax, and a flail chest. These entities should always be considered in any patient with severe respiratory distress.

An initial look at the patient, after complete undressing, should give the examiner several pieces of information about the patient's respiratory status. The following questions should be answered. Is the patient making respiratory efforts, and if so, how strongly and how rapidly? Is the patient awake and able to protect his airway from aspiration? Is air actually exchanging via the nose and mouth? Is respiratory noise present (i.e., gasping, stridor, or wheezing)? Is the chest wall moving symmetrically on both sides, or is there splinting or paradoxical movement? Are there any surface markings, wounds, abrasions, or ecchymoses indicative of the area or extent of trauma? Is the patient breathing easily, or are the accessory muscles being used? What are the relative durations of inspiration and expiration? Is the patient comfortable lying supine, or is there a need to sit upright or in some other position to maximize ventilation?

If the patient is apneic, or is making ventilatory effort, but the airway is totally obstructed, immediate attention must be directed to it. First, the mouth should be opened and suction applied to the back of the throat. If a "cafe coronary" is a possibility and the patient is unconscious, insertion of two fingers over the tongue to the area of the glottis will usually disclose whether any foreign body is present and allow its easy removal. In the conscious patient in respiratory distress, insertion of anything into the nose or mouth usually exacerbates the distress and should be avoided, unless a specific therapeutic maneuver, such as endotracheal intubation, is being carried out.

Once secretions or foreign bodies are removed, or their presence excluded, the jaw should be displaced anteriorly, either by grasping the symphysis and lifting, or by using both hands and lifting forward on the mandibular angles. If the airway can be opened, a well-fitted mask can be used to ventilate the patient using positive pressure and 100 percent oxygen for 2 to 3 minutes. If it is not possible to establish ventilation with a mask, one should immediately intubate the patient via the oral route with a No. 6 or No.7 cuffed endotracheal tube. The physician who is not an anesthetist and who intubates patients infrequently, should use a large straight blade for the laryngoscope. Miller or Wisconsin blades are preferred for these allow the epiglottis to be lifted out of the way, so that the vocal cords can be directly visualized during insertion of the endotracheal tube.

In more than 99 percent of patients, airway access via oral intubation of the trachea is successful. However, the occasional patient with severe maxillofacial injury, bleeding, distortion of anatomy, or foreign body, requires emergency tracheostomy. When necessary, a cricothyroidotomy should be done between the laryngeal cartilage and the cricoid. This is preferred over a classic tracheostomy made through the second or third tracheal rings. Access to the cricothyroid membrane is much faster and easier, as it lies nearer the surface and requires minimal retraction for exposure. Concern about subglottic stenosis or vocal cord dysfunction following this procedure has been shown in recent series not to be a significant problem. A transverse incision, 2 to 3 cm long, is made directly over the cricothyroid membrane, with the patient's neck extended. The membrane is incised transversely over the anterior third of the tracheal circumference, and a curved clamp is inserted and spread to define the opening. A 5–7 mm (ID) curved (60°) tracheostomy tube is inserted, and the cuff is inflated. The tube should be immediately secured around the neck with tracheostomy cord.

The question often arises as to whether endotracheal intubation or tracheostomy, both of which require neck extension for optimal performance, should be attempted in the unconscious patient where a cervical spine fracture is a possibility and where roentgenographic studies have not been obtained. In such circumstances it is necessary to decide which is the greater threat to the patient—the obstructed airway or the possible cervical spine fracture. The airway virtually always has priority, because the possiblity of cervical cord injury is relatively remote. However, if circumstances allow, and the patient is not facing a life-threatening situation, cervical spine injury should be excluded first. Even if intubation is indicated, the maintenance of axial traction by an assistant, while the tube is inserted, minimizes the chance of cord injury, even if an unstable fracture is present.

Airway problems that are not severe enough to require immediate intubation, but nevertheless which are significant, should be reassessed every few minutes. In general, the tendency is to wait too long before intubating patients, and when patients are in obvious distress or when respiratory rates exceed 35 respirations per minute, intubation is indicated. Injuries that result in swelling or hematoma of the tongue and floor of the mouth are particularly hazardous. These cause airway obstruction and render the patient extremely difficult, if not impossible, to intubate. The continuous presence of an anesthesiologist is preferred when a patient exhibits respiratory distress or has a major thoracic injury. This is preferable even if the patient is not thought to need intubation at the time. The initial 1 to 2 hours after injury are critical, and failure to monitor airway problems closely frequently leads to preventable mortality. This is particularly apparent when patients get sequestered in radiology suites for extended periods.

If the degree of airway impairment is not such that it requires immediate intubation, the examiner should proceed with the remainder of the pulmonary assessment. A careful visual assessment is important at the outset to define areas of splinting or paradoxical movement. The thorax should be palpated carefully for crepitus or rib instability, or, if the patient is awake, to define those areas where palpation elicits pain. This is most easily done by initially compressing the sternum toward the spine, followed by compression of both hemithoraces medially with the examiner's hands on each side of the chest. Rib fractures are the most common injury seen after blunt trauma, and their diagnosis is predominantly clinical. If a rib is fractured, there is point tenderness at the fracture site, and pressure on the rib at a distant location will reproduce the pain. X-ray films should be used to define multiple rib fractures, but multiple views, needed to rule out all possible fracture sites, are not necessary. It is useful to remember that costochondral fractures do not show up on x-ray films but are commonly present. These must be diagnosed by the physical exam. The trachea should be palpated and its position relative to the sternal notch noted. The clavicles and scapula should also be palpated for tenderness or deformity.

If respiratory distress is present, the chest should be auscultated to determine if breath sounds are reduced on one side. However, if the patient is not in any respiratory distress, I do not spend time on auscultation at this point in the assessment. It should be noted that, although physical diagnosis texts describe marked differences in breath sounds on the two sides of the chest as being a diagnostic criterion for pneumothorax, the practical usefulness of this observation is limited. The differences in breath sounds may be subtle, and in a noisy trauma room, impossible to distinguish. Thus auscultation should be recognized as being only of limited value and should never be the sole determinant of treatment or nontreatment of a pneumothorax.

At this point in the evaluation, a physician should have a fairly good idea of the thoracic pathology present, based on the examination and the mechanism of injury, and should be in a position to answer the following questions. Is it confined to one hemithorax? Does it cross the midline, with the concomitant risk of major vascular or cardiac injury and perforation of the esophagus or trachea? Is there subcutaneous emphysema, suggesting tracheal or bronchial disruption? Are there obvious rib fractures, and if so, approximately how extensive are they? Is there good reason to suspect that there is a pneumo- or hemothorax? Often, the final answer to many of these questions must await the chest roentgenogram, as physical diagnosis is, at best, inexact. However, with a comprompromised patient, there may not be time to see the roentgenogram, and therapy must be undertaken on the basis of the physical findings and likely injury. The patient in severe respiratory distress, who is not relieved by tracheal intubation, should have chest tubes placed prior to any roentgenographic examination, as they may be lifesaving. If injuries appear confined to one side, initially a unilateral chest tube should be placed, or if lateralization is not possible, bilateral tubes should be inserted (see chapter on *Hemopneumothorax*, for details of technique).

Normally, there is time to obtain a chest roentgenogram. If at all possible, this should be taken with the patient in an upright position to better define intrapleural fluid. If a pneumothorax is suspected, both expiratory and inspiratory films will help to confirm it in difficult cases. If a hemo- or pneumothorax is present, a large bore siliconized straight chest tube (size 36 or 40 F) should be inserted laterally between the anterior and posterior axillary folds at the level of the nipples or above. The tube should be directed posteriorly and superiorly so that it lies behind the lung and evacuates both fluid and air. In trauma patients there is no place for the use of right-angle tubes or for insertion of tubes in the anterior second interspace, as these lead to complications in placement; right-angle tubes have no advantages over straight tubes placed laterally.

BLOOD VOLUME AND CARDIAC STATUS

The next priority is to assess the degree of shock and to decide on the type and size of intravenous catheters to be placed, and the type and volume of fluid replacement to be used. An evaluation of the degree of shock must always be considered in light of the time elapsed since injury. If, for example, the injury occurred 15 minutes before and the patient is in profound shock, massive bleeding is occurring and several large-bore intravenous access lines are needed. Conversely, if the injury occurred 2 hours before and the degree of shock is mild, the rate of bleeding is not immediately life-threatening, and less aggressive volume restitution is needed.

The indicators that are commonly used for assessment of shock in the emergency setting are as follows:

1. Blood pressure
2. Pulse rate
3. Skin perfusion (color, temperature, moisture)
4. Urine output
5. Mental status
6. Central venous pressure

Each of these will be discussed in regard to their appropriate use.

Blood Pressure

Although blood pressure is the time-honored parameter used to define volume loss, this appears to be less accurate and sensitive than pulse rate, skin perfusion, or urine output. The response of blood pressure to intravascular depletion is nonlinear. This is because compensatory mechanisms of increased cardiac rate and contractility, and venous and arteriolar vasoconstriction provide excellent compensation for the first 15 to 20 percent of intravascular volume loss in the healthy young adult. After about 20 percent volume loss, the blood pressure begins to decline; In the average patient, blood pressure will be in the 60 to 80 mm Hg range with 30 percent volume loss and in the 30 to 50 mm Hg with 40 percent volume loss. Therefore, as volume loss becomes more severe the decline in blood pressure is more precipitous. In the elderly patient who cannot compensate by the aforementioned mechanisms, the decline in blood pressure begins at 10 to 15 percent volume loss and proceeds to the point of arrest by 40 percent loss. The nonlinear behavior of blood pressure has two disadvantages: declines in blood pressure are a relatively insensitive sign of early shock, and in the infrequently monitored patient, blood pressure may appear stable for an initial period and then, rather suddenly, appear to "crash."

The other deficiency related to blood pressure monitoring is the lack of an absolute "normal". A patient who is normally hypertensive may be in profound shock when his systolic pressure is 120 mm Hg, whereas the healthy young athlete may be entirely normal with a systolic pressure of 90 mm Hg.

Pulse Rate

Pulse rate is the second commonly used indicator, and is more sensitive than blood pressure readings. The value of this indicator is significantly limited by the lack of specificity. This is because the emotionalism, the pain, and the excitement surrounding the trauma situation may result in tachycardia without hypovolemia. However, if tachycardia is sustained above levels of 120 beats per minute, this should be considered an indicator of hypovolemia until proven otherwise. In young patients the heart rate may accelerate to 160 to 180 beats per minute when accompanied by severe volume depletion. The older patient is unable to accelerate to this degree and only rarely will sustain rates greater than 140 beats per minute.

Skin Perfusion

Skin perfusion is generally underappreciated as an indicator of hypovolemia, yet is the sign I place the most confidence in, when initially evaluating the patient. The early physiologic compensation for volume loss is vasoconstriction of the vessels to the skin and muscle. This is manifested by paleness and coolness of the skin, which develops quite rapidly. The release of epinephrine, which also accompanies hypovolemia, causes sweating. Thus, in such a situation, palpation of the patient's trunk immediately reveals coolness and moisture. The lower extemities are the first to manifest the vasoconstriction, and palpation over the kneecaps or the feet provides the best "early warning" of impending shock. These signs of skin perfusion can be used with confidence in all age groups.

Urine Output

The fourth indicator of hypovolemia is urine output, and any patient with significant trauma should always have an indwelling urinary bladder catheter inserted as soon as possible. This enables the monitoring of urine volume every 15 minutes. After skin perfusion, this is the second most reliable indicator of volume loss, and is only slightly less sensitive. The second level of compensation of the body to hypovolemia is visceral vasoconstriction, and this results in decreased flow to the gut, liver, and kidney. Urine output immediately reflects decreases in renal blood flow; hence, its value as an indicator. A minimally adequate urine volume is 0.5 ml per kilogram per hour, and resuscitative fluids should be administered rapidly until this level is reached. If urine output exceeds 1 ml per kilogram per hour, the fluid administration rate can be decreased. During resuscitation or surgery, the urine output is measured on an ongoing basis; overall this is the best indicator of the adequacy of volume restitution.

Mental Status

Alteration in mental status is the fifth indicator of hypovolemia. This is rarely seen because it is present only with preterminal degrees of hypovolemia. Compensatory mechanisms maintain flow to the myocardium and brain with great tenacity; hence, one does not see cerebral hypoperfusion until blood pressure is in the 30 to 50 mm Hg systolic range or below. The alteration usually seen is agitation and mental confusion, which causes the patient to become irrational, anxious, and uncooperative. Because, in the emergency setting, such states are also commonly produced by alcohol or other drugs it may occasionally be hard to distinguish alterations attributable to hypovolemia from those attributable to drugs. This is particularly true when both may be present.

Central Venous Pressure

The last parameter, central venous pressure, is not a good indicator of hypovolemia, since the normal levels of 3 to 8 mm Hg are relatively hard to distinguish from hypovolemic levels of 0 to 5 mm Hg. This is particularly so when, the examiner is initially estimating the pressure by inspection of external jugular neck veins. The importance of this indicator is to distinguish hypovolemia from the other two traumatic causes of shock which require fundamentally different treatment; these are cardiac tamponade and tension pneumothorax. When a patient presents in shock with penetrating trauma in the precordial area, there is no way of knowing from external inspection whether the patient is hypovolemic or in cardiac tamponade, yet rapid and correct treatment is absolutely dependent on making the distinction. In this setting, if a central venous catheter is inserted, the central venous pressure, as judged by inspection of the external jugular neck veins or by actual measurement, is the only test that provides immediate and unambiguous discrimination of the two conditions. With hypovolemic shock the central venous pressure is less than 5 mm Hg, whereas a similar degree of cardiogenic shock requires a central venous pressure of 25 mm Hg or greater. It is easy to make this distinction by external inspection of the neck veins. This should always be the next observation made when it is determined that a patient is in shock.

The presence of moderate or severe shock demands immediate treatment without waiting for the complete assessment of the patient. The urgency of placement, the size, and the number of intravenous lines is dictated by the degree of shock and the apparent rate of bleeding. Patients who are hemodynamically stable, who exhibit no signs of shock, and who have apparently minimal injury, need only a percutaneous catheter of approximately 18-gauge size. If a patient is hemodynamically stable, but a more major injury is suspected, a large bore percutaneous line, either 16- or 14-gauge, is started. If shock is present to any degree, a large bore percutaneous catheter plus a cutdown is placed. If shock is profound and injuries are massive, two or three cutdowns are placed.

When doing cutdowns, I prefer to use the saphenous vein at the ankle for rapid access, and to use an 8-French feeding tube or cut-off intravenous extension tubing as the intravenous catheter. The second most favored site is the antecubital crease, where either the basilic or cephalic vein is available. These veins accept large catheters. As a third alternative, the saphenous vein at the fossa ovalis can be used. In this case the catheter is threaded into the femoral vein. The two latter sites offer the advantage that the catheter can be threaded centrally in order to obtain central venous pressure readings; however, they require slightly more time to place.

The use of large bore catheters, introduced percutaneously into central veins such as the subclavian or internal jugular, are often advocated in the trauma patient, but I feel this has several hazards. The greatest is iatrogenic pneumothorax, that may add further to the critically ill patient's problems. The incidence of this complication, even with elective placement of subclavian lines is 5 to 10 percent, and this is bound to be higher in the emergency setting. If the patient already has a chest tube in place, placement of a subclavian or internal jugular line should obviously be on the same side, as it is protected to a degree.

The second problem is that large central veins are collapsed when the patient is in shock, and are harder to puncture cleanly. Putting the patient into the Trendelenberg position, before placing the line may not be feasible, and if respiratory problems are present, this position may exacerbate them.

The need for multiple large-bore intravenous access in the rapidly bleeding patient cannot be overemphasized. Once the patient is on the operating table with drapes in place, it is too late to get rapid access. If the patient has a massive bleeding site in the abdomen, he will predictably "crash" when the abdomen is initially opened and decompressed, and it usually takes a few minutes to identify and control the bleeding site. Unless the anesthetist can pump blood rapidly during this time (approximately 1,000 ml every 5 minutes) the patient may arrest from hypovolemia. This happens no matter how controllable the injury may be. This problem must be anticipated, because it is too late to start putting in lines after the abdomen is opened.

After intravenous lines are placed, one must decide on the resuscitative fluid to be administered; the initial choice, prior to blood availability, is a balanced salt solution. This can be given either alone or in conjunction with colloid solutions. Either crystalloids or colloids can be used effectively to resuscitate the hypovolemic patient, if given in the appropriate quantities. Although a great deal has been written about the beneficial or detrimental effects of one or the other on pulmonary function, it is my opinion, based on my own studies as well as on a thorough review of the literature, that there is no difference in the effect of either if given to equivalent hemodynamic end points.

The major difference in these solutions is economic: a balanced salt solution typically costs $2.00 per L, whereas plasma or an albumin containing substitute typically costs over $100 per L. If both produce equivalent effects, it is difficult to justify the more expensive product.

There is a difference in the resuscitative effects of the solutions. This has been shown in multiple studies. The difference relates to intravascular retention, which is greater with colloid solution. Balanced salt solutions equilibrate rapidly with the interstitial space and hence have a greater volume of distribution than colloids. As a result, two to three times as much balanced salt solution as colloid solution is required for equivalent intravascular filling. However, if this extra amount is given, the hemodynamic effects are equivalent, and there are no ill effects from the extra salt solution other than increased peripheral edema. As mentioned before, it has been shown in clinical studies that there is no increase in pulmonary interstitial fluid and no tendency to pulmonary edema as a result of crystalloid usage.

Whichever fluid is chosen, it should be administered in sufficient quantity to rapidly restore the patient's intravascular volume status to normal. This will be evidenced by the disappearance of signs of shock, the return of vital signs to normal, and a urine output of 0.5 to 1.0 ml per kilogram per hour. The correction of shock should not require more than the first 10 to 15 minutes after the patient's arrival at the Emergency Department. If shock cannot be corrected immediately or if it recurs after initial correction, this provides the best evidence for ongoing blood loss and the need for definitive surgery.

Red cells are the second component of the intravascular replacement needed to provide adequate oxygen carrying capacity. Packed cells or whole blood can be used, though in the acute emergency setting my own preference is for whole blood. This has much lower viscosity and can be more quickly and easily transfused. When cross-matching is not possible, I prefer type specific blood, though type O blood is also used in many centers and appears to have minimal risk. Sufficient red cells are normally given to maintain the hematocrit at 30 percent, though much lower levels are typically tolerated in previously healthy young patients. In patients who have major cardiac dysfunction or low fixed cardiac outputs, it is essential to maintain hematocrits at higher levels, at least 35 to 40 percent.

INITIAL NEUROLOGIC EVALUATION

Neurologic assessment begins during the initial contact with the patient. It is immediately evident whether the patient is conscious or comatose, and if conscious, whether there is alteration of the normal mental state. Attempts to take the history indicate the patient's mental status. Usually only a few questions are required to tell whether he is normal, confused, agitated, or inappropriate. The dominant element of CNS assessment in the trauma patient, both initially and on a continuing basis, is the level of consciousness. There are multiple ways of defining this, but I find it most useful to use five levels. These are normal, obtunded, appropriately responsive to pain, inappropriately responsive to pain, and unresponsive. The first of these is self-explanatory and defines the awake, alert patient who answers questions appropriately. The second category is broad and generally defines the patient who is responsive to verbal stimuli, but in whom responses are inappropriate or mentation is sluggish. The third category defines a patient who does not respond to verbal stimuli, but withdraws from a painful stimulus. the fourth category defines patients who do not attempt to withdraw from the source of pain, but do respond by movement of some type, either of another part of the body, or by extensor posturing. The last group are those who make no movement in response to pain but who retain brain stem functions.

An important point to mention is that CNS injury does not cause hypotension until brain stem function is lost; by the time this occurs the patient is universally unsalvageable. Therefore it is important never to blame hypotension on neurologic injury. Rather the assumption should be made that there is a source of blood loss in addition to the neurologic injury. The only exception to this occurs in patients with spinal cord injuries and paraplegia. These patients may develop postural hypotension because of a failure of sympathetic tone peripherally. In these patients the hypotension is usually corrected by intravascular volume administration.

In the patient with any degree of mental impairment, it is essential that mental status be initially documented and then repeatedly assessed at 15 to 30 minute intervals. Most of the treatable intracranial lesions produce deteriorating levels of consciousness during the first 1 or 2 hours of observation; failure to detect these may lead to delay in treatment with associated poorer outcome. Patients who have altered mental status attributable to drugs usually improve during the first few hours of observation; thus ongoing assessment is critical to distinguish those with organic disease from those with pharmacologic alterations.

The second part of the neurologic assessment is the definition of lateralizing signs. These are sought most commonly in the pupillary reflexes. This is because increased intracranial pressure is usually manifested first by sluggishness or loss of the pupillary response to light. Less commonly, the extraocular movements are impaired. Lateralization should be further defined by examining the extremities and by determining whether movement and strength of arms and legs are full and equal. Moving the unconscious patient is contraindicated when fractures may be present, but in a conscious patient, pain experienced at the fracture site prevents any attempt at movement.

SECONDARY ASSESSMENT

DONALD D. TRUNKEY, M.D.

The unstable trauma patient usually declares himself shortly after the initial resuscitation. If the patient's condition remains unstable, operative intervention to control hemorrhage or evacuate mass lesions within the cranial vault is imperative to effect patient salvage. If, on the other hand, the patient becomes hemodynamically stable and is not deteriorating neurologically, a secondary examination and assessment should be carried out. A rapid but thorough examination from head to toe, including all systems, must be done. The surgeon must be thorough, since a missed injury may go unrecognized for many more hours. Particular emphasis should be placed on a complete neurologic and orthopaedic examination; it should be remembered that few patients have permanent disability from torso trauma, whereas a missed neurologic or orthopaedic injury may lead to permanent disability and an unacceptable outcome.

NEUROLOGIC EXAMINATION

Ideally, a neurologic examination is performed in the field or during transportation to the emergency department, but if not, it definitely should be performed as soon as possible after the patient's arrival in the emergency department. This cursory clinical examination is the most important assessment of a neurologic injury, and it may be all that is required to establish the need for exploratory burr holes and decompressive craniotomy. The essentials of the emergency examination include assessment of (1) hemispheric function (e.g., the Glasgow Coma Scale); (2) brain stem function testing by testing cranial nerves, motor activity, and respirations; and (3) assessment of spinal cord integrity by motor activity, sensation and bulbocavernosus reflex tests (Table 1). Obvious or suspected cervical spine fracture should be treated by maintaining axial orientation using Gardner-Well tongs or other means of traction.

If the patient's condition stabilizes as a result of resuscitation, further diagnostic tests such as CT scanning or arteriography may be warranted. This decision should be governed by both the patient's clinical course and repeated neurologic examinations. If the patient deteriorates rapidly, the clinician must assume the presence of a mass lesion. A decision must be made either to take an additional 15 to 20 minutes to obtain a CT scan or to proceed immediately with burr holes and decompressive craniotomy.

MAXILLOFACIAL TRAUMA

Maxillofacial trauma is associated with two lifethreatening conditions—airway obstruction and hemorrhage. During the secondary assessment, the retropharyngeal area should be examined carefully for any deviation of the trachea and for signs of upper airway obstruction.

Because of the generous blood supply to the facial area, hemorrhage can be a significant problem. Bleeding lacerations can be controlled temporarily with interlocking sutures. Nasopharyngeal and pharyngeal hemorrhage may require intubation to prevent aspiration of blood. In general, maxillofacial trauma without airway obstruction or massive hemorrhage does not require immediate treatment. Treatment can be delayed for a period of days while other injuries are treated and stabilized.

THE CHEST

During the secondary examination, the clinician should perform careful palpation of the entire chest cage, feeling each rib, the sternum, and clavicles. Point tenderness is usually indicative of underlying fractures. Tracheal shift should

TABLE 1   Correlation Between Clinical Signs and Levels of Brain Function

Anatomic Region	Neurologic Sign
Cerebral hemispheres	Verbral responses Purposeful movements

Brainstem	Reflex motor movements:
	    decortication
	    decerebration

Reticular activating system	Eye opening
Midbrain CN* III	Reactive pupils
Pons CN V + VII	Corneal reflex
CN VIII, VI, III + MLF	Doll's eyes and ice water responses
Medulla	Breathing Blood pressure

Spinal cord	Deep tendon reflexes
	Rectal exam
	    sphincter tone
	    bulbocavernosus reflex

* CN = Cranial Nerve

be noted, and careful auscultation of both hemithoraces should be performed. The presence of percussion tympany should be tested. The spinous processes should be palpated and any pain or deformity noted. Finally, the examiners should listen to heart sounds, noting in particular their character and whether or not they are muffled or diminished. The patient's pulse pressure should be checked as well.

THE ABDOMEN

The abdomen is a notorious diagnostic trap for even the most experienced clinician; in approximately 40 percent of patients with significant hemoperitoneum, there are no clinical manifestations. In fact, in most instances intraperitoneal hemorrhage usually presents as unexplained hypotension, a falling hematocrit, or a rising white count, and with signs and symptoms of associated injuries such as lower rib fractures or pelvic fractures. Clinicians who look for abdominal distention as a clinical sign of internal blood loss may have waited too long since, in a typical 70-kg individual, a 1-cm change in the radius of the abdomen may account for as much as 3 L of blood loss. Serial abdominal examinations, along with hematocrit determinations and white cell count, are mandatory in the immediate post-injury period. For patients requiring surgery for other injuries, such as orthopaedic or neurologic injuries, peritoneal lavage or CT scanning of the abdominal cavity should be considered. A rectal examination should be performed as part of the primary assessment; if not, it should certainly be performed during the secondary assessment. The clinician should note the location and size of the prostate, sphincter tone, and the presence of pathologic reflexes such as the bulbocavernosus reflex.

FRACTURE MANAGEMENT

Patients with major fracture injuries should arrive in the emergency room with splints in place. Unsplinted fractures should be splinted as soon as possible after initial resuscitation to prevent further blood loss and neurovascular damage, to reduce pain, and to prevent continued microembolization. A Gram stain and culture of open fractures should be performed. Open fracture wounds should be wrapped temporarily in clean dressings in preparation for irrigation and debridement in the operating room. If the patient's condition stabilizes during the resuscitation, roentgenograms should be obtained of all body areas where fractures are suspected. All peripheral pulses should be assessed and noted. A diminished pulse, particularly compared with the pulse in the other extremity, usually mandates further evaluation by arteriography or digital subtraction arteriography.

OCCULT HEMORRHAGE

The clinician must be aware of the likely locations of blood loss. Each hemithorax may contain 2 L of blood. For this reason, a chest film is essential before proceeding to the operating room and can be extremely helpful to the surgeon in determining the surgical approach. Another highly suspect area of hidden blood loss is the abdomen. Distention is a late and unreliable sign. If the patient is in shock and the chest film is normal, and if there are no external signs of bleeding, it must be assumed that there is intra-abdominal hemorrhage. The pelvis is considered part of the abdomen and can conceal large amounts of blood. The thigh may contain 4 to 6 units of whole blood after a major fracture or crush injury. In some circumstances, the pneumatic antishock garment (PASG) may be useful in controlling hemorrhage from the pelvis or femur, at least temporarily. This is particularly true in trauma cases in rural areas where prehospital time is increased because of distance factors. If the patient arrives in the emergency room with a PASG already in place, it is imperative not to remove it until there is venous access to the circulation, and the surgeon is ready to treat this specific injury. The pneumatic antishock garment is best removed in the operating room, with the patient prepped and anesthetized.

SPECIAL DIAGNOSTIC TESTING

DONALD D. TRUNKEY, M.D.
MICHAEL P. FEDERLE, M.D.

BLOOD AND URINE TESTS

Hematocrit

All patients subjected to major trauma should have their peripheral blood hematocrits determined, although surgery should not be delayed if the results are not immediately available. The hematocrit is determined either by centrifuging a specimen of blood in a capillary tube or by a Coulter counter.

The hematocrit remains unchanged for several hours after acute hemorrhage in the patient who is not given intravenous fluid replacement. In patients who are given fluid replacement, the hematocrit falls rapidly and in proportion to the amount of blood lost—approximately 3 points for every unit of blood lost. The hematocrit eventually falls the same amount in patients who bleed chronically. In patients who are not resuscitated, equilibration by transcapillary refill is usually attained within 72 hours.

In most instances, a hematocrit is determined on the first sample of blood after the primary intravenous line has been established. Subsequent serial determinations are more valuable than a single determination. This test is particularly useful in following the condition of patients with occult hemorrhage such as hemoperitoneum.

Urinalysis

All patients subjected to major trauma should also have a urinalysis, but again, surgery should not be delayed if the results are not immediately available. Microscopic examination of the urine reveals the presence or absence of red blood cells. Immersing a reagent strip—a plastic strip impregnated with several compounds that give color reactions with specific substances—in the urine measures urine pH and detects protein, glucose, ketone bodies, bilirubin, and occult blood.

Reagent strips can also detect myoglobinuria in patients with either severe crush injuries or burns involving muscles. The reagent for hemoglobin on the strip cross-reacts with myoglobin. This cross-reactivity, along with the insolubility of hemoglobin in ammonium sulfate, allows the physician to test for myoglobinuria. Eighty percent ammonium sulfate is added to an aliquot of urine to precipitate out any hemoglobin in the specimen. The aliquot is then centrifuged, and the supernatant is tested with the hemoglobin part of the reagent strip. A positive reaction suggests myoglobinuria. Both positive and negative reactions should be confirmed by electrophoretic and immunochemical methods.

Urine can also be checked for drugs and other toxic substances. The surgeon should be wary in interpreting toxicology screens; a positive screen for drugs in an irrational, belligerent patient may suggest drug ingestion, or the patient's behavior may be caused by subdural hematoma. The physician's task is to identify patients with correctable lesions.

Serum Glucose

Blood glucose concentrations should be measured in every patient who has been subjected to trauma, again with the understanding that surgery should proceed even if the results are not available. Severe hyperglycemia is usually detected on urinalysis as glucosuria. Hypoglycemia is not measured by examination of the urine, and tragedy may result if an insulin reaction, which may have contributed to the trauma, is missed.

White Blood Count

Under normal circumstances, peripheral blood contains 4,000 to 10,000 white cells per microliter (μl). The total white count can be determined by lysing red cells and counting nucleated white cells manually in a counting chamber or by an automated technique, the most popular of which is the Coulter counter. More important than the total white count is the differential white count, which gives the proportion of different cell types that comprise the total number of white cells. Of primary importance in the patient who has sustained trauma is the "shift to the left," which reflects an absolute increase in the number of neutrophils, particularly the more immature forms. Serial white count determinations are of more value than single determinations in working up the trauma patient. The development of neutrophilia or the appearance of a shift to the left may give the clinician early clues to an inflammatory response, usually in the peritoneal cavity, as the cause of early mobilization of neutrophils.

Serum Amylase

Amylase, an enzyme secreted by both the pancreas and the salivary glands, splits starch into its component sugars. Damage to either the glandular cells or the ductal systems may cause amylase to enter the blood stream. Amylase activity is measured by one of two methods, both of which depend on the ability of amylase to digest a starch solution. In the Somogyi method, sugars are measured colorimetrically, and normal values are 40 to 140 units per deciliter. The second method utilizes a starch dye substrate, and the amount of liberated dye is measured. This method gives lower values, the upper limits of normal being 25 units per deciliter.

Elevated serum amylase, especially when levels are persistently more than 300 Somogyi units per deciliter, suggests pancreatic injury. The pancreas can be seriously damaged, however, and the serum amylase level may be normal. In addition, transient serum amylase levels can be high in patients with an undamaged pancreas. Thus, for the most part, we do not rely on serum amylase concentrations in assessing the trauma patient.

Other Blood Tests

Other laboratory blood tests that should be considered but not requested routinely on trauma patients include serum electrolytes (sodium, potassium, bicarbonate, chloride), blood urea nitrogen, creatinine, and liver function tests. Approximately 40 ml of whole blood should be obtained as soon as the first intravenous line has been inserted. Ten milliliters of blood should be sent immediately for typing and crossmatching. The remainder is kept in reserve for the aforementioned tests when they are indicated, either by history or subsequent events. Ten milliliters of blood is kept aside for toxicology and blood alcohol determinations, which are done when the history warrants it.

Arterial Blood Gases

Arterial blood gases, which are obtained anaerobically from the femoral or radial artery, include the partial pressure of oxygen (Po_2), the partial pressure of carbon dioxide (Pco_2), and blood pH. The arterial Po_2 is indicative of the amount of oxygen passing from inspired air into the blood. It is influenced by ventilatory capacity, pulmonary perfusing surfaces, distribution of pulmonary blood flow, and the adequacy of pulmonary and systemic circulation. The Pco_2 is a more accurate measure of ventilation, since carbon dioxide diffuses more readily across alveolar surfaces than does oxygen. Blood pH values accurately reflect the body's acid-base balance, but they do not by themselves tell the clinician whether an abnormality is the result of metabolic or respiratory causes. In the severely traumatized patient, the pH is most commonly below 7.4 and reflects a metabolic acidosis secondary to the accumulation of hydrogen ions. The metabolic acidosis may be altered by compensatory respiratory alkalosis if the patient is spontaneously ventilating, and by the resuscitation procedure itself. Resuscitation is often attempted with balanced salt solution that contains variable amounts of base. Isolated measurements may give the physician some index of the ventilatory status or perfusion, but serial measurements give more reliable information.

RADIOLOGY

Chest Films

Every trauma patient should have a chest film early in the course of his resuscitation. Except for the patient who has had an emergency room thoracotomy, no trauma patient should go to surgery, no matter how urgent the case, without a chest film.

A portable film is more than adequate. The radiologic technologist should be available when the critically injured patient is brought in. A film cassette can be laid under the patient when he is initially being rolled over to examine his back, or when he is being transferred from the ambulance stretcher to the hospital guerney. Obtaining the film should take no more than 15 seconds. If the patient has to be taken to the operating room immediately, the film can be developed while the patient is being transported. The interpretation of the film can be called to the surgeon in the operating room while he is preparing the patient for surgery.

The information obtained from the chest film can be life-saving. A patient in hypovolemic or cardiogenic shock, without an obvious source of extracavitary blood loss, either must be bleeding into his left chest, right chest, or abdomen or must have cardiogenic shock due to myocardial failure, pericardial tamponade, a tension pneumothorax, or a ruptured hemidiaphragm with displacement of abdominal viscera into the chest. A chest film can confirm the diagnosis and direct the surgeon to the appropriate body cavity. The time spent in obtaining the film saves time in the long run.

The chest film may show a number of abnormalities that may be hard to detect on physical examination. Hemothorax or simple pneumothorax can be missed in the rushed atmosphere of a noisy emergency room, but will be obvious on a chest roentgenogram. A chest film of a patient with a ruptured left hemidiaphragm may not show abdominal viscera in the left chest; it may only show an abnormal position of a nasogastric tube. Aortic or intrathoracic great vessel ruptures are almost always associated with at least some abnormality of the mediastinum or the aortic knob; they may also be associated with fractures of the posterior portion of the first or second ribs, apical capping, displacement of the mainstem bronchi, or deviation of the nasogastric tube within the esophagus. A pulmonary contusion typically shows a lung infiltrate within 1 hour of the injury. Ruptures of the tracheobronchial tree often show mediastinal air. An acute pericardial tamponade may show an enlarged heart shadow, but usually no abnormality is seen on the chest film. Rib fractures may be demonstrated on the chest film, or they may not, even with rib details.

Cervical Spine Films

All hemodynamically stable patients with major craniofacial trauma or with physical signs of a cervical spine injury warrant roentgenograms of the cervical spine. The most important view to obtain is the lateral film. The seventh cervical vertebra must be visible on film, since many cervical fractures involve that vertebra. It is often necessary for two medical attendants to be in the radiology suite when the film is being obtained, one to maintain the patient's head in an axial orientation while the other pulls down on the patient's upper extremities to expose the seventh vertebra.

The lateral film demonstrates misalignment in most patients with an unstable cervical spine. The anterior or posterior borders of the spinal canal may be out of line; the atlas and odontoid may be displaced; or the vertebral bodies may be compressed or fractured. The lateral film may also indicate the need for more views, such as odontoid, anterior-posterior, oblique, or flexion-extension films.

Abdominal Films

In contrast to the chest roentgenogram, the plain film of the abdomen usually does not contribute much to the therapeutic management of trauma patients. However, in multiply injured patients, if time permits, an abdominal film should be obtained in the radiology suite when other film studies are being obtained. The film may show fractures of the lumbar vertebrae or of the transverse process; both types of fractures indicate that strong forces were applied to the abdomen and back. Scoliosis indicates retroperitoneal trauma and bleeding, causing spasm of the paraspinous muscles. The same injury may obliterate the psoas margins or the kidney shadows. Air around the duodenum indicates retroperitoneal rupture of the duodenum. The roentgenographic signs of bleeding in the peritoneal cavity, such as fluid in the paracolic gutters or obliteration of the properitoneal fat line, become positive only with blood loss that is so large that the physician should be able to detect it easily on physical examination. In cadavers, as an example, less than 800 ml of intra-abdominal fluid is undetectable on plain films of the abdomen.

Genitourinary Films

The excretory urogram, cystogram, and urethrogram are the mainstays for preliminary evaluation of injuries to the genitourinary tract. An intravenous pyelogram should be obtained in any stable patient with hematuria, which is defined as more than 100 red blood cells per high-powered field in an unspun specimen. An intravenous pyelogram should also be obtained, even in the absence of hematuria, in stable patients with severe blunt trauma or with penetrating injuries near a kidney or ureter.

A cystogram should be obtained in any patient with hematuria and a history of severe lower abdominal or pelvic trauma, particularly the inebriated patient with lower abdominal blunt trauma. A urethrogram should be obtained in any patient with a suspected urethral tear as manifested by gross penile blood or when difficulty is encountered in passing a Foley catheter.

The pyelogram can be obtained by administering 100 ml of contrast material intravenously to the adult patient early during the course of resuscitation. The first plain film of the abdomen usually gives most of the information that is needed. The cystogram can be obtained by infusing 150 ml of contrast material through the Foley catheter into the bladder; the infusion should be by gravity. An anterior-posterior view and either an oblique or a lateral view of the bladder should be obtained; a single-view cystogram misses 40 percent of bladder ruptures. The urethrogram can be obtained by gently injecting 30 ml of contrast material into the urethral meatus. If a Foley catheter is already in place, some detail of the urethra can be obtained by injecting contrast material into the urethra around the catheter.

Contrast studies of the genitourinary tract can delineate many abnormalities. The excretory urogram shows the number of functioning kidneys—a nonvisualized kidney usually indicates absence of the organ or interruption of its blood supply. The degree of contrast material extravasation gives an index of parenchymal damage.

The ureters usually are not seen in their entirety with the single-film urogram. In blunt trauma, this nonvisualization usually is not important because ureteral ruptures are rare. In contrast, in trauma that penetrates near a ureter, an effort should be made to see the entire structure. Lacerations of the ureter may be small and easily missed. Bladder ruptures are frequently posterior; hence, the need for oblique or lateral views.

Cranial Computed Tomography

Computed tomography (CT) of the head should be obtained (1) in any hemodynamically stable patient with a suspected depressed skull fracture, (2) in any stable patient with a severe neurologic deficit, and (3) in any patient stable or even moderately unstable with a worsening neurologic status. Not every obtunded, inebriated patient needs CT as long as he has no neurologic deficit other than the obtundation. If the obtundation persists for more than several hours, however, CT should be obtained—drunkenness should lighten with time, not stay the same, and it certainly should not worsen. CT of the head is definitive for diagnosis of depressed fracture, epidural hematoma, subdural hematoma, intra-cerebral hematoma, and cerebral edema. CT has made cerebral arteriography for trauma obsolete and plain films of the skull less important. If the patient has a neurologic deficit, he should have CT. If the patient has no neurologic deficit, usually no radiologic study is needed.

Abdominal Computed Tomography

Computerized tomography of the abdomen can help to evaluate hemody-namically stable patients who have been subjected to blunt trauma of the lower chest or abdomen, especially patients with equivocal indications for celiotomy, or patients who are difficult to evaluate because of obtundation or spinal cord damage. CT can detect intra- and retroperitoneal bleeding and can also identify the damaged organ. CT is most accurate in assessing those organs—the liver, spleen, kidneys, and pancreas—which are most likely to be damaged by blunt trauma. It is also accurate in detecting retroduodenal air or edema associated with duodenal disruption and free intraperitoneal air associated with rupture of the small or large intestine.

Arteriography

A thoracic aortogram should be obtained in any hemodynamically stable patient who has a suspected disruption of the thoracic aorta or of the great ves-sels. Suspicion should arise if the patient has a decreased blood pressure in the left arm or exhibits a widened mediastinum or obliteration of the aortic knob on chest film. Other indications are listed in the section on chest film.

In the stable patient, selected arteriography may be used to evaluate sus-pected arterial injuries in the neck and in the extremities. Suspicion of arterial injury should be aroused by penetrating injury near an artery, hematoma, bruit, decreased distal pulses, diminished peripheral perfusion, or compromised neu-rologic function associated with a penetrating injury. Severe blunt trauma to the region of the knee also is suspect. If arteriograms are not obtained in patients with suspected injuries to large arteries, i.e., the carotid, brachial, femoral, and popliteal, the vessels should be explored.

In stable patients with penetrating injuries to the base or upper one-third of the neck, arteriography is preferable to exploration. These vessels are difficult to expose, and arteriography can be helpful in the planning of an operation. In penetrating injuries to the middle third of the neck and to the extremities, either arteriography or exploration can be used. Exploration of these wounds is preferred (1) if the patient is unstable, (2) if the hematoma is expanding, or (3) if the ex-tremity distal to the injury is ischemic. Exposure of the vessels of the middle third of the neck or of the extremities is usually straightforward, and no time should be lost with arteriography.

Radionuclide Scanning and Sonography

Echocardiography is occasionally useful in ruling out a pericardial tamponade in the stable patient. Otherwise, radionuclide scans and sonograms have little to offer in the assessment of the trauma patient; they lack anatomic resolution and have limitations in comprehensive imaging of abdominal and retroperitoneal structures. They are occasionally useful in the evaluation of agitated patients with artifact-impaired CT evaluation and in the follow-up of known visceral injuries.

DIAGNOSTIC PERITONEAL LAVAGE

H. DAVID ROOT, M.D., Ph.D.

Early, prompt, and complete assessment of the severely injured trauma victim is of the utmost importance so that appropriate therapy may be chosen and instituted before the onset of hemorrhagic shock or peritonitis. Hemorrhagic shock, especially if recurrent, is associated with a mortality of approximately 25 percent. It can also be responsible for host compromise which facilitates the development of sepsis, the major cause of death in trauma victims who reach an emergency room alive. A patient who is subjected to more than one episode of hypovolemic shock within the first 4 hours of injury may reach a stage when resuscitation is difficult, if not impossible.

GENERAL CONSIDERATIONS

Early detection and treatment of internal bleeding can minimize the number of units of blood required to treat these patients, thereby decreasing the risk of hepatitis, transfusion morbidity, and mortality. Compromise of host defenses by hypovolemic shock has been demonstrated and measured in the human model, as well as in the laboratory. It has been well demonstrated that an episode of hypovolemic shock compromises the patient's resistance to infection at any site, be it pulmonary, genitourinary, or within serous cavities. Moreover, it has been well demonstrated that the mortality and morbidity from ruptured bowel, in particular the duodenum and colon, increase dramatically if the time from injury to treatment is greater than 8 hours. The mortality rate in duodenal injury averages 5 percent if treatment is rendered within 6 hours of injury, but rises to 75 percent if treatment is delayed by more than 24 hours.

On the other hand, an unnecessary laparotomy presents added risks to the patient, exacts a physiologic toll from the trauma victim, and inflicts increased medical care costs, discomfort, and loss of wages. Therefore, there is need for prompt, thorough, accurate, and safe assessment of the trauma victim as early as possible in the post-injury course.

Prior to the introduction of diagnostic peritoneal lavage (DPL) in 1965, trauma victims with blunt abdominal injury faced a number of severe problems; the diagnosis of intra-abdominal bleeding or ruptured viscera was often delayed or overlooked, and unnecessary laparotomies were performed in response to confusing clinical signs and symptoms. The incidence of missed liver injuries was reported to be as high as 45 percent in a series from St. Paul Ramsey Hospital. Mortality and morbidity rates from delayed detection of ruptured small bowel in blunt trauma victims have been as high as 20 percent and 25 percent, respectively. There were few radiologic signs that could be utilized consistently to detect visceral injury due to blunt abdominal trauma. Pelvic fractures were detectable by plain films, but the extent of associated injury could not be detected radiographically in these patients. Seeming stability of the hematocrit of the peripheral blood is not a reliable early sign of intra-abdominal bleeding, nor is an elevated white blood cell count reliable in the trauma victim. Clinical examination of the patient was reliable only if the patient developed cardinal signs of intra-abdominal bleeding such as a grossly expanding abdomen with profound and recurrent hypovolemic shock or tenderness.

Evaluation for peritoneal signs is often confused in the blunt trauma victim because of central nervous system alterations secondary to drug intoxication, head injury, or spinal cord injury. Pain from fractured ribs as well as fractured pelvis may be referred to the abdomen, making it difficult to evaluate the degree of peritoneal irritation or resistance to palpation. Several series have reported that, in a patient with blunt injury to the abdomen, overall accuracy of the physical examination is about 59 percent, with problems of false-positive and false-negative results. Ongoing clinical evaluation of the patient is extremely important, but may not be accurate enough to detect bleeding and ruptured viscera before profound shock and/or peritonitis becomes evident clinically.

DIAGNOSTIC PERITONEAL LAVAGE

Diagnostic peritoneal lavage (DPL) has been found useful, accurate, and sensitive in the hands of many trauma surgeons, as reported by institutions throughout the United States and Europe. The stated accuracy is approximately 98.5 percent; the incidence of false-negative results is approximately 0.5 to 1.0 percent and that of false-positive results is approximately 1 percent, depending on the experience and skill of the person performing the DPL. The current procedure has evolved from the original technique of simply introducing a catheter with many side holes into the peritoneal cavity through an infra-umbilical incision. There have been several modifications of the equipment and technique, e.g., entry through the umbilicus and direct percutaneous puncture with a short Teflon cannula through a large-bore needle. Evaluation of the returning fluid has evolved from simple visual detection of the presence of gross blood or purulent-appearing material in the returning dialysate fluid to the determination of red cell and white cell counts by hemocytometer.

My technique for performing diagnostic peritoneal lavage is as follows: With the patient supine, and a Foley catheter in the bladder, the abdomen is prepped with an appropriate cleansing solution around and below the umbilicus. Sterile technique is used to drape with skin towels. With a solution of 1 percent Xylocaine consisting of 0.5 cc of 1:1000 epinephrine in 10 cc of Xylocaine, the skin, subcutaneous tissues, and linea alba are anesthetized through a 22-gauge needle. Prior detection of known allergies is important. A site is chosen approximately 2 inches below the umbilicus for a vertical skin incision approximately 2 cm in length, but proportional to the depth of subcutaneous fat. Blunt dissection is carried down through the subcutaneous tissue to the linea alba. Short right-angle retractors can be of help in exposing the linea alba. All bleeding in the subcutaneous tissues is carefully controlled to minimize false-positive results. The linea alba is further anesthetized with the lidocaine/epinephrine combination. A small stab wound (large enough for the catheter) is made in the linea alba with a No. 11 blade. The sides of the incised fascia are grasped with an Allis clamp or hemostat and countertraction is applied in an anterior direction. The peritoneum is punctured with the No. 11 blade. With careful hand control to prevent a sudden thrust, the peritoneal lavage catheter with a central metal obturator is introduced into the peritoneal cavity. As soon as the peritoneum is penetrated, the obturator is withdrawn approximately one inch. While continuous traction is applied on the fascia in an anterior direction, the catheter is gently advanced inferiorly into the pelvis on either side. If resistance is met, the catheter is carefully withdrawn and may be introduced in a lateral or superior direction into an area of free peritoneal cavity. The catheter is aspirated with a syringe. If free blood is withdrawn, the test is positive. Free blood was evident in about 75 percent of the trauma victims studied who had a positive result. Mid-line scars are to be avoided. Peritoneal lavage can be carried out with a similar technique in the upper quadrants or in a supraumbilical area.

If no free blood is aspirated, lactated Ringer's solution, 20 cc per kilogram, is rapidly run into the peritoneal cavity. For practical calculation, 1,000 cc is used in the adult and 500 cc is used in the child. A 1.6 percent dialysate solution or normal saline may be used as well. Solutions containing only glucose are to be avoided. The bags of fluid are elevated on an IV stand several feet above the patient, and the connecting catheter introduces the fluid through the peritoneal lavage catheter. If the patient experiences pain or discomfort as the fluid is instilled, it is probable that the catheter is not in the peritoneal cavity but is instead in the rectus sheath or subcutaneous space. The fluid is run in as rapidly as possible. The tubing is left connected. A patient in stable condition should be turned to one side and then the other for approximately 30 seconds on each. This facilitates mixing of the fluid in the peritoneal cavity. The fluid bags or bottles are then placed on the floor and the fluid is then siphoned back into the bags from the peritoneal cavity. It is important that at least 75 cc of fluid is returned into the bags, but it is unnecessary to retrieve more than 200 cc from the peritoneal cavity.

The appearance of the fluid as it comes back through the tubing into the bag is carefully noted. If it is bloody, the test is positive. If it is salmon-pink and doubtful, two means of evaluating it are possible: (1) A paper with typewritten print is held behind the tubing and the print examined through the fluid in the tubing. If the print is legible, the test is probably negative. (2) Borderline or questionable fluid should be sent to the laboratory for a red cell count on an aliquot. The fluid is thoroughly mixed before a sample is taken for a red cell count. A reading of 100,0000 per milliliter of red cells is considered positive.

A white cell count should also be done, mixing the fluid thoroughly and obtaining a hemocytometer count. If the white cell count is over 500 cells per milliliter, it is positive. A smear should be examined for bacteria or enteric content, either of which is considered a positive result. A leukocyte count is *not* of help if it is negative, and less than 3 hours has elapsed between the time of injury and the time of the peritoneal lavage. According to recent findings, approximately 3 hours should pass before the polymorphonuclear cells begin to migrate from the capillaries of the peritoneal cavity into the peritoneal fluid. A white cell count of 500 or more per milliliter was found to be significant in the experimental work. The presence of a positive result indicates the need for laparotomy in these patients.

If, on the other hand, the returning fluid is more than 75 cc and is crystal clear, this finding is considered to be a true negative result. The catheter is then withdrawn and a simple suture closure of the infraumbilical skin incision is made. If the stab wound in the linea alba is just large enough to accommodate the DPL catheter, there is no need to put a suture in the linea alba opening. If the stab wound is larger, a single stitch in the linea alba may be appropriate to prevent any subsequent herniation. Sterile technique is important. A Bandaid over the closed incision is all that is necessary.

If the patient requires a laparotomy for a positive test result, carrying the midline incision through the site of the DPL procedure is appropriate and is not associated with any known increase in morbidity and mortality.

Complications of Diagnostic Peritoneal Lavage

The complications of peritoneal lavage are those attendant upon misadventures with insertion of the catheter. If the catheter is forcefully introduced through an old abdominal incision, bowel may be perforated by the catheter. Undue pressure with an obturator may damage regional intra-abdominal tissue such as the omentum, mesentery, bowel, iliac arteries or veins, aorta or vena cava. Mild inflammation may be noted around the skin incision subsequently, but it is rare for a wound infection to occur at the DPL site. It is important that the bladder be emptied with a Foley catheter in place before the DPL is done, so that bladder injury is avoided. A rare persistent urachal sinus or persistent vitelline duct may be encountered, but this is extremely unusual. Evidence or history of umbilical discharge is an indication that the DPL should be done above the umbilicus or in either upper quadrant.

In a patient with a fractured pelvis, the DPL should be done promptly, before dissection of the retroperitoneal hematoma is extended up to the umbilical level. Although false-positive results have been predicted when the DPL is carried out below the umbilicus, if the linea alba is sought and catheter insertion is performed through it, a false-positive result is unusual in a patient with a fractured pelvis. If the surgeon is concerned about this, a supraumbilical site of catheter introduction is appropriate. Evidence of blood in the preperitoneal tissues is significant. Careful attention to detail can minimize the incidence of false-positive and false-negative results, as well as complications from this procedure. The catheter that is introduced with a central obturator through an intact linea alba requires more force for introduction and therefore is more likely to penetrate some intra-abdominal viscus than is the catheter introduced through a small stab wound in the linea alba with anterior countertraction against the thrusting force of the catheter.

Wound Trauma

Utilization of DPL technique in patients with gunshot wounds of the abdomen is not wise. A gunshot wound that has probably penetrated the peritoneum warrants a laparotomy. Utilization of DPL in stab wound victims is gaining advocates, the initial series being worked out by Thal and associates at Parkland Hospital. The policy is as follows: If the patient has a stab wound that may have penetrated the peritoneal cavity, the wound is explored under local anesthesia in the emergency room with the intent of proving the peritoneal penetration. If penetration is found, but there is no compelling clinical indication for laparotomy such as exuding blood or enteric content, or shock, a DPL is performed. If positive, the patient undergoes laparotomy; if negative, the patient is observed in the hospital.

Diagnostic Concerns

There are warnings to be heeded concerning overdependence on DPL. DPL is *not* accurate for patients with retroperitoneal visceral injuries, such as duodenal, pancreatic, renal, ureteral, bladder, or extraperitoneal colon injuries. It is only helpful in detecting the presence of abnormal fluids and content of the peritoneal cavity. In cases of protracted delay in which there is an extraperitoneal septic focus, a secondary leukocytosis in the peritoneal cavity is possible and can produce a positive result in DPL. It has been found that in patients with a ruptured diaphragm, the incidence of false-negative DPL results is about 30 percent. Therefore, extra care is advised in reading the chest film and examining the diaphragm for evidence of abnormalities. Obliteration of a clear shadow of the diaphragm or unexplained mediastinal shadow should trigger further investigation with contrast studies of the esophagus and stomach. An unusual circumstance of a completely contained subcapsular hematoma of the spleen or liver has been reported and recorded at our own institution. The incidence of such nonbleeding, nonleaking, completely self-contained hematomas is unknown. Those that rupture manifest themselves several hours to days after the initial trauma episode. Therefore, it is important to maintain careful clinical vigilance over the patient, and if clinical signs change, the DPL can be repeated through a site somewhat inferior to the initial one. If the clinical indications are clear-cut, the patient should undergo laparotomy for evidence of hypovolemia. Since only about 50 percent of patients with free blood in the peritoneal cavity show signs of peritoneal irritation, dependence on physical examination alone is treacherous.

The future of peritoneal lavage, in combination with other diagnostic techniques, such as angiography, CT scanning, and ultrasound scanning, demands ongoing evaluation and assessment. We need to refine our diagnostic approaches to these patients, so that the patient with a self-limiting small amount of bleeding from a superficial crack in the liver will not be subjected to an unnecessary laparotomy. Further refinements need to be studied so that the diagnostic accuracy approaches 100 percent for detecting significant visceral injury requiring surgical intervention.

TRAUMA PRINCIPLES

TREATMENT PRIORITIES

DONALD D. TRUNKEY, M.D.

Priorities of care, whether in the prehospital or hospital setting, are predicated on common sense. The determinants of priorities are severity of injury, hemodynamic stability, and the ability to deliver prompt, definitive surgical care. The overriding concern is not only to minimize mortality, but also to maintain a functional human being. In general, resuscitation and treatment are always directed primarily at the brain, followed by the cardiopulmonary viscera including the airway, the abdominal viscera, the extremities including both vascular and orthopaedic injuries, and finally, maxillofacial injuries.

PREHOSPITAL PRIORITIES

Approximately 80 percent of all injuries are not life-threatening or permanently disabling. In many instances, this can be determined by triage criteria including trauma severity scores (see chapter on *Triage of Patients to Trauma Centers*) mechanism of injury, and most importantly, experience. In general, patients with these injuries can be transported to an appropriate hospital within a reasonable time and do not require code 3 status. The remaining 20 percent are at risk for loss of life or permanent disability and demand rapid transport, ideally to the nearest center capable of providing *immediate*, definitive surgical care. Approximately 50 to 55 percent of prehospital deaths are secondary to head injury, which also accounts for at least 50 percent of in-hospital deaths. One study has shown that in patients with space-occupying lesions, the time interval from injury to surgical decompression is critical. The patients treated by decompression within 2 hours of injury had a better prognosis than patients treated by decompression between 2 and 4 hours following injury. Even more striking is the high mortality that occurs when decompression is delayed for longer than 4 hours following injury. The same study also showed a linear relationship between the amount of disability and delay in surgical care. In the prehospital setting, the only definitive management necessary in the unconscious, head-injured patient is establishment of an airway, preferably by endotracheal intubation. Other treatment modalities have not been proved efficacious.

Prehospital treatment of life-threatening hemorrhage is more controversial, but in general, no treatment should be undertaken that prolongs the prehospital time unnecessarily. The treatment of fractures can be initiated during extrication and completed during transportation. Protection of the spine is necessary throughout extrication and prehospital transport.

HOSPITAL PRIORITIES

Priorities in the emergency room are determined by whether the patient's condition is unstable, both hemodynamically and neurologically, or whether his condition can be temporarily stabilized. In the unstable, head-injured patient, airway management and volume resuscitation should be carried out as quickly as possible, a rapid, directed CT scan should be obtained, and decompression of any space-occupying lesion should be carried out as rapidly as possible. To expedite this, the head can be shaved in the emergency room while the patient is being resuscitated. If a lesion requiring surgery is not found on CT, consideration of a burr hole with intracranial pressure (ICP) monitoring to better manage the patient should be strongly considered. If the patient has concomitant hemodynamic instability, volume resuscitation should be carried out and a chest roentgenogram obtained. This will help the general surgeon to decide whether a thoracotomy or exploratory laparotomy to control hemorrhage is necessary at the same time as a craniotomy. In these unstable situations, resuscitation in the emergency room should be limited to 15 minutes at most, and no other diagnostic studies except CT scan and chest film are necessary. Other diagnostic roentgenograms and a more complete physical examination must await completion of the first portions of surgery, which are life-saving.

If the patient arrives in a hemodynamically stable condition, or if his condition becomes stable shortly after arrival, a more deliberate approach is indicated. A complete secondary examination is carried out, focusing attention on orthopaedic and neurologic injuries, since these are most commonly associated with permanent disability. Roentgenograms and other tests should also be directed toward diagnosis of these injuries. If serial hematocrit, white cell count, or physical examination suggests the possibility of hemorrhage there are, in general, three possible sources: the thorax, the abdomen, or the thigh. Two of the three can be ruled out fairly easily. Chest film is invaluable as a diagnostic procedure and can often direct the surgeon toward the appropriate cavity. Physical examination of the thigh should immediately inform the examiner if there is fracture and subsequent occult hemorrhage within the thigh compartment. If the chest and thigh do not have significant injury, the occult bleeding is assumed to be occurring into the retroperitoneum or peritoneal cavity. The appropriate management is immediate surgical exploration.

Value judgments must often be exercised during the initial resuscitation and therapeutic planning. For example, the patient who has a widened mediastinum on roentgenogram must be assumed to have other sources of injury and blood loss. For all intents and purposes, it is virtually impossible to be subjected to enough kinetic energy to lacerate the thoracic aorta and not have damage elsewhere in the body. In most instances, rupture of the thoracic aorta does not occur immediately, particularly if blood pressure can be controlled. If the patient is hemodynamically unstable, exploratory laparotomy is indicated prior to aortogram. After the abdomen has been explored, an aortogram can be obtained while the patient is still under the anesthetic. If the chest film reveals a widened mediastinum and the patient is hemodynamically stable, an aortogram should be obtained. If this is positive, CT scan of the abdomen, peritoneal lavage, or exploratory laparotomy should be carried out before repair of the thoracic aorta. In most instances, repair of a ruptured thoracic aorta demands a right lateral decubitus position, making it necessary to establish that there is no intra-abdominal injury before such positioning. In patients who have both torso injury and vascular injury in an extremity, priorities are determined by the patients' hemodynamic stability. If the patient is unstable, the torso injury takes precedence, recognizing that saving the life may sacrifice the limb. However, control of the vascular injury may be necessary before exploration of the torso injury. If the patient is hemodynamcially stable, CT scan of the abdomen, peritoneal lavage, or rapid mini-laparotomy may be performed before repairing the vascular injury in the extremity. In general, all orthopaedic injuries should undergo stabilization and internal or external fixation after the patient has had repair of the torso or head injuries. This principle allows rapid mobilization of the patient in the intensive care unit during the postoperative period. Exceptions to this general rule are patients who are hypothermic or hemodynamically unstable after torso or head surgery. Repair of their orthopaedic injuries should be delayed for 12 to 24 hours until stability can be achieved and the patient rewarmed.

OPERATIVE PRIORITIES

The trauma patient must be prepared and the drapes positioned over a large area so that the surgeon can gain access to any body cavity expeditiously and can properly place drains and chest tubes, if needed. The entire anterior portion and both lateral portions of the torso should be painted with povidone-iodine and draped, so that the surgeon can work in a sterile field from the neck and clavicle cephalad, to the groins caudad, and from table top to table top laterally. Prepping should not involve more than a few minutes and is preferably carried out prior to anesthesia induction so that, should deterioration occur, immediate laparotomy or thoracotomy can be carried out. This prepping and draping of the torso should not interfere with concomitant craniotomy.

For rapid access and wide exposure of the abdomen, the midline incision is the best choice. Only rarely are transverse or oblique incisions appropriate for trauma surgery. Surgeons should be prepared to extend the midline incision up the sternum, as a sternum-splitting incision, or into the right or left chest if necessary. Repair of chest injuries that requires access to posterior mediastinal structures such as the left subclavian artery may necessitate the "trap door" incision, i.e., lateral extension along the clavicle with removal of the medial portion of the clavicle and extension into the third or fourth intercostal space.

When the presence of abdominal injury is questionable or its site uncertain, it is usually best to start with an upper midline incision that extends from just below the xiphoid to just above the umbilicus. The incision can be centered on the umbilicus if the injury is presumed to be in the lower abdomen. However, most of the complicated problems lie in the upper abdomen, hence the xiphoid to umbilical exploratory incision.

When intra-abdominal injury is encountered, the incision should routinely be extended below the umbilicus to the pubis if the injuries appear major.

An abdomen filled with bright red blood usually indicates an arterial injury. The patient should be eviscerated so that each corner of the abdomen can be rapidly inspected, and packs should be placed temporarily to absorb the free blood. All quadrants of the abdomen and the mesentery should be inspected on the first pass. This can be done within a minute or two, so that the major source of hemorrhage can be located and dealt with first. The application of packs controls bleeding from many arterial injuries, and if the injury can be controlled by pack or direct pressure, this should be done while volume is restored. Initially, the injury should not be directly exposed because the vascular system may suddenly decompress, and rapid bleeding in a previously hypovolemic patient frequently leads to cardiac arrest.

If the injury appears to be arterial and in the upper abdomen, the possibility of injury to the visceral portion of the aorta or one of its major upper abdominal branches should be considered and proximal control undertaken. If a hematoma extends to the level of the diaphragm, the left chest should be opened and the aorta encircled. If the aortic hiatus is free of hematoma, the gastrohepatic ligament should be divided, and the aorta should be encircled as it emerges through the crura of the diaphragm.

Minor injuries and minor sources of hemorrhage should not distract the surgeon who is dealing with major ongoing hemorrhage, particularly venous hemorrhage. Venous bleeding may not be obvious since it occurs under low pressure and may not be as dramatic, or as evident, as arterial hemorrhage. Almost all venous bleeding can be controlled by the judicious application of packs, a measure that allows time for restoration of volume. If, during the initial exploration, retraction downward of the dome of the liver results in massive venous hemorrhage, injury to the hepatic veins or intrahepatic cava should be strongly suspected, and the appropriate operative approach considered. It may be necessary to insert an intracaval shunt or to have the assistant directly compress the liver parenchyma while direct ligation or repair of the hepatic veins is carried out. Tractotomy may be necessary before the injury can be visualized.

After initial control of hemorrhage has been achieved with clamps or packs, an attempt should be made to control fecal soilage prior to definitive surgery.

Obvious holes in small bowel or colon can be temporarily controlled by a running chronic suture or by Babcock clamps.

After neurosurgical and torso injuries have been treated, a decision must be made regarding the management of associated orthopaedic and maxillofacial injuries. If the patient is hemodynamically unstable or hypothermic, it may be prudent to document the various fractures, temporarily splint them, and take the patient to the intensive care unit for further volume resuscitation and warming. A planned return to the operating room within 24 hours is then scheduled. During the second operation, orthopaedic and maxillofacial injuries are treated, and a secondary exploratory laparotomy for abdominal toilet is carried out. On the other hand, if the patient is hemodynamically stable and has not sustained significant hypothermia after treatment of neurosurgical and torso injuries, orthopaedic injuries should be definitively treated while the patient is still under the same anesthetic.

INTENSIVE CARE PRIORITIES

During the past 15 to 20 years, it has become apparent that the primary purpose of the trauma intensive care unit is to treat and support organ dysfunction as it arises. Most often this is due to sepsis or the injury itself. Further discussion of the primary goals is beyond the scope of this section.

Priorities of intensive care fall into five categories, (1) direction of care, (2) mobilization of the patient, (3) expeditious removal of all tubes, (4) nutrition, and (5) acute rehabilitation. It is imperative that direction of care be under the guidance and direction of one individual, preferably that individual who has directed the emergency and operative care. Such an individual should ensure continuity of care and direct the many consultants necessary to evaluate organ function and provide all of the support services.

Early mobilization of the acutely injured patient in the postoperative period cannot be overemphasized. This minimizes organ failure, restores anabolism, and minimizes disability. Removal and replacement of all tubes placed in the emergency room, except the endotracheal tube, should be accomplished within 24 hours after injury. Tubes placed in the emergency room tend to be contaminated and only serve as a source of sepsis. In general, all tubes should be viewed as a wick between the environment and the patient's interior. Early removal minimizes the risk of contamination.

An early decision should be made regarding supplemental nutrition, preferably within 48 hours of the injury. If the patient is incapable of taking normal enteral nutrition, the first consideration should be placement of a feeding tube and provision of the required protein-calorie nutrition via the enteral route. If this is not possible, the secondary choice should be intravenous parenteral nutrition. Optimally, during the initial surgery, subsequent nutrition should be considered, and the placement of a feeding jejunostomy or hyperalimentation line performed as early as possible. The primary goal is to achieve positive nitrogen balance with a minimum of complications.

The final priority is acute rehabilitation, which should be started as soon as possible after the injury. In the unconscious patient, this includes skin protection and passive motion of joints. As soon as the patient is able to cooperate, a trapeze bar and active physical therapy by nurses or trained specialists should be routine, not only in the intensive care unit, but also as the patient progresses to ward care.

A more complex area for rehabilitation is the psychological aspect, which is more difficult to quantitate, but is, nevertheless, a major problem in the post-injury period. Family support is essential, and professional psychologists or psychiatrists should be utilized when any psychiatric dysfunction is evident. Many patients, but particularly those who are innocent victims of random violence, have severe emotional sequelae that interfere with family relationships and normal activities. This post-traumatic stress disorder has thus far received minimal attention, and no specific therapies to prevent or treat it can be recommended.

WOUND BALLISTICS

MARTIN L. FACKLER, M.D., F.A.C.S.

Gunshot wounds are treated competently by most surgeons, even if they have little knowledge of wound ballistics. The damage to the tissues is usually obvious. Physical examination and roentgenograms of the wounded part, realization that all gunshot wounds are contaminated and contain some necrotic tissue, and common sense should be all the information the surgeon needs in most cases to make the necessary treatment decisions.

WOUNDING MECHANISMS

Understanding the mechanisms by which a gunshot disrupts tissue is the foundation of rational treatment. The penetrating projectile crushes the tissue it strikes, forming a "permanent cavity," or hole edged by frayed tissue remnants. Tissue surrounding the bullet path is stretched radially outward by bullet passage; the dilatation of the walls of the bullet hole is called the "temporary cavity." The maximum tissue displacement by the temporary cavity follows bullet passage by a few milliseconds. To what extent the tissue returns to its former state and position depends, for the most part, on its elasticity. The temporary cavity stretch is nothing more than a localized area of "blunt trauma"; keeping this in mind helps one to determine the relative vulnerability of various body parts to this mechanism of injury. Wounds from different weapons vary only in the amount and location of crushed and stretched tissue along the projectile path.

WOUND PROFILES

At the Letterman Army Institute of Research, a technique was developed for measuring the amount and location of the crushed and stretched tissue caused by a given projectile. The entire missile path is caught in one or more $25 \times 25 \times 50$ cm blocks of ordnance gelatin. The studies show that a 10 percent solution at 4 °C mirrors the wound dimensions in living, anesthetized, swine muscle. Biplanar roentgenograms of the blocks reveal the projectile fragmentation pattern. The data are presented in a standard pictorial form called the "wound profile." Figures 1, 2, and 3 show wound profiles illustrating different tissue damage patterns caused by projectiles with different characteristics.

Handguns

Most projectiles striking tissue at a speed below 900 ft per second (274 m per second) produce wound profiles similar to the one made by a 45-caliber automatic pistol (Fig. 1). The predominant mechanism of tissue injury is crush. There is some temporary cavitation, but tissue displacement is so small that there is no clinically detectable damage. Most of the common 22s, 32s, and 38s fit into this category. Bullet shape and construction make little difference at this velocity.

Rifles Loaded with Full-Metal-Jacketed Ammunition

Most full-metal-jacketed bullets striking tissue at speeds between 2,000 ft per second (610 m per second) and 3,000 ft per second (914 m per second) produce wound profiles similar to the one made by the 7.62 NATO rifle bullet (Fig. 2). No deformation of the bullet occurs unless bone is struck. After traveling some distance through tissue, the bullet yaws and makes a 180-degree turn around its transverse axis, completing its path traveling backward. The distance traveled point-forward, before marked yaw begins, is a recognized characteristic of the particular bullet. The 7.62 NATO round (see Fig. 2) begins its yaw after about 16 cm; the Russian AK-47 (familiar to those who served in Vietnam) does not yaw until after approximately 26 cm of point-forward penetration. Rifle bullets are usually longer than pistol bullets, and so at maximum yaw (traveling sideways) they can crush up to three times as much tissue as when traveling point-forward. As marked yaw usually occurs over less than one-third of the bullet's total penetration, the relative increase in crushed tissue is small. The large temporary cavity caused by the yawing bullet is the notable feature of this class of projectile. Just as a diver makes a large splash if he hits the water at a large "yaw" angle, the nonstreamlined yawing projectile causes more disturbance in passing through tissue. This is manifested as a larger tissue displacement or stretch.

Rifles Loaded with Soft-Point or Hollow-Point Bullets

Most bullets of the "expanding" variety (designed for hunting rather than military purposes) produce a marked increase in crushed tissue or permanent cavity formation (Fig. 3). Soft-point or hollow-point bullets are designed to deform on striking soft tissue. The bullet begins to flatten its tip within a few centimeters of penetration; bullet diameter increases and its length shortens. The diameter of the flattened forward part expands about 2 to 2½ times the original bullet diameter, and the bullet ends up resembling a mushroom (the expansion

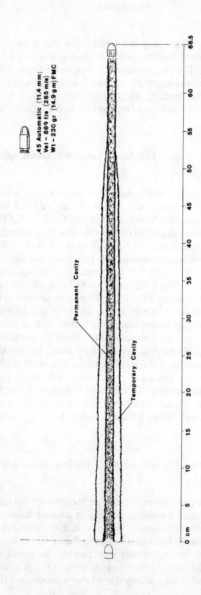

Figure 1 Wound profile of the 45 ACP pistol. The predominant wounding mechanism is tissue crush. This is typical of most handgun wounds seen in the large city hospitals.

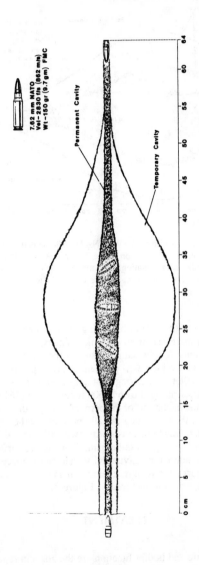

7.62 mm NATO
Vel—2830 f/s (862 m/s)
Wt—150 gr (9.7 gm) FMC

Permanent Cavity

Temporary Cavity

Figure 2 Wound profile produced by the 7.62 NATO rifle with full-metal-jacketed military bullet.

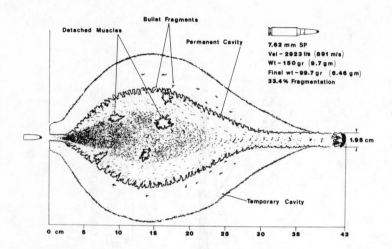

Figure 3 Wound profile of the 7.62 NATO rifle loaded with a soft-point bullet. This civilian version of the 7.62 NATO is called the 308 Winchester. Bullet fragmentation is the major cause of the massive increase in tissue destruction seen here as compared to Figure 2.

process is often referred to as "mushrooming"). The amount of tissue struck (cross-sectional area) increases up to six times. The new blunt shape causes a marked temporary cavity for the same reason as the yawing bullet.

The major cause of the increased permanent cavity pictured in Figure 3 is fragmentation of the bullet. Bullet fragmentation effects increase with striking velocity and, for bullets striking at over 2,500 ft per second (762 m per second), fragmentation causes the major part of the permanent tissue disruption. As pieces of the bullet break off, they are flung radially outward by the centrifugal force of bullet rotation. Each fragment crushes its own path through tissue, ending up as far as 8 cm from the original bullet path. This tissue, perforated multiple times, is stretched by temporary cavitation which causes pieces of muscle to be detached. The synergy between fragmentation and temporary cavity stretch causes the massive destruction pictured in Figure 3.

TREATMENT

Preservation of life and bodily function are the goals in repairing or limiting the damage done by gunshot. Recommendations made here are not meant as absolute rules; common sense and clinical conditions may dictate exceptions. Contrary to popular opinion, information on the striking velocity or energy of the wounding bullet is *not* necessary to make treatment decisions. All gunshot wounds are treated according to the same principles, regardless of striking velocity. The often repeated maxim, "high-velocity gunshot wounds need radical debridement," has *no* valid scientific support. As bullets in flight are not sterile, a cephalosporin antibiotic should be started as soon as the patient with gunshot wound is seen, and this regimen should be continued for 3 to 5 days.

Ideally, removal of all devitalized tissue would give the body defenses the best environment for healing the wound, but removal of *all* devitalized tissue is never accomplished even in the most meticulous of operations. (How does one attain hemostasis without causing some devitalization?) It has been documented in the clinical experience of large city hospitals that handgun wounds through skin and muscle heal well if left solely to the body's defense mechanisms. However, the simple excision of entrance wounds with small skin elipse allows the physician to look at the bullet hole in the muscle and determine whether there is any apparent reason to carry the exploration further. It also affords drainage and can be closed in 3 or 4 days simply by taping the skin edges together, a procedure that takes little time and adds no morbidity. Small exit wounds are treated in a similar fashion. Exit wounds may be large and gaping with pieces of detached skin and muscle *if* the bullet fragmented, or they ocasionally may be stellate due to the stretch of temporary cavitation alone. In either case, wide open wounds should ensure good drainage. Obviously nonviable or partially detached tissue should be removed, and the wounds should be left unsutured and covered with a dry gauze dressing. Wound healing can then be monitored by daily dressing changes.

The Chest

Gunshot wounds that penetrate the pleural cavity and cause a hemopneumothorax should be handled with chest tubes. The need for thoracotomy is dictated by the clinical course. On occasion, when a tangential gunshot wound of the chest wall is inflicted by a weapon with the potential for a large temporary cavity (see Figs. 2 and 3), a pulmonary contusion can develop even without penetration of the bullet into the pleural cavity. These contusions may be apparent on the first chest film or may not become apparent until later. They are treated in the same way as pulmonary contusions caused by any other form of blunt trauma, but the physician should be alert to the possibility of diagnosing these occult contusions and beginning early treatment.

The Abdomen

Laparotomy is recommended for all penetrating gunshot wounds of the peritoneal cavity. The preoperative roentgenogram that shows multiple bullet fragments is an indication of extensive tissue destruction (see Fig. 3). The civilian trauma surgeon's experience with fragmenting rifle bullets is limited, but the experience in Vietnam gave military surgeons the opportunity to become familiar with these wounds. Contrasting the wounds produced by a shot through the abdomen with the M-16 (this bullet causes wide tissue destruction because the bullet fragments) with the Russian AK-47 (whose steel-jacketed bullet does not fragment unless bone is struck), one typically observes the following:

1. The M-16 causes actual gaps in small bowel continuity up to 7 cm long; these are handled by cutting across the bowel where it appears normal (about 1 cm from the wound edge usually) and doing an anastomosis.
2. The AK-47 typically causes small perforations of the bowel (less than 1 cm in diameter—exactly like a handgun wound). These are handled by resection and anastomosis.

The amount of damage done by the bullets is vastly different; in one case approximately 9 cm of bowel was lost, compared to less than 3 cm in the other case. *Some may find it surprising that the amount of bowel the surgeon excised during debridement was the same in both cases.*

The same wound management principle applies to blood vessels and other tissues; one cuts across tissue where it appears normal. There is no valid reason to excise an extra 1 or 2 cm in deference to the weapon's velocity or energy. The liver (like other solid abdominal organs) is one place where the stretch of a large temporary cavity alone (see Fig. 2) causes massive tissue disruption. This is another example of the blunt trauma effect of temporary cavitation, and it is an instance in which the physician does not have roentgenographic identification of bullet fragmentation to indicate extensive tissue disruption. However, this poses no clinical diagnostic problem since the abdomen is being explored anyway, and the damage will become apparent. Gunshot wounds of the colon are excised in the same manner as those in the small bowel, but the ends are brought out as a double-barreled colostomy.

The Extremities

For wound tracts that pass near major arteries, either exploration or arteriogram is indicated to determine the status of the vessel. If bone is struck, there may be increased damage due to bone fragments acting as secondary missiles. Localization of bone fragment position by roentgenography helps to determine how much extra tissue damage has occurred as each fragment sliced and crushed its way through muscles to get to its final position.

The best method of handling the extremity wound caused by gunshot that has not hit the bone and is well away from major vessels (for instance, a shot through the anterolateral aspect of the upper thigh with 15 cm of muscle perforated) has been the subject of much debate in wound ballistics circles. If the wound was caused by a ''high-velocity'' rifle, many would argue that the wound tract must be completely explored and/or excised. This is no small operation and can cause considerable long-term morbidity. Comparing Figures 1 and 2 shows the fallacy of using projectile velocity or energy to make clinical decisions. Projectile energy is an approximation only of *potential* destructiveness; *actual* tissue disruption is what must be treated. Looking at the first 15 cm of missile travel in Figure 2, we can see that both the crush and the stretch of tissue are less than for the same first 15 cm in the path of the handgun wound shown in Figure 1. The velocity of the rifle bullet was four times that produced by the handgun. Fragmentation of the bullet shows up well on roentgenogram and points out the areas of actual tissue disruption that should be explored. In the absence of radiologic evidence of bullet fragmentation, exploration of the entire path of these wounds may cause more damage than was done originally by the bullet. Incisions should be made parallel to the long axis of the extremity, and muscles should be divided in the same direction. (This is mentioned only in an attempt to counter any false impressions given by animal dissection demonstrations in which the tissue disruption was demonstrated by cutting across the major muscle bundles rather than properly splitting them in the direction of their fibers.)

Short-range (up to 20 ft, i.e., 6 m) shotgun blasts are probably the most challenging treatment problem of all gunshot trauma. The multiple perforation effect described for fragmenting bullets has its ultimate example in the massive tissue destruction associated with these wounds. The devitalized tissue and other debris (which may include pieces of cardboard wadding) need to be removed, hemostasis attained, and the wound left open for later reconstruction. Surgical management of neurovascular bundles of extremities that are injured by shotgun blasts is a problem. Doing a primary arterial graft across the gap, after the devastation has been cleaned up, generally does not work well. An extra-anatomic graft may be considered, if conditions permit, or sometimes immediate amputation of the extremity is the best solution. These large tissue defects can tax the ingenuity of the surgeon in both the initial treatment and the later reconstruction.

FORCE IN BLUNT TRAUMA

DONALD D. TRUNKEY, M.D.

Blunt injury can be caused by direct impact deceleration, shear forces, and rotary forces. Direct impact or forced compression is probably the most common cause of significant injury, and the severity can be estimated if one knows the force and duration of impact, as well as the mass of contact area in the patient. Table 1 demonstrates the most common sites of body injury from motor vehicle accidents. Ejection, steering assembly impact, windshield impact, instrument panel impact, and rear collision account for the majority of these.

Most investigators agree that there is a direct correlation between degree of injury and velocity forced compression. There may be differences in severity of injury depending on what part of the torso is injured. For example, the thorax appears to sustain less damage from direct compressive forces than does the abdomen. This is no doubt due to the protective nature of the chest wall as well as the compressibility of the lung.

Postmortem examinations of cadavers have shown that decelerating impact against an object such as a steering column at approximately 16 miles per hour may be associated with fracture of four to six ribs. Contributing factors include age, deceleration time, and failure to wear a seat belt. More recent retrospective analyses of live patients confirm these earlier studies.

Deceleration injuries are most often associated with high-speed motor vehicle accidents and falls from high altitudes. Tables 2 and 3 show the relative weights of organs at different speeds and as a function of distance fallen. As the body decelerates, the organs continue to move forward at maximum velocity, tearing vessels and tissues from points of attachment. Rotary forces also tend to cause tearing injuries from a tumbling type of action.

Shear forces tend to produce degloving types of injuries such as may occur when the patient is run over by a large vehicle. As the vehicle passes over the body, the skin and subcutaneous tissues are pushed ahead, and nutrient blood supply is torn from the inferior muscular sources. Subsequent extensive soft tissue loss is common following such injury. Low-velocity, high- compression injuries to the abdomen may also cause shear force injury to solid parenchymatous organs such as the liver or spleen. In contrast, high- velocity, low compression injuries are probably secondary to bursting.

Blunt trauma, particularly of low velocity and under certain conditions, can result in a crush syndrome, that is, swollen necrotic muscle confined within a fascial compartment. The crush or compartment syndrome can be caused by direct impact on the muscle or by continuous pressure, which produces tissue ischemia and necrosis. The continuous pressure can be generated by obtunded patients lying on their extremities in an awkward position; the pressure can also

TABLE 1   Incidence of Torso Injury in Motor Vehicle Accidents*

	Driver Non-fatal (%)	Fatal (%)	Non-fatal (%)	Fatal (%)
Face, teeth	21	20	28	10
Larynx, trachea, bronchi	4	35	--	--
Sternum	22	5	--	--
Vertebral column	9	20	10	25
Ribs	36	20	40	25
Flail chest	29	40	19	35
Lung	33	40	15	30
Pneumothorax	23	25	19	40
Hemothorax	34	35	21	45
Heart and pericardium	13	60	15	40
Aorta and major vessels	5	40	11	85
Diaphragm	5	65	8	20
Liver	17	55	5	35
Spleen	13	55	5	35

* These percentages primarily reflect dashboard injuries in unrestrained occupants. Modified from Besson and Saegesser: Color Atlas of Chest Trauma and Associated Injuries. Oradell, New Jersey, Medical Economics Books; 1983.

TABLE 2   "Apparent Weight" of the Organs of the Human Body During a Violent Impact

Actual Organ Weight (kg)	Apparent Weight (kg)*		
	36 km/hr	72 km/hr	108 km/hr
Spleen (0.25)	2.5	10	22.5
Heart (0.35)	3.5	14	31.5
Encephalon (1.5)	15	60	135
Liver (1.8)	18	72	162
Blood (5.0)	50	200	450
Whole body (70)	700	2,800	6,300

* At 36 km/hr, the inertial weight of the body and its parts is increased tenfold over resting weight; at 72 km/hr the increase is fortyfold; at 108 km/hr the increase is ninetyfold. From Besson and Saegesser: Color Atlas of Chest Trauma and Associated Injuries. Oradell, New Jersey, Medical Economics Books; 1983.

TABLE 3 Relation of Distance Fallen to Velocity at Impact

Duration of Fall (secs)	Distance Fallen (ft)	Velocity at Impact	
		(ft/sec)	(mph)
1	16.1	32.2	21.9
2	64.4	64.4	43.9
3	144.9	96.6	65.8
4	257.6	128.8	87.8
5	402.5	161.0	109.8
6	579.6	193.2	131.7

Modified from Besson and Saegesser: Color Atlas of Chest Trauma and Associated Injuries. New Jersey, Oradell, Medical Economics Books; 1983.

be generated by severe muscular exertion, metabolic disturbances, and toxicity syndromes.

The pathophysiology of compartment syndrome begins with local compression of muscle, decreased capillary flow, damage to capillaries and arterioles, and eventually ischemic necrosis of the compressed muscle. This, in turn, leads to increased permeability of capillaries. Fluid leaks into the interstitium, compartment pressure builds up, and a compartment tamponade occurs. This syndrome may occur rapidly as a result of severe injury causing hemorrhage, increased pressure within the compartment, and rapid onset of ischemia.

The symptoms and signs of early compartment syndrome include pain and tense swelling in the affected extremity. Skin edema is frequently minimal. If tissue damage is extensive enough, the patient develops a third space loss of plasma, resulting in increased hematocrit, progressive hypovolemia, and oliguria.

The sequelae of the compartment syndrome are muscle necrosis, nerve damage, and paralysis. If myoglobin and hemoglobin are released into the plasma and precipitate in the renal tubules, tubular necrosis may result.

Treatment includes early fasciotomy, excision of necrotic tissue, and volume resuscitation. An alkaline pH in the urine should be maintained by giving bicarbonate, and diuresis should be promoted by administering mannitol to the patient.

ANTIBIOTIC USE

E. PATCHEN DELLINGER, M.D.

Infection is a major cause of death and disability following trauma. Of patients who die more than 2 days following trauma, the majority die of infectious complications. Trauma predisposes to infection in a number of ways. The obvious prerequisite for most infections is the disruption of mechanical barriers that normally prevent access of bacteria to sterile sites in the body. Bacterial contamination may be either exogenous, from sources in the environment, or endogenous, coming from the gastrointestinal tract or female genital tract. Bacterial contamination is a prerequisite for infection, but it is not the sole cause. Nonmechanical host defense mechanisms are also disturbed by major traumatic injury. Disturbance of normal tissue perfusion, either locally or systemically, and impairment of oxygenation, either alone or combined with perfusion abnormalities, significantly increase the incidence and severity of infection. Prompt attention to adequate airway maintenance and fluid resuscitation dramatically influences these risk factors. Techniques of local wound management also greatly affect the subsequent risk of infection. The details of these techniques are described in the chapter on *Wound Management*.

PRINCIPLES OF ANTIBIOTIC PROPHYLAXIS

The appropriate use of preventive or prophylactic antibiotics, in conjunction with the previously mentioned treatment principles, may significantly decrease post-traumatic infections. If antibiotics are used without proper attention to these principles, they are unlikely to provide any benefit.

The theoretic work that established the principles of prophylactic antibiotic use was done in animals many years ago. This work showed that a reduction in the number and severity of infections could be obtained through the administration of antibiotics during a finite period following bacterial contamination of tissues. The greatest protection was obtained when antibiotics were present in tissues before bacterial contamination had occurred. This concept has since been verified in a wide variety of clinical settings by trials that have compared antibiotic administration with placebo for scheduled surgical procedures. The data concerning duration of antibiotic administration are less clear. Modern practice has tended to shorten the duration of antibiotic administration for scheduled surgical procedures. Abundant evidence supports the efficacy of a single preoperative dose of an antibiotic.

In the case of trauma patients, less information is available and more controversy exists. Common wisdom has held that, in the setting of trauma, antibiotics should be administered for a prolonged period to counteract the disadvantage of starting antibiotic administration only after bacterial contamination has occurred. This principle, although frequently discussed, has rarely been studied.

Published studies clearly indicate that antibiotic use decreases the development and severity of infection following penetrating abdominal injuries with intestinal perforation and following open fractures.

WOUNDS WITHOUT ENDOGENOUS CONTAMINATION

Soft tissue wounds may be divided into two categories: those with relatively little exogenous contamination, such as a laceration caused by a clean kitchen knife, and those subject to heavy exogenous contamination, such as wounds caused by farm machinery or human bites or those containing foreign material. These wounds may also be classified according to the physical nature of the injury. A simple, sharp laceration has minimal surrounding tissue damage. A complex laceration caused by blunt injury or by tearing has additional surrounding tissue damage, bleeding, and interruption of blood supply, all of which increase the risk of infection. Simple lacerations, from relatively clean objects, that are closed within 4 hours have a low infection rate and do not warrant prophylactic antibiotics. With complex lacerations and blunt injuries, the physical handling of the wound and the resuscitation of the patient have far more to do with subsequent infection risk than does antibiotic use. It is possible that antibiotic use in this setting reduces the risk of infection, but no controlled trials support this opinion.

If antibiotics are to be effective, adequate tissue levels of antibiotics must be achieved as soon as possible, certainly in less than 4 hours from injury. A parenteral antibiotic with activity against *Streptococcus* and *Staphylococcus* should be given; one gram of nafcillin, oxacillin, or cefazolin is appropriate. The antibiotic can be repeated again in 4 hours. It is highly doubtful that further administration adds any additional protection. Frequent examination of the wound for signs of infection and early appropriate treatment by drainage is preferable to prolonged antibiotic administration, which may simply mask signs of infection, causing delay in diagnosis. It is almost certainly useless to provide a patient with a written prescription for an oral antibiotic after suturing a laceration in the emergency room.

In cases of puncture wound, the physician must rule out damage to such functional tissues as nerves, tendons, vessels, and bowel and assess the probability of endogenous contamination. If this has been done, there is little in the way of physical attention to the wound that is beneficial. It is logical to administer one or two doses of nafcillin, oxacillin, or cefazolin to these patients. The effectiveness of this practice is unknown, and the prescription of additional antibiotics is not warranted. All wounds, but especially puncture wounds, require inquiry into the tetanus immune status of the patient. Tetanus prevention is accomplished solely by both active and passive immunization. Antibiotics play no role in tetanus prevention.

Open Fractures

Open fractures combine bony and soft tissue damage with skin laceration and the potential for exogenous contamination. The overall infection rate is clearly related to the degree of soft tissue damage surrounding the fracture and especially to the extent of vascular injury. Adequate fixation of the bony fragments, sufficient debridement of the soft tissues, and restoration of perfusion are the factors that determine the patient's risk of infection. Within this context, several large series have demonstrated that appropriate antibiotic use can further reduce infection rates. The most common practice is to administer cefazolin, 1 g IV every 6 hours, beginning as soon as possible after injury and continuing for 3 to 5 days. Nafcillin or oxacillin would probably be equally effective; a much shorter course of antibiotic administration might be effective, but this has not been studied.

Basilar Skull Fractures

In patients suffering basilar skull fractures with cerebral spinal fluid (CSF) leak, there is a small but definite risk of developing meningitis. The cause of infection in such cases appears to be communication from the sinuses or the middle ear with the subarachnoid space, and the most common pathogens are *Pneumococcus* or *Haemophilus influenzae*. Since reports of this complication first appeared, some neurosurgeons have advocated the administration of preventive antibiotics, either for 5 days following the diagnosis of a basilar skull fracture or for the duration of the CSF leak. No data exist regarding the efficacy of this practice. In fact, theory suggests that it would be preferable not to use antibiotics in this setting. Preventive antibiotics can be effective when a short duration of contamination exists, and antibiotics effective against the pathogens can be used during this interval. In settings where the risk of infection continues over an extended time, preventive antibiotics do not work. Instead, they result in the generation of resistant bacteria that then cause infections more difficult to treat. In the case of patients with basilar skull fractures, it is preferable to monitor them closely for early signs of meningitis and institute early diagnostic procedures and aggressive treatment should such an infection occur.

WOUNDS WITH DEFINITE ENDOGENOUS CONTAMINATION

Wounds that penetrate the gastrointestinal tract anywhere between the mouth and the anus expose sterile tissues to major endogenous contamination. This is also true of the female genital tract. Infection risk varies dramatically according to the circumstances of injury, the extent of associated injuries, and the initial resuscitation of the patient. Trauma-related infections occur in 10 to 60 percent of patients with the average close to 20 percent. In this setting, strong evidence supports the contention that early administration of antibiotics is beneficial and that adequate coverage of both aerobic and anaerobic pathogens is important. My practice is to administer antibiotics in the emergency room as soon as an injury with a high probability of involving the gastrointestinal (GI) tract is detected. I begin with 2 g of cefoxitin intravenously. An alternate, effective choice would be gentamicin, 2 to 2.5 mg per kilogram IV, combined with clindamycin, 900 mg IV. At laparotomy, if no bowel injury is discovered, no further antibiotics are needed.

Until recently most trauma centers have continued antibiotics for 3 to 5 days following injury when penetration of the bowel was confirmed at laparotomy. Several recent reports have indicated acceptable results with 24 to 48 hours of antibiotic administration. My own practice is to administer high doses of antibiotics (2 g of cefoxitin intravenously every 4 hours) for only 12 hours. If blood loss exceeds 5 units during the operative procedure, an additional dose of antibiotics should then be given.

After antibiotics are stopped, the patient is closely observed in the postoperative period for signs of infection. All patients who undergo laparotomy for traumatic injury experience fever and leukocytosis during the first 5 days following injury. This includes the 80 percent of patients who recover without any infectious complications. For this reason, the mere presence of fever or elevated white count is not an indication for antibiotic administration. When an infection is diagnosed, it usually requires a procedure such as opening the wound or draining an intra-abdominal abscess, in addition to antibiotics. Early use of antibiotics before diagnosis is most likely to delay diagnosis without preventing the infection.

WOUNDS WITH NO IMMEDIATE ENDOGENOUS OR EXOGENOUS CONTAMINATION

Wounds such as closed fractures, blunt chest injuries, and injuries to the liver, spleen, kidneys, pancreas, or bladder cause neither exogenous nor endogenous contamination. In the absence of other known contamination or active infection in the injured organ, none of these injuries requires antibiotic administration. When such injuries require operative intervention, the indications for antibiotic use are the same as for elective operations on the same organs. Common practice dictates the administration of cefazolin immediately before and for 12 to 24 hours following open fixation of fractures. None of the other injuries has ever been demonstrated to benefit from prophylactic antibiotic administration.

OTHER POST-TRAUMA INFECTIONS

Chest Tubes

Many patients require chest tubes following penetrating or blunt trauma to the chest. Because of the circumstances under which these tubes are placed, this procedure may carry an increased risk of infection compared to elective chest tube placement. It is preferable to observe adequate sterile precautions at the time of tube placement rather than use antibiotics to compensate for poor sterile technique. If a hospital appears to have a problem with chest tube infections, the administration of 1 g of cefazolin IV at the time of chest tube placement may be beneficial. There is no reason to administer additional antibiotics; greater effort should be devoted to preventing infection at the source by improved sterile technique in tube placement and care of the suction and drainage equipment.

Pulmonary Contusion

Some authorities advocate prophylactic antibiotic administration for patients with pulmonary contusion or adult respiratory distress syndrome. Such patients are at increased risk for pulmonary infection from endotracheal intubation and impairment of local pulmonary defense mechanisms. However, the risk of infection is always present and is not reduced by antibiotic administration. The most likely result of prophylactic antibiotics in these patients is the development of infection with resistant organisms.

Aspiration

Trauma patients, particularly those with head or facial injuries, are in danger of aspirating gastric contents, oral secretions, or blood. Aspiration may be followed by pulmonary infection, termed aspiration pneumonia. Early findings of infection on chest film, combined with fever and leukocytosis, are most likely the result of chemical injury to the lung rather than subsequent infection. This chemical injury, however, does impair local defenses and may predispose the patient to subsequent infection with bacteria introduced at the same time. No precise treatment plan for such patients exists. Many physicians start antibiotics in this setting in order to treat aspiration pneumonia expectantly. The efficacy of this practice is unproven. My choice for such a patient is the immediate administration of cefazolin, 1 g IV, followed by two more doses at 6 and 12 hours. This covers most oral and gastric flora in the nonhospitalized patient. If a brief contamination has occurred, infection may be prevented. If not, close observation of the patient should detect subsequent bacterial infection and permit adequate culture and sensitively testing of pulmonary secretions, uninfluenced by precipitous antibiotic administration.

Since infection is a serious complication of trauma and occurs in such a significant number of these patients, the temptation to use antibiotics extensively is great. Despite the large number of patients treated for injuries in the United States, there is a paucity of solid information to guide us in this area. Evidence suggests that the most effective means of preventing infection is by adhering to the basic principles of resuscitation and tissue injury management. The optimal restoration and support of normal physiology accomplishes these goals. Indiscriminate use of antibiotics may induce a false sense of security, mask early signs of infection, and promote development of resistant bacteria.

When antibiotics are used, the earliest possible administration with high doses for a short duration provides the greatest likelihood of success. Immediate parenteral administration should be used. In the trauma setting, oral administration delivers antibiotic levels that are too little, too late. For wounds with exogenous contamination, cefazolin or oxacillin is adequate. If the exogenous contamination occurs in an environment such as a farm where gram-negative rods and/or anaerobes are likely to reside, coverage should be broadened to the same regimen as is used for endogenous bowel contamination. My personal choice is cefoxitin, 2 g IV. A reasonable alternative would be gentamicin, 2 to 2.5 mg per kilogram IV, combined with parenteral clindamycin, 900 mg.

GENERAL PRINCIPLES OF MANAGEMENT

ANESTHESIA

RICHARD B. WEISKOPF, M.D.
HENRY BARRIE FAIRLEY, M.B., M.S.

The purpose of this chapter is to familiarize the reader with the role of the anesthesiologist as it is practiced in a trauma center, to acquaint the non-anesthetist clinician with the clinical problems and therapeutic options faced on the "other side of the screen," and to provide a relatively brief framework for those anesthetists who only occasionally are required to anesthetize trauma victims.

ANESTHESIA FOR MINOR TRAUMA

Trauma that does not require surgery of a major body cavity (abdomen, thorax, cranium) and has neither caused significant blood loss nor created other major alterations of systemic physiologic function may be considered to be minor from surgical and physiologic perspectives. Occasionally, the risks connected with the administration of an anesthetic may be substantial; these include potential loss of the patency of the patient's airway and the consequences of any important coincidental disease(s), particularly if inadequately treated. The required anesthetic techniques and agents differ between the elective (prepared) patient and the emergency patient with, for example, uncontrolled hypertension, cardiac failure, or fluid and electrolyte disturbance. Therefore, the risks of proceeding immediately with administration of an anesthetic must be balanced with the urgency of the need for surgical correction. There will be times when an interim period is inappropriate (e.g., severe, multiple trauma), and there may be occasions when surgery may be forgone (e.g., minor tendon laceration in a respiratory or cardiac cripple).

Problems surrounding airway management are the single largest cause of anesthetic morbidity and mortality. All anesthetic and surgical plans must take full cognizance of this problem. Trauma patients must be regarded as having a "full stomach," i.e., the stomach may contain significant amounts of food or fluid, or both. Patients who have been traumatized frequently give unreliable histories with respect to most recent alimentation. In addition, trauma may decelerate or halt gastrointestinal processes. Options for handling this problem are discussed later in this chapter. The risk inherent in proceeding with anesthesia and surgery with a patient with a "full stomach" may vary with the patient and the injury; no rule can be given, other than the need for careful evaluation of the relative merits of delaying or proceeding with surgery. *The option of regional anesthesia* (to be discussed) *does not guarantee airway protection, and thus does not solve the problem.*

Choice of Anesthesia for Minor Trauma

The surgical site of many minor injuries may be adequately anesthetized by local infiltration, a regional anesthetic, or block of peripheral nerves with a local anesthetic, or by a general anesthetic. Available data fail to show a difference in mortality between general and regional anesthesia. Other considerations frequently narrow the options.

Regional anesthesia is not a satisfactory solution for dealing with the hazard of the full stomach. Excessive associated sedation, accidental intravascular injection of local anesthetics, cuff failure during an intravenous regional anesthetic (Bier block), or the use of excessive amounts of local anesthetic (to be discussed) may cause unconsciousness and convulsions with resultant emesis or regurgitation and subsequent aspiration.

Because of the potential for airway infringement, with the exception of the smallest, most superficial lacerations, no injury of the face or neck that requires surgical correction should be regarded as a "minor" anesthetic procedure (to be discussed).

Use of Local Anesthetics

All local anesthetics can achieve toxic blood concentrations. The plasma concentration achieved depends on the site of injection, the amount of drug injected, the presence or absence of a vasoconstrictor mixed with the local anesthetic, and the patient's size, blood volume, hepatic function, and general physical status. Table 1 lists commonly used local anesthetics and their maximal doses in an otherwise healthy, fit patient. *As a patient's physical state deteriorates, the maximal safe dose of local anesthetic decreases.* Table 1 must be considered a *guideline.* Following various types of regional anesthesia, plasma concentrations of local anesthetics vary in descending order after intercostal nerve block, epidural block, axillary block, and subcutaneous infiltration. In general, toxicity of local anesthetics is additive; as maximal dosage is neared, switching to another local anesthetic does not offer any advantage. The addition of a potent vasoconstrictor (epinephrine 1:200,000) decreases blood flow to the site of injection and thereby decreases uptake of the anesthetic, by the blood, thus decreasing plasma concentration and prolonging the neural blockade. Table 1 assumes that epinephrine 1:200,000 is added to the local anesthetic. However, it is pointed out that as relatively largely volumes of solution are injected, the patient may exhibit signs and symptoms of excessive epinephrine administration. If a vasoconstrictor is not added to the local anesthetic (e.g., because of concern regarding resultant tachycardia or hypertension in a patient with heart disease), the maximal amount of local anesthetic agent should be reduced by at least one-third. The addition of epinephrine to the local anesthetic is also valuable as a diagnostic tool that provides early indication of an intravascular injection. A test dose of 3 ml of the local anesthetic containing 1:200,000 epinephrine is injected prior to the injection of the contemplated complete dose. If the heart rate does not increase and there are no manifestations to suggest intravenous administration of the anesthetic in the ensuing 1 or 2 minutes, it can be assumed that the drugs were not administered intravascularly, and the remainder of the injection at that site can proceed. The practitioner is referred to texts on regional anesthesia for descriptions of techniques and complications of individual nerve blocks, blocks of plexi, and major regional blocks.

ANESTHESIA FOR MAJOR TRAUMA

Initial Evaluation and Management

Airway and Gas Exchange

All seriously traumatized patients should receive oxygen during transport to and upon arrival in the emergency room because many physiologic sequelae

TABLE 1 Doses of Commonly Used Local Anesthetics*

Local Anesthetic	Maximal Safe Dose (mg/kg)	Adequate Concentration for Subcutaneous Infiltration	Maximal dose (ml) of Adequate Concentration in 70-kg Patient†
Chloroprocaine	20	1%	140
Cocaine‡	2		
Bupivacaine	3	0.25%	84
Procaine	15	1%	105
Lidocaine	7	0.5%	100
Tetracaine	2	0.1%	140

* Amounts assume a healthy fit patient and addition of epinephrine, 1:200,000, to local anesthetic (except cocaine).
† Each 20 ml of these solutions contain 0.1 mg epinephrine; subcutaneous infiltration of 60 ml of solution may result in signs and symptoms of administration of excessive quantities of epinephrine.
‡ Cocaine is not recommended for subcutaneous infiltration. It is included in this table because of its usefulness as a topical mucosal anesthetic.

of trauma result in arterial hypoxemia while the patient is breathing air. The chest should be auscultated bilaterally, and if there is any question of a possible chest injury, roentgenograms should be obtained immediately. Hemothoraces or pneumothoraces should be relieved by placement of large-bore chest tubes. If systemic arterial blood pressure is unobtainable, the trachea should be intubated immediately and the lungs ventilated with 100 percent oxygen as part of the initial emergency room resuscitation sequence (rapid intravenous fluid administration and, if necessary, thoracotomy and aortic cross-clamping). Fixed, dilated pupils do not necessarily indicate irreversible central nervous system damage and do not contraindicate early aggressive management. If an esophageal obturator has been previously inserted, it should not be removed until the airway is protected with a cuffed endotracheal tube, because of the likelihood of regurgitation of gastric contents and the possibility of subsequent aspiration. Masks attached to esophageal obturators may be removed by squeezing components at the mask orifice. Patients who are markedly hypotensive despite rapid intravenous infusion also require early intubation to support gas exchange and protect the airway, since cerebral ischemia commonly causes muscular flaccidity and regurgitation of gastric contents. It is difficult to time endotracheal intubation of an awake, hypotensive patient in the emergency room; the decision requires experience and judgment. Intubation frequently is accomplished without drugs or with the aid of topical anesthesia alone. If anesthesia is necessary for intubation of the trachea, we use a ketamine-succinylcholine sequence (to be described).

Facial Fractures and Upper Airway Injuries

Airway assessment is the first priority in this group of patients. Massive facial injuries may result in nasal obstruction, oropharyngeal edema, or hematomata of such magnitude that immediate tracheotomy or cricothyroidotomy is necessary in the emergency room. In all other cases, the rate of swelling in the upper airway must be evaluated. The principle is to ensure maintenance of a patent airway and to avoid limitation of available techniques by "sudden" airway obstruction. In patients with major fractures of the mandible and maxilla (LeFort III) in whom massive edema has yet to occur, oral intubation is preferred and, if required, is usually easily accomplished. In the most obtunded, the trachea may be intubated without anesthesia. If this situation is misjudged, vomiting may occur and strong suction with a large-bore sucker must be immediately available. Blind nasal intubation following major facial injury is discouraged because of the hazard of potential false passages into nasal sinuses and the cranial vault and the possibility of dislodging loose bone and tissue. It is unusual for an alert, cooperative patient with facial injuries to require intubation in the emergency department. However, if endotracheal intubation is necessary, the options for its accomplishment following direct laryngoscopy are (1) topical anesthesia of the tongue and hypopharynx by alternately spraying a local anesthetic and advancing the laryngoscope, or (2) general anesthesia preceded by preoxygenation, cricoid pressure, thiopental or ketamine, and succinylcholine. Fractures of the mandible alone usually do not cause airway or intubation difficulties when the larynx is normal.

Injuries of the larynx may cause rapid respiratory obstruction and require immediate tracheotomy. In less urgent situations, a history of trauma to the head and neck, stridor, hoarseness, and crepitus in the neck are all suggestive of laryngeal injury. Deceleration is the most frequent cause of a fractured larynx, which is often associated with a fracture of C6 or C7. Three useful tests for evaluation of laryngeal fracture are (1) a check of the ability of the patient to make a high-pitched "e" sound, which requires mobile cricoarytenoid joints, normal tense cords, and functioning intrinsic laryngeal neuromuscular mechanisms; (2) indirect laryngoscopy; and (3) radiography of the larynx, especially, a computerized tomographic CT scan. If uncertainty exists, fiberoptic laryngoscopy may be performed under topical anesthesia. If laryngeal injury is suspected, all possible information should be accumulated prior to induction of general anesthesia. Attempts at endotracheal intubation may cause mucosal stripping and bleeding, displacement of fractured cartilage into the airway lumen, and laryngeal obstruction.

When a fractured larynx is present, laryngofissure and repair of mucosal lacerations and cartilage fractures are frequently carried out. Classically, a tracheotomy under local anesthesia is performed first. Alternatively, endotracheal intubation through the glottis may be attempted, but only in the presence of the most benign preoperative findings and when laryngeal visualization is excellent. If a tracheotomy is necessary in an uncooperative child, a small dose of ketamine may be used as a supplement to local anesthesia; however, airway obstruction may ensue.

In all cases of possible airway compromise, when it is uncertain whether a patent airway can be maintained, that is, if airway obstruction could occur, the procedures should be carried out in an operating room with equipment and personnel ready for immediate tracheotomy.

Head Injuries

A high percentage of unconscious patients with recent head injuries require intubation for one or more of the following indications: (1) to alleviate airway obstruction, (2) to prevent aspiration, or (3) to ensure hyperventilation for the purpose of minimizing intracranial pressure. If it is decided not to intubate the trachea of a patient who has a fresh head injury, this individual must be observed closely; personnel who are able to intubate the patient's trachea must be readily available. Sudden rapid deterioration commonly occurs within the first few hours, and therefore a single evaluation is not sufficient. When possible, cervical films should be obtained prior to intubation, although, in our experience, cervical fractures are rare in patients who require intubation for a head injury. If it is suspected that the neck is unstable, a cervical collar is applied, and oral intubation may be attempted using an endotracheal tube with the distal 3 to 5 cm bent in the shape of a "hockey stick" by means of a lubricated stylet. If oral intubation appears technically straightforward, we do not hesitate to use muscle relaxants while applying cricoid pressure, following a period of preoxygenation. During laryngoscopy and intubation, the surgeon should hold the patient's head applying axial traction, and warn of any impending excessive extension. Alternatives to direct laryngoscopy are blind nasal intubation (which may be easy in the hyperventilating patient) or, if the former cannot be accomplished, and time permits, intubation over a fiberoptic laryngosope or fiberoptic bronchoscope. If all else fails, tracheotomy may be necessary.

Barbiturates, other hypnotics, or muscle relaxants may be required to control restlessness, either to permit CT scanning or angiography, or to prevent an increase in intracranial pressure owing to straining caused by the irritation of an endotracheal tube. The resultant decreased ability to conduct a neurologic assessment should not be an overriding consideration. Either a surgical decompression is indicated by the radiologic findings or, if not, a catheter may be inserted to accurately monitor intracranial pressure.

Fluid Resuscitation

In any patient in whom a major injury is suspected, at least two large-bore intravenous cannulae should be inserted, one of which should be located centrally (superior vena cava or right atrium). These cannulae should be at least 16 gauge and preferably larger. It is not unusual to need 3 or 4 large-bore cannulae to rapidly and adequately restore circulating blood volume of a major trauma victim. One should not depend on lower extremity lines for infusion in patients in whom disruption of iliac veins or the inferior vena cava is a possibility. Placement of a central venous catheter is essential to properly manage the fluid volume resuscitation. A catheter should be placed in the bladder in all patients; however, for many reasons, urine output should not be the primary guide for fluid management. Patients who have decreased skin perfusion with resultant pallor and coolness, narrow pulse pressure, tachycardia, and orthostatic hypotension are likely to have lost in excess of 20 to 25 percent of their blood volume (normal blood volume in the adult is approximately 75 ml per kilogram body weight). Cardiac output will have decreased in approximate proportion to blood loss. Deterioration of mental status indicates a more severe loss of blood volume, usually in excess of 40 percent. Vigorous fluid resuscitation must be started. To help keep track of infused volume, it is useful to sequentially number each new bag of fluid. Blood volume should be restored so that central venous pressure measures several mm Hg. We use a balanced salt solution for this purpose. Three or more liters may be required if the previously described signs are present. If a pneumatic antishock garment (MAST or G suit) has been inflated around the victim's abdomen and lower limbs, thereby increasing peripheral vascular resistance, a variable amount of intravascular volume may also have been shifted centrally. Thus, the measured central venous pressure will not be an accurate reflection of total intravascular volume. With careful observation of hemodynamic status, the suit should be deflated, one compartment at a time, only when volume replacement has started, the central pressure is at least 6 mm Hg, and immediate surgery can be performed if necessary.

Premedication Agents

Premedicants should not be used routinely. Sedatives, hypnotics, and narcotics should be administered to hypovolemic patients only with extreme caution. Agents without effective antidotes should be avoided. Although narcotics are effective in relieving pain and anxiety, they dilate peripheral blood vessels and may produce further hypotension with resultant cerebral ischemia adding to the sedative effect of the narcotic. This may result in regurgitation of gastric contents and aspiration. Intramuscular cimetidine is sometimes advocated as a means of decreasing gastric acidity in emergency surgery patients. This is not universal practice and we do not rely on this approach, nor do we rely on metoclopromide to speed gastric emptying.

Operating Room Management

Preparation of Equipment

In order to provide expeditious care for victims of major trauma at a moment's notice, a completely ready operating room should be available at all times. The anesthesiologist should have the following recently checked equipment in place: (1) anesthesia machine, (2) volume-controlled ventilator, with appropriate values preset, (3) suction, (4) laryngoscope with spare blades and endotracheal tubes with stylets, (5) appropriate drugs (a nondepolarizing muscle relaxant, succinylcholine, intravenous induction agent) drawn into labeled syringes, (6) two intravenous infusion sets with pumps and blood warmers, filled with balanced salt solutions, (7) devices for externally pressurizing bags of fluid or blood, to increase their rate of administration, (8) material required for placement of an arterial line, (9) warming blanket and a device to provide heated humidified inspired gases, (10) defibrillator with internal and external paddles, and (11) calibrated equipment to monitor arterial blood pressure, central venous pressure, neuromuscular blockade, temperature, and electrocardiograph.

Choice of Anesthetic (Regional or General)

For the more major injuries, particularly in the presence of cardiovascular instability or injuries of the abdomen or thorax, we prefer general anesthesia to regional. Spinal anesthesia does not permit control of ventilation, and the resultant sympathetic block abolishes important homeostatic responses to hypovolemia. Additionally, in patients with abdominal injuries, preoperative uncertainty regarding the extent of the necessary exploration and procedures precludes limited block levels. On the other hand, infiltration anesthesia or regional blocks can be extremely useful for the management of the more minor peripheral injuries, provided attention is paid to the maximum safe dose of the selected local anesthetic agent relative to the patient's body size and physical status (discussed above).

Induction and Maintenance of General Anesthesia

During induction of anesthesia, aspiration of gastric contents into the lungs may follow passive regurgitation or active vomiting. When diaphragmatic relaxation occurs secondary to cerebral ischemia, heavy sedation, or anesthesia, passive regurgitation may occur as a result of the difference in pressure between the abdomen and the thorax. Several hours of delay in scheduling surgery and administration of metoclopramide may decrease the probability of food remaining in the stomach, but this is never totally reliable and may be contraindicated by the urgency of the injury. A low gastric acidity and/or an empty stomach cannot be assumed for extended periods following trauma. To prevent gastric contents from reaching the pharynx and being aspirated, the following steps should be taken.

1. In all cases of intestinal obstruction, ileus, or gastroduodenal perforation or bleeding, a nasogastric sump tube should be placed and the stomach aspirated immediately prior to induction (although this does not ensure an empty stomach).
2. The probable ease of laryngoscopy and oral intubation should be assessed. If an extraordinarily difficult laryngoscopy and endotracheal intubation is anticipated, alternative approaches should be considered (to be discussed).
3. Prior to proceeding further, powerful suction must be available.
4. To minimize the increase in intragastric pressure subsequent to administration of succinylcholine, a small dose of a nondepolarizing muscle relaxant is administered (e.g., 4.5 mg of d-tubocurarine chloride or 1.5 mg of pancuronium) 3 to 5 minutes before the succinylcholine. The patient is given

100 percent oxygen to breathe through a tight-fitting face mask. This preoxygenation is carried out for at least 3 minutes of quiet breathing, time permitting. If time does not permit, four or five maximum inspirations may suffice. Anteroposterior pressure is then applied with two fingers on the cricoid cartilage (compressing the upper esophagus against the cervical vertebral column) (Sellick maneuver), and a rapidly acting intravenous hypnotic and muscle relaxant (usually succinylcholine) is administered intravenously.

Laryngoscopy, tracheal intubation, cuff inflation, and checks of tube location are carried out before cricoid pressure is removed. Endotracheal tube placement is confirmed by (1) observation and auscultation of the chest and absence of sounds in the stomach in response to positive pressure ventilation, and (2) by palpation of the endotracheal tube cuff between the cricoid and the suprasternal notch on injection into the cuff of an additional 5 to 10 ml of air. If—following the foregoing sequence of full preoxygenation, precurarization, cricoid pressure, a single induction dose of an appropriate intravenous induction agent, and succinylcholine—intubation of the trachea cannot be accomplished and the patient is not grossly hypotensive, the actions of the intravenous agent and succinylcholine should be allowed to terminate (approximately 5 minutes) and the patient allowed to awaken. Alternate approaches can then be considered. If laryngoscopy and intubation are expected to be difficult, other options are, in order of preference (1) awake intubation (nasally or orally) following topical anesthesia (if necessary with a fiberoptic laryngoscope), and (2) tracheotomy under local anesthesia. In many acute injuries of the jaw and neck, in which the state of the pharynx is in doubt, we prefer direct laryngoscopy and oral intubation as a first step. Then, if nasal intubation is required, a nasal tube may be advanced under direct vision with the larynx in full view and the airway protected. This permits full evaluation of the injury prior to nasal intubation.

Whenever possible, hypovolemia is corrected before the patient is transported to the operating room and anesthesia is induced. If correction is not possible because of the nature and extent of the injuries (that is, the rate of hemorrhage exceeds maximal capability to restore intravascular volume), it may be necessary to induce "anesthesia" in the hypovolemic patient. If the patient is unconscious or severely obtunded, intubation of the trachea should be accomplished without drugs or with neuromuscular blocking agents alone. If the patient is conscious despite being uncorrectably hypovolemic, some mode of anesthesia should be provided prior to initiation of surgery.

In the presence of hemorrhagic hypotension and decreased venous return, no anesthetic technique or agent reliably maintains homeostatic mechanisms and hemodynamic function. This is true of those anesthetic agents that, during normovolemia, result in cardiovascular depression as well as those agents that may result in cardiovascular stimulation, also during normovolemia (e.g., ketamine). Very small doses of ketamine (0.35 to 0.7 mg per kilogram intravenously) can be useful for inducing "anesthesia" in hypovolemic, hypotensive conscious patients. In a hypovolemic patient, the indirect stimulatory responses may not be elicited, and ketamine's direct action of myocardial depression may result in cardiovascular decompensation. The maximal depressant effect is seen 5 minutes after administration. The anesthetist should expect cardiovascular decompensation following administration of any anesthetic agent to a hypovolemic patient. Once intubated, the patient should be mechanically ventilated to free the anesthesiologist's hands. Evidence is lacking that either respiratory acidosis or alkalosis is beneficial during massive hypovolemia. We therefore attempt to maintain normocapnia, which has the added advantage of not confusing interpretation of acid-base status. A scheme for induction of anesthesia in major trauma victims is provided in Figure 1.

Following induction of anesthesia, only oxygen and neuromuscular blocking agents are administered until the hemodynamic situation is stabilized and systemic blood pressure rises to a mean of 50 torr. At that point cerebral perfusion should be adequate, and it is then appropriate to consider the administration of other anesthetic agents. The goal is to provide analgesia or amnesia with minimal cardiovascular disturbance. Since the clinical situation is still in great flux and conditions may deteriorate, in principle, agents that are easily removed or whose actions are readily terminated should be used. Cyclopropane and ether are contraindicated because of the risk of explosion in a setting with a multiplicity of personnel and electrical equipment. Furthermore, cyclopropane decreases survival time in shocked dogs. Halothane, enflurane, or isoflurane may be cautiously added in small concentrations (for example, 0.1%) to the background of 100 percent oxygen and the cardiovascular effects noted. All the inhalation agents are direct myocardial depressants and may result in significantly decreased myocardial performance and hypotension if added too rapidly or in too great a concentration. Recent data suggest that isoflurane and halothane may provide better tissue oxygenation than enflurane during hypovolemia. However, because isoflurane may cause hypotension and tachycardia, its use in a patient with large fluid volume shifts may lead to a diagnostic dilemma; we therefore avoid its use in these circumstances. Thus, our anesthetic vapor of choice is halothane. The anesthetist must pay extremely close attention to the variable clinical situation and be prepared to cease administration of all inhalation agents should hypotension ensue.

Nitrous oxide should not be used for these patients. Although nitrous oxide is a superior analgesic, it is frequently depressant in the hypotensive, hypovolemic patient. Recent data suggest that during hypovolemia the cardiovascular and metabolic consequences of administration of nitrous oxide is no different from the administration of halothane. Since nitrous oxide must be used in relatively high concentrations, this adds to the potential for hypoxia because of decreased inspired oxygen concentration. Furthermore, nitrous oxide increases the volume of any previously unrelieved pneumothorax and increases bowel distention, potentially adding technical difficulty to the surgery. We avoid the use of narcotics here, because once given they cannot be removed as can the inhalation agents, and because data suggest that endogenous opioids have deleterious

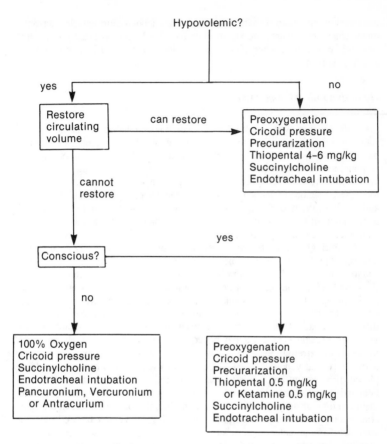

Figure 1 Scheme for induction of anesthesia in major trauma victims

actions during shock. The use of naloxone to reverse narcotic action may be only partially successful because of hypoperfusion at the site(s) of action and because the antagonist has a shorter duration of action than the agonist. Using this approach, some patients may recall some intraoperative events, especially if anesthesia is not instituted as mean systemic arterial pressure rises to 50 torr.

In selecting a muscle relaxant for continued use during the procedure, d-tubocurarine is avoided because of its propensity to release histamine, resulting in further hypotension. The vagolytic properties of pancuronium observed during ordinary circumstances may not be significant in the setting of greatly increased sympathetic activity. Among the nondepolarizing muscle relaxants, metocurine, atracurium, and vecuronium have the least cardiovascular actions, although atracurium, when given in large doses, can cause histamine release and hypotension.

Hemodynamic Management

After the airway is secured and ventilation is established, the hemodynamic status of the patient remains the primary issue. The hemodynamic status of the patient changes rapidly because of the rapidity and intensity of physiologic response to hemorrhage (increased sympathetic system activity; increased renin-angiotensin system activity; increased vasopressin secretion, peripheral circulatory effects, actions of acidic metabolites, direct hypoxic effects, and fluid shifts) and the multiplicity of therapeutic maneuvers in the acute situation. Anesthetic agents alter all these processes and thereby further complicate the physiologic response, diagnosis, and therapy.

Accordingly, accurate beat-to-beat blood pressure monitoring is an important aspect of the acute management of the major trauma victim. For this reason and to allow repeated, rapid sampling of arterial blood for measurement of Po_2, Pco_2, and pH, an indwelling arterial cannula should be placed as early as feasible in the operating room sequence and connected to a pressure transducer for continuous measurement of blood pressure. Percutaneous insertion may be difficult in a patient whose systemic arterial blood pressure is unobtainable or is very low; a surgical cut-down may be required. The arterial line should be placed in the upper extremity because it may be necessary to cross-clamp the thoracic aorta. A central venous (superior vena cava or right atrial) cannula should be placed, time permitting, while the patient is in the emergency room. If the patient arrives in the operating room without a centrally located catheter, its placement is a high priority and should be accomplished soon thereafter. In the operating room, introduction through an internal jugular vein is favored over the approach from an antecubital or subclavian vein, both because of the ease and rapidity of insertion through the former and because of the accessibility of this route while surgery proceeds. To permit continuous accurate assessment of central venous pressure, and for rapid verification of position, the cannula should be connected to a pressure transducer and the wave-form visually displayed. Measurements obtained by the use of hydraulic manometers are unreliable. It is essential to obtain accurate reference of zero pressure for the CVP. This is conveniently accomplished by placing a length of intravenous line connecting tubing, filled with saline, from the transducer to a point on the patient's midaxillary line. Opening the transducer to this line, while it is closed to all other ports, establishes a correct zero point. It will not be necessary to alter the height of the transducer should patient position or OR table height be altered. The correct zero reference may be reestablished by again opening the transducer to the zero line with other ports closed. The preponderance of victims of major trauma are young and do not have heart disease; thus right-sided cardiac filling pressure, as reflected by central venous pressure, usually correlates well with left-side cardiac filling pressure. Placement of a pulmonary arterial line in the early care of the massively injured patient is neither necessary nor advisable; time is better spent tending to issues of higher priority.

If need arises for intraoperative assessment of left-sided filling pressure, a left atrial catheter may be inserted directly if thoracotomy has been performed. Direct observation of filling of the heart is also useful in the evaluation of the patient's volume status. The early stages of resuscitation of the massively bleeding patient require continuous communication between the surgeons and the anesthetists as to the nature and extent of the injuries and the hemodynamic indices. If it is necessary to cross-clamp the aorta to provide adequate blood flow to the brain and heart in the presence of massive hypovolemia and marked hypotension, subsequent removal of the clamp may result in hypotension owing to circulating volume filling a previously empty, acidotic vascular tree. Consequently, reperfusion should be established gradually by partial unclamping as hemodynamics permit, with addition of volume or base (to be discussed), or both, as required.

Intraoperative Fluid Resuscitation

The amount of fluid volume to be administered is guided by the systemic blood pressure and cardiac filling. Fluids are administered as rapidly as possible until the central venous pressure is in the normal range for an anesthetized patient (8 to 10 torr) or the systemic blood pressure is in the normal range.

Much research and discussion have surrounded the issue of which fluid to administer. The clinician may currently choose from whole blood, red blood cell suspensions (packed, washed, or frozen), salt solutions (crystalloid), protein-containing fluids (colloid), or other osmotically active agents, such as dextran and starch. Whole blood is the fluid of choice despite some deficiencies of banked blood. The advantages of whole blood are (1) it has the ability to transport as well as to on- and off-load oxygen and carbon dioxide, (2) it contains most clotting factors in adequate supply, and (3) it is a good buffer at physiologic pH. The disadvantages of banked blood include (1) low storage temperature (4 °C) with high thermal capacity, (2) decreased clotting factors V and VIII, (3) lack of functional platelets after 24 hours of storage, (4) low pH, (5) high potassium concentration (although it returns to normal with restoration of red cell sodium pump activity), (6) decreased red cell survival, (7) presence of citrate, (8) risk of transmission of hepatitis, cytomegalic virus, and AIDS, (9) decreased red cell 2,3-diphosphoglycerate (DPG) concentration, resulting in high hemoglobin affinity for oxygen, and (10) presence of red cell membrane antigens, which requires typing and crossmatching of the patient's blood with the blood to be transfused. However, the U.S. Army had highly favorable experience in Viet Nam using unmatched low anti-A and low anti-B titer group O blood, and the need for crossmatch for patients who have neither been pregnant nor received prior transfusion has been eliminated, provided antibody screening is negative.

Blood banks fractionate most whole blood into its component parts, separating plasma from red blood cells. Consequently, anesthetists may need to rely on packed red blood cells ordinarily spun to an hematocrit of approximately 70 percent. Many blood banks now remove more plasma, replacing it with an additive solution. Viscosity is decreased, but so are clotting factors. Packed cells should be reconstituted to an approximately normal hematocrit prior to transfusion to decrease viscosity and thus ease administration. Sodium chloride, 0.9 percent, is the only fluid recommended by the American Association of Blood Banks for use for this purpose. However, we have reconstituted many thousands of units of packed cells during the past 7 years, using a balanced salt solution containing magnesium instead of calcium, without a single instance of clot formation. Because packed cells contain little plasma, some of the advantages of whole blood are diminished. The quantity of clotting factors is decreased. Oxygen transport is not affected, however, and the CO_2 transport capability is only somewhat decreased as is buffering capacity.

Although devices available for collecting, washing, and transfusing the patient's own shed blood can be successfully utilized in elective surgery, no such device is available which meets the specific needs of the situation surrounding intraoperative care of the major trauma victim. These devices require a significant degree of operator attention and take several minutes to process a unit of cells, and the result is a product that contains *no* platelets or clotting factors. Calcium is present only if it has been added to the suspension medium. Furthermore, many major victims have intestinal injury, which, when present, precludes the transfusing of shed blood because of the risk of bacterial contamination. Therefore, we do not recommend the use of these devices in the initial operating room management of major trauma victims.

Despite considerable laboratory and clinical investigation, there is no firm evidence that the use of microfilters for blood administration is beneficial. The resistance of these greatly impedes rapid blood administration, and we therefore do not recommend their use in this setting.

Note that when extremely rapid infusion of viscous fluid is required, there are considerable differences in resistance to flow between various types of infusion equipment and blood warmers. Stopcocks offer high resistance because their internal diameter is smaller than that of intravenous tubing, and therefore they should not be used. Warming of banked blood not only is essential to prevent severe hypothermia (to be discussed), but greatly decreases blood viscosity and thereby allows for its more rapid administration.

Inevitably, until the trauma victim's blood is typed, fluids other than blood must be administered. Current evidence indicates that in this regard colloid is of no advantage over crystalloid and, in fact, may be detrimental. Given the expense of the former and the availability and ease of the administration of the latter, there seems to be little, if any, reason to administer colloid in the acute resuscitative period. We prefer a balanced salt solution that does not contain calcium, which we also use for reconstitution of packed cells (previously discussed). Resuscitative fluids undergoing research and development include perfluorochemicals (fluorocarbons) and stroma-free hemoglobin, either in solution or encased in layers of lipid. The oxygen content of fluorocarbons is proportional to the partial pressure of oxygen in the fluid and reaches an acceptable level only at very high Po_2. Furthermore, fluorocarbons are extremely expensive, have extraordinarily long half-lives, are stored frozen, require at least 30 minutes for defrosting, must be mixed prior to use, are administered slowly, decrease leukocyte chemotaxis, and have a significant incidence of allergic response. Relying on their use for resuscitation from major trauma is inappropriate.

Recently, it has become possible to prepare hemoglobin with little, if any, stromal element, thus eliminating renal toxicity and offering the advantage of high oxygen content at normal Po_2. Furthermore, hemoglobin so prepared can be stored in its crystalline form at room temperature for prolonged periods of time, and since no red cell membranes and antigens are present, standard blood typing is unnecessary. Phosphorylation and cross-linking the molecules have extended the products's intravascular half-life to approximately 24 hours and increased its P_{50} to an approximately normal value. Stroma-free hemoglobin has been shown to be superior to albumin in supporting myocardial function. Should testing demonstrate efficacy and safety, stroma-free hemoglobin may find its place in the earliest phases of resuscitation of the massively bleeding patient.

Persistent Hypotension Despite Apparently Adequate Fluid Administration

This situation is observed at some stage in the operating room management of many patients who have sustained extremely major injuries. The first checks should be of the accuracy of the monitoring system.

The zero setting and calibration of transducers should be checked. It is useful to have placed a blood pressure cuff on the limb that has been cannulated for the arterial pressure. The occlusion pressure can then be used to validate the measured intra-arterial pressure. Possible causes of the continuing hypotension must then be reviewed. These include undetected hemorrhage; hemothorax, pneumothorax, or pericardial tamponade; acidosis; hypothermia; air or fat embolism; or an error in administration of ventilation or anesthesia. Hypocalcemia may be present in extreme cases of hypoperfusion, hypothermia, and massive transfusion.

If correction of all other problems (to be discussed) is ineffective in restoring systemic pressure, we empirically administer calcium chloride, 0.5 to 1 g intravenously, since ionized calcium measurements are not readily available. However, frequent, repeated doses of calcium are not recommended because of the danger of producing ventricular tachycardia or fibrillation, which may be refractory to all therapy. Calcium and other pressors including epinephrine, norepinephrine, dopamine, and dobutamine have diminished effectiveness in the presence of acidosis.

Myocardial failure in a previously healthy young trauma victim is distinctly uncommon unless the patient has had direct myocardial injury or prolonged myocardial hypoxia. However, if all other possible causes of persistent hypotension have been excluded or treated, additional fluids may be administered until the central venous pressure is 20 to 25 torr. If arterial pressure does not respond, as a *last resort*, pressor agents (dopamine or dobutamine, 3 to 12 µg per kilogram per minute intravenously initially) may be infused. It must be pointed out that *pressors must not be used in place of restoration of adequate circulating blood volume*. An unusual cause of myocardial failure following perforating chest injuries is coronary air embolism, which may be diagnosed by direct observation of the coronary arteries. The question of the existence of a "myocardial depressant factor" in hypovolemic shock is controversial. In addition to hemorrhage, metabolic acidosis and hypothermia are the two most common secondary aggravating factors in the massively bleeding traumatized patient.

Acid-Base Balance

Poor tissue perfusion results in decreased availability of oxygen at the end of the mitochondrial electron transport chain, which results in tissue accumulation of lactic acid. Hepatic uptake of lactate from blood is impaired during severe reductions of hepatic blood flow or during severe hypoxia. It is not clinically convenient to measure lactic acid concentrations. However, its appearance in the blood results in an increase in base deficit. Base deficit may be rapidly estimated from measurements of arterial Pco_2 and pH, by use of Siggaard-Andersen's nomogram, Severinghaus's slide rule, or automated blood gas equipment using equations developed by the latter. Arterial blood gases and pH should be measured as soon as possible. The treatment of acidosis secondary to hypovolemia is volume replacement. If volume is restored and perfusion is satisfactory, the acidosis becomes corrected as the liver extracts lactate from the blood and the tissues cease lactate production. Thus, treatment of acidosis per se is not required. However, acidosis can result in persistence of hypotension despite adequate restoration of circulating blood volume. Myocardial performance deteriorates at pH below 7.2. Ideally, the magnitude of the acidosis should be measured. If data are not yet available, it is safe to administer $NaHCO_3$ as a therapeutic test. It is unusual to observe clinically important cardiovascular effects of metabolic acidosis at base deficits less than 10 mEq per liter, and in this setting acidosis of considerably greater magnitude is common. Whole-body base deficit is usually calculated from the formula 0.3 base excess (BE; mEq per liter) × body weight in kilograms. Thus, 200 or more mEq of $NaHCO_3$

may be required to correct a clinically important metabolic acidosis. Since cardiovascular instability is usually present when administration of $NaHCO_3$ is indicated, a calculated dose of bicarbonate does not provide exact correction. Frequent, repeated evaluation is necessary. Pco_2 and pH should be measured at 37 °C and not corrected to the patient's temperature based on evidence that, over a wide temperature range, vertebrate plasma pH is closely related to the pH of water and the ionization of imidazole. In any event, over the clinical range, computation of base excess is nearly independent of temperature.

It is not clear whether measured Po_2 should be corrected to the patient's temperature or reported at 37 °C. However, temperature correction is necessary for computation of alveolar-arterial difference in oxygen tension ($AaDO_2$). Furthermore, in the hypothermic patient, if temperature correction results in error, it is on the side of patient safety.

Hypothermia

Poor perfusion, opening of major body cavities, and administration of fluids of temperature less than body temperature inevitably result in hypothermia. Hypothermia presents multiple dangers. Myocardial function decreases with temperature. Myocardial hypothermia is poorly tolerated in the clinical setting of decreased myocardial preload and prolonged poor myocardial perfusion. As myocardial temperature falls to approximately 30 °C, arrhythmias become common. Refractory ventricular fibrillation frequently occurs when myocardial temperature falls an additional 1 to 3 centigrade degrees. Hypothermia adds to the coagulation defects (to be discussed) by causing sequestration of platelets. This phenomenon is reversible with rewarming. Additional problems of hypothermia include alteration of drug action and half-life, and confusion of interpretation of blood gas, pH, and acid-base data.

Temperature should be measured continuously by a thermistor or thermocouple placed in the esophagus, just behind the heart, or by the use of the thermistor of a thermodilution pulmonary artery catheter, if one has been inserted. These sites are preferred to those that are more distal because of the life-threatening hazard of myocardial hypothermia. Rapid changes in myocardial and blood temperature are reflected slowly at other sites, which are less central, such as the rectum.

Although it may not be possible to maintain normothermic conditions in the massively bleeding, traumatized patient, it is possible to prevent severe hypothermia. All administered intravenous fluids should be warmed. Some commercially available devices can warm blood effectively without adding important resistance to flow, thus allowing for high flow rates. A plugged-in, connected, circulating-water warming blanket should always be in place on the operating table. The device should be set at 40 °C and switched on at first notice of a patient's likely transport to the operating room, since most of these devices require 10 to 20 minutes to reach operating temperature. Warming blankets, although useful, are of less than optimal value because of poor peripheral circulation during massive hypovolemia. Heated inspired humidity is of greater value in preventing serious hypothermia, since nearly all the right heart output is exposed as a thin layer to the inspired heat in the pulmonary circulation. If the foregoing measures fail, warm crystalloid solution should be placed in the chest or abdominal cavities. Since we have been routinely using heated inspired humidity and warming all administered blood and intravenous fluid for all major trauma victims, the practice of filling body cavities with warm saline has become unusual.

Coagulation

A bleeding diathesis following massive blood loss and replacement is not uncommon. Causes are lesions of banked blood, hypothermia, consumption coagulopathy, and platelet dysfunction. The most frequent cause of a coagulopathy in the massively bleeding trauma patient is dilutional thrombocytopenia and/or platelet dysfunction. Platelet function is severely impaired within minutes of storage at 4 °C, with survival limited to less than 48 hours. Many blood banks remove platelets from blood after its collection. Thus, nearly all blood transfused is free of functional platelets, creating a dilutional thrombocytopenia. Furthermore, hypothermia causes platelet sequestration.

The coagulopathy of massive transfusion occurs commonly when between one and two times the estimated blood volume has been administered. Treatment of the dilutional thrombocytopenia or platelet dysfunction is accomplished by administration of platelets. Ten units of platelet concentrates should be administered if further significant transfusion is anticipated or generalized bleeding is apparent. Most hospital blood banks do not stock platelets; thus they may need to be ordered well in advance. Additional units of platelets are required if hemorrhage is not controlled. Since the plasma in which platelets are suspended contains quantities of coagulation factors similar to that of fresh frozen plasma (except for somewhat decreased but nevertheless hemostatic levels of factors V and VIII), administration of fresh frozen plasma may be unnecessary if platelets have been infused.

Development of a consumptive coagulopathy (possibly resulting from release of tissue thromboplastin) further depletes the diluted platelets and already decreased clotting factors.

Concentrations of coagulation factors V and VIII decrease with time in stored blood. Fortunately, only 5 to 30 percent of normally present quantities of these factors are necessary for surgical hemostasis. Furthermore, the liver can rapidly produce large quantities of factor VIII once circulation has been restored. Fresh frozen plasma contains all coagulation factors, but no platelets. A decrease in coagulation factors is an unusual cause of the coagulopathy of massive trauma and transfusion. If a decrease of coagulation factors is diagnosed as a cause of the coagulopathy, 2 units of fresh frozen plasma should be adminstered.

Although precise diagnosis of a coagulation defect requires laboratory tests such as bleeding time, prothrombin time, activated partial thromboplastin time, and fibrin split product levels, logistics may preclude their use. The most convenient method for determining the etiology of a bleeding disorder in the victim of major trauma is to observe the coagulation time. Few, if any, intraoperative coagulopathies of trauma victims cannot be appropriately managed by this regimen. If a solid clot does not form in a glass tube within 15 minutes, decreased clotting factors are implicated. If the clot forms but does not retract, thrombocytopenia is the likely cause. If the clot lyses, fibrinolysis is likely.

Calcium is bound by citrate, the anticoagulant of banked blood. However, hypocalcemia has not been demonstrated as a cause of the bleeding diathesis of massive transfusion. We do not administer calcium routinely as prophylaxis against coagulation defects. However, we do administer calcium to treat the myocardial effects of hypocalcemia (previously discussed).

We transfuse fresh whole blood (stored less than 24 hours) exceedingly rarely, only as a last resort, when all other modes of therapy for a coagulopathy of trauma and/or massive transfusion have failed. However, it should be noted that if appropriate diagnosis and therapy of the coagulopathy of trauma and/or massive transfusion have been followed, there is no rationale for the administration of fresh whole blood.

The Patient with Multiple Injuries

Frequently, priorities must be allocated in order to determine not only which injuries require immediate intervention (e.g., correction of major hemorrhage, cardiac tamponade, subdural hematoma), but also whether to continue operating after the most life-threatening problems have been corrected. This latter decision frequently involves injuries such as facial and long bone fractures. Considerations include:

1. Outcome considerations that dictate urgent surgery.
2. Physiologic status. At the time when the decision is being made as to whether to proceed with less urgent surgery, an assessment should be made of the patient's response to injury, anesthesia, and surgery. Factors to be considered include (a) the magnitude of the proposed procedures, including probable duration and blood loss, (b) hemodynamic stability and acid-base status, (c) pulmonary gas exchange and mechanics, (d) blood volume replacement and coagulation status, and (e) temperature. Prolonged major, non-life-saving procedures involving substantial potential blood loss should not be contemplated in any patient who is not hemodynamically stable, who has impaired lung-thorax mechanics (e.g., from pulmonary edema or contusion, distend-

ed abdomen, bronchospasm) or whose $P(A-a)O_2$ is greater than 250 to 300 mm Hg when the FiO_2 is 0.99. If blood volume replacement has exceeded the patient's blood volume, proceeding with additional, prolonged surgery for injuries that are not life-threatening is relatively contraindicated. An obvious coagulopathy is an absolute contraindication to proceeding with non-life or limb-saving surgery. Inability to maintain the patient's temperature at 33 °C or greater is also a contraindication to proceeding.

3. Prolonged anesthesia. There is no generally applicable information relating outcome to length of anesthesia, independent of the magnitude of the surgical procedure. Therefore, of itself, this should not be a consideration.

4. Evolving intracranial injury. A conscious patient who has an obvious head injury but not lateralizing signs may require urgent surgery for hemorrhage at site(s) other than the cranium. During anesthesia, it is not possible to detect an increase in intracranial pressure, except in the extreme, unless a cannula to monitor intracranial pressure has been inserted. Absence of pupillary changes is not a reliable index of satisfactory intracranial pressure. In such cases, the decision to proceed with less urgent surgery requires special consideration. In outline, there are four options (a) proceed, based on neurosurgical opinion that the extent of the original head injury was trivial; (b) permit the patient to awaken from anesthesia in order to allow further neurosurgical assessment; (c) maintain anesthesia and proceed to CT scan; or (d) insert a cannula to monitor ICP and determine whether to pursue further radiologic evaluation, carry out intracranial exploration, or proceed with other surgery.

5. Sustaining anesthesia excellence. Usually it is in the best interest of the patient for the same anesthesia personnel to remain with the patient from induction to emergence and, in many cases, for the subsequent postoperative period, especially if the patient's condition is unstable. An exception is when, in prolonged operations, due to tiredness it is difficult to sustain vigilance and to make objectively based decisions. If multiple procedures involving various surgical teams are proposed, it may be appropriate to involve an anesthesia "team," members of which can take a break or, if necessary, be replaced. If this is deemed necessary, provision *must* be made for continuity, i.e., sufficient overlap to permit a clear understanding of the injuries, surgical and anesthetic course, and the patient's responses.

Special Problems

Thoracic Injuries

Any one of three injuries—pulmonary, aortic, or cardiac—may require special action by the anesthesiologist.

Pulmonary Injuries. It is not uncommon for alveolar pressure to exceed pressures in adjoining perforated pulmonary vessels, causing systemic air embolism. Occasionally, a massive bronchial air leak may prevent effective mechanical ventilation. Placement of a double-lumen endotracheal tube provides maximal control of this problem and also prevents hemorrhage from one lung into the other. If it is not possible to place a double-lumen endotracheal tube, endobronchial intubation may be accomplished using a long endotracheal tube. This is more applicable for left-sided leaks, since the anatomy of the tracheal bifurcation renders right main bronchial intubation more probable. Since one-lung ventilation is likely to result in a degree of hypoxia, owing to shunting of blood through the unventilated lung, these maneuvers are only short-term, emergent expedients. Inhaled agents should include only oxygen and anesthetic vapor until measurements of systemic arterial Po_2 are obtained.

Aortic Injuries. Prolonged suprarenal clamping of the aorta may increase myocardial afterload and cause renal and spinal cord ischemia. The higher the clamp, the greater the likelihood of resultant left ventricular failure from the great increase in afterload. These problems may be minimized by the placement of a shunt if control below the aortic injury is feasible. However, if distal control is not feasible and a shunt is not placed, an agent such as sodium nitroprusside may be required to decrease myocardial afterload and permit volume loading while the aortic clamp is in place. Arterial pressure monitoring should be from the right arm if injury to the arch of the aorta is suspected. If time permits, left ventricular filling pressure should be monitored.

Cardiac Injuries and Tamponade. Rapid surgical correction is essential. Needle aspiration of traumatic cardiac tamponade does not often alleviate the hemodynamic problem. Intravenous fluid should be administered to achieve and maintain high cardiac filling pressure. Although theoretically important, this is only a short-term, temporizing measure. There is no anesthetic agent that allows for the maintenance of venous return and cardiac output in the presence of hemodynamically important cardiac tamponade. Anesthesia should not be induced until the patient is prepared and the surgeons are ready to initiate surgical measures to decompress the pericardium *immediately* on induction of anesthesia.

Spinal Injuries

The approach to securing an airway has been discussed elsewhere in this chapter. Although use of succinylcholine is contraindicated several days after a denervation injury, there is no evidence of muscle membrane instability in the first few hours. Thus, if otherwise indicated, succinylcholine may be used. Patients in halo traction who require anesthesia for other injuries should be intubated, while awake, under topical anesthesia, either orally or nasally. If necessary, a fiberoptic bronchoscope should be used. "Spinal shock" may result from acute spinal cord injuries, especially those that are cervical or high thoracic.

Large volumes of intravenous fluid may be required to maintain adequate cardiac filling and systemic arterial blood pressure. Central venous pressure should be monitored, and continuous infusion of an alpha-adrenergic agent (e.g., phenylepherine) may be used to compensate for the sympathetic denervation, provided cardiac filling and urine output are maintained.

Head Injuries

After securing the airway and providing the required resuscitation, the goal is to achieve and maintain normal or low intracranial pressure while maintaining acceptable systemic hemodynamics. This may be difficult. Intracranial pressure is decreased as much as possible by administration of mannitol or furosemide, induction of hypocapnia ($PaCO_2$ 25 torr), and maintenance of a low venous pressure. A mechanical ventilator wave-form with rapid inspiratory flow rate may assist in minimizing intrathoracic pressure. Barbiturates and narcotics are used to minimize autonomic response to intubation and incision. They are probably preferable to the anesthetic vapors because of their less unfavorable effects on intracranial pressure. However, there is no strong evidence to support large-dose barbiturate therapy for brain protection in this setting. Marked hypotension imediately following intracranial decompression is common. Treatment consists of administration of fluids and, if necessary, the judicious use of a pressor, such as ephedrine, to replace the sudden decrease of sympathetic activity. We routinely establish arterial and central venous pressure monitoring as soon as possible after induction of anesthesia. A coagulopathy is occasionally seen. The etiology of this disseminated intravascular coagulation-like picture is not clear, but probably relates to the release of brain thromboplastin. Neurogenic pulmonary edema following head injury may be seen in rare instances. Myocardial failure is not the etiology of this disorder, and therefore treatment with inotropic agents is not appropriate. Facilities must be available for intraoperative application of positive end-expiratory pressure.

The Open Globe

Facial injuries may include trauma to the globe of the eye. Loss of vitreous humor, iris, and lens may result in permanent blindness and require evisceration. To minimize this possibility, every effort is made to avoid raising intraocular pressure. Intraocular pressure and intracranial pressure are controlled by similar factors, but in addition, active contraction of orbital and extraocular muscle may "squeeze" the globe. Induction of anesthesia must be smooth, and there must be neither "squeeze" of eye muscles nor straining during surgery. The fasciculations that follow administration of succinylcholine cause a transient increase in intraocular pressure, but its clinical importance is uncertain. It is not known whether administration of a small dose of a nondepolarizing neuromuscular blocking agent prevents the increase in intraocular pressure caused by succinylcholine. Nevertheless, our preference includes the use of "precurarization," followed by a large dose of thiopental, and succinylcholine; or, if a smaller dose of thiopental would be safer, substituting a large dose of pancuronium (0.15 mg per kilogram), vecuronium (0.15 mg per kilogram), or atracurium (0.6 mg per kilogram) for the succinylcholine. Either way, the profound myoneural block is maintained and is monitored with a nerve stimulator. The ventilator is adjusted to maintain hypocapnia.

The Immediate Postoperative Period

At the end of surgery, for all but the most massive trauma, when hypovolemia has been corrected and the hemodynamic status is stable, the temperature is greater than 34 °C, and pulmonary gas exchange is satisfactory, it is usually appropriate to extubate the patient's trachea and to administer oxygen in the recovery room. Because of the danger of possible regurgitation and aspiration of gastric contents, the patient should not be extubated until awake with intact upper airway reflexes.

After major trauma, the condition of many patients remains unstable in a number of ways, including blood volume and hemodynamics, temperature, acid-base balance, and coagulation. In some instances, pulmonary edema is present as a result of pulmonary trauma or secondary to previous cardiac ischemia or massive fluid load. Intracranial pressure may require monitoring. Intensive care is necessary, but the process of transfer is not simple and involves a lapse of time before the patient is settled in the intensive care unit (ICU) with all monitoring systems functioning and the ICU staff conversant with the ongoing problems. There are various ways to meet this situation, but the guiding principles are as follows:

1. Establish and maintain as much monitored stability as is feasible in the operating room, that is, do not take a "blind leap" to the ICU with a hypovolemic, hypotensive patient whose blood gas levels and acid-base status are unknown. If necessary, stay in the operating room long enough to correct these defects.

2. Use portable electronic monitoring and mechanical ventilation equipment for the move to the ICU and ensure that these are functioning well before leaving the operating room. In patients with severely impaired cardiorespiratory status, a change to manual ventilation may result in a sufficient change in intrathoracic pressure to cause increased hypotension or intracranial pressure, or to permit a change in lung volume with resulting deterioration in oxygen exchange.

3. Forewarn the ICU to prepare the necessary ventilation and monitoring equip-

ment and any other urgently required therapy, such as blood products, so that they are in place and ready upon arrival of the patient.

4. On arrival, establish continuity of ventilation and blood pressure monitoring as first priority. Stay with the patient until all monitoring and support systems are re-established and the ICU staff is familiarized with the patient's circumstances and orders.

WOUNDS

JURIS BUNKIS, M.D.
ROBERT L. WALTON, M.D.

Most wounds resulting from trauma are relatively minor injuries and can be treated in an emergency room, with the patient returning home after treatment. The care of all wounds, however, is governed by the same biologic principles, and the essence of treatment in each case is proper wound care based on biologic principles—*not* on spinal reflexes, anecdotal empiricism, or handbook dogma.

The phenomenon of healing is manifested by various cellular and intercellular events including epithelization, wound contraction, and collagen synthesis. Wounds heal at their maximum rate only when allowed to do so. An understanding of the basic principles of wound healing and management is necessary to allow the surgeon to make the right decisions in order to obtain a superior result. The practical management of wounds should be based on knowledge of the nature of the injury, functional anatomy, and the reparative process.

WOUND ASSESSMENT

A pertinent history and physical examination are essential. As with any injury, priorities are given to life-threatening conditions. Regardless of wound appearance, attention must first be directed toward establishing adequacy of airway, ventilation, and circulation. The history should be obtained from the patient or, if unattainable, from a reliable witness. The mechanism of injury should be determined to shed light on the nature and extent of the injury. Is the injury due to an automobile accident, a fall, a stab, or a gunshot wound? Was a pen knife or machete employed? Is the wound due to a bullet from a small-caliber, low-velocity handgun or to a powerful, short-range shotgun blast? Did the patient fall from 3 or 30 feet? is the injury due to a relatively clean plate glass window or a barnyard pitchfork? How much time has elasped since the injury? How much blood was lost at the scene? What symptoms—e.g., hemoptysis, dyspnea, hematuria, paresthesia–has the patient experienced?

Alterations in the body's capability to respond to injury may alter the healing process. Stress, diabetes mellitus, malnutrition, bleeding disorders, and immunotherapy or steroid therapy represent systemic factors that may impede wound healing. The presence of other local factors (e.g., peripheral vascular disease, prior radiation therapy, or cutaneous eruptions) that may affect the healing process should also be determined by the surgeon.

A thorough physical examination should be performed. Present comments will be limited to examination of the wound, but one must remember to begin the examination with an overall assessment of the patient's nutritional status, vital signs, and other aspects of his general condition.

The examining physician must first ascertain the location of the injury. A stab to the neck, thorax, or abdomen presents a different set of potential problems that does a superficial laceration of the buttocks. Deep lacerations of the extremities also frequently involve important underlying structures. The evaluation and management of deep wounds of the head and neck, extremities, chest, and abdomen are discussed in separate chapters of this book.

The depth of injury—as determined by loss of function of the injured part as well as injury to underlying nerves, blood vessels, ducts, tendons, bones, and joints–should be noted. The location, extent and cause of the wound indicate which laboratory or radiologic studies are needed.

Gross contamination of the wound or the presence of foreign bodies should be noted, as should the viability of tissues and the possibility of tissue loss.

Careful examination of the wound is imperative for proper diagnosis and management. Such examination is possible only in an appropriate facility equipped with adequate lighting and instrumentation. Frequently, this necessitates taking the patient to the operating room, but universal guidelines cannot be established owing to the variability of standards between different emergency departments. Except under conditions of significant vascular compromise, a tourniquet is helpful in providing a dry field for the controlled evaluation of extremity wounds. Needless to say, sterile technique and gentle handling of tissues are mandatory.

Definitive wound evaluation cannot be performed in an uncooperative patient. It may be necessary to consider restraints, sedation, general anesthesia, or even a delay of the evaluation until more favorable conditions (e.g., sobriety) can be obtained. If anesthesia is given for this purpose, a thorough functional (including neurologic) examination should be performed when possible, prior to administration of the anesthesia.

WOUND CLASSIFICATION

Tissue injury is caused by mechanical forces. Shear, tensile, and compressive forces, alone or in combination, produce predictable patterns of tissue injury. Knowledge of the nature and magnitude of mechanical forces that produced the injury allows the surgeon to predict the extent of tissue damage. The predictability of certain injury patterns has allowed classification of wounds into specific categories: abrasions, lacerations, contusions, avulsions, amputations, degloving, and bursting injuries.

Lacerations result from shear forces applied to the skin by sharp objects. Relatively little energy is required to produce such lacerations, and a minimal amount of tissue is injured. Consequently, the general demands for wound healing are easily satisfied, and wound infections are relatively infrequent.

Tensile forces can tear soft tissue. When tensile force exceeds the elastic yield of tissue, stretching and eventual separation of the parts occur. The extent of injury is greater than in simple lacerations because the amount of energy absorbed by the soft tissue is larger. Such injuries may produce intimal damage in surrounding blood vessels, with subsequent thrombosis and ischemia to the injured parts. The structural integrity of nerves, muscles, ligaments, and tendons may also be disrupted. Such an injury places a greater demand on the biologic process of repair, decreases wound defense mechanism, and enhances susceptibility to infection.

Soft tissue compression between two opposing forces results in the greatest amount of tissue damage. Hemorrhage occurs in the soft tissues, with subsequent ecchymosis and hematoma formation. Edema affects capillary blood flow and prolongs the inflammatory phase of wound healing. Intimal damage to blood vessels may result in thrombosis and tissue necrosis. If the forces of compression are of significant magnitude, actual separation of the skin and soft tissue can occur to produce a "bursting" or "degloving" injury. Such wounds are markedly impaired in their ability to heal.

Wounds can also be classified, according to the expected level of bacterial contamination, into the following categories: clean, potentially contaminated, or contaminated. A thyroidectomy incision produced under sterile operating room conditions represents an example of a clean wound. Potentially contaminated wounds include those in which a hollow viscus (e.g, gallbladder, trachea, ureter, appendix) has been entered, but gross spillage of infected contents has not occurred. Other examples of potentially contaminated wounds include stab wounds with a kitchen knife and lacerations with glass or other relatively clean objects. Contaminated wounds contain quantitative bacterial counts exceeding 10^5 bacteria per gram of tissue, and the high probability of wound infection exists if such wounds are closed primarily. A puncture wound made with a dirty pitchfork, human bites, and wounds that have sustained gross spillage of infected secretions fall into this category.

For therapeutic purposes, superficial wounds can be classified as being either tidy or untidy. Tidy wounds are caused by sharp objects, result in minimal tissue injury and contamination, and can usually be closed under favorable circumstances. Untidy wounds, however, are manifested by extensive soft tissue injury or contamination and require major intervention to allow satisfactory wound healing. Management of untidy wounds may be influenced by the extent and location of the injury. A surgeon may be able to surgically convert an untidy wound to a tidy one, and thus permit immediate closure.

ANESTHESIA

Satisfactory anesthesia often must be provided to ensure the patient's comfort while the wound is being assessed and treated. The age and mental status of the patient, as well as the extent of the wound, dictate whether a local, regional, or general anesthetic is preferable. Local or regional anesthesia requires the cooperation of patient, surgeon, and, if present, anesthesiologist.

Frequently, a supplemental tranquilizing agent may be beneficial in an anxious patient. Diazepam (Valium) provides good sedative and amnesic effects, but minimal respiratory and circulatory effects, at the usual dose of 5 to 10 mg. In addition, diazapam increases the threshold to lidocaine-induced seizures. It can be given orally or intravenously. If given intravenously, the injection site should be flushed with normal saline to avoid tissue irritation from the diazepam. Intramuscular administration, which frequently results in erratic absorption, should be avoided.

A "pediatric cocktail" containing meperidine (Demerol), 2 mg per kilogram, chlorpromazine (Thorazine), 1 mg per kilogram, and promethazine (Phenergan), 1 mg per kilogram, is a useful supplement for the pediatric population during suturing of lacerations or other potentially painful procedures. Such a "cocktail," however, should not replace a gentle, personal approach to the patient.

Local anesthesia is recommended for most minor wounds. The anesthetic agent may be infiltrated directly into the wound to reduce the discomfort associated with injection. Infiltration directly into the wound risks spreading potential infection and should be avoided in heavily contaminated wounds. The pain associated with cutaneous injection is due in part to the stretching of sensory nerve endings in the dermis. This can be minimized by using smaller, more concentrated volumes of anesthetic and slower infiltration rates. The least amount of anesthetic that will provide adequate anesthesia should be employed to minimize distortion of important landmarks, particularly when dealing with facial lacerations. In certain critical situations (e.g., in approximating the vermilion border), the key anatomic structures may be approximated with a single 6-0 monofilament suture prior to instillation of any anesthetic solution. Alternatively methylene blue tattoos can be placed at critical anatomic points prior to injection of the anesthetic agent to allow subsequent accurate alignment.

Hemostasis is frequently achieved following injury by vasospasm, platelet plugging, and fibrin clot formation. Lidocaine and similar anesthetic agents cause vasodilation, which may result in rebleeding. The addition of epinephrine to the local anesthetic solution will overcome this tendency. An epinephrine concentration of 1:80,000 provides as much vasoconstriction as a 1:200,000 solution, but more dilute solutions are virtually ineffective. A 1:200,000 solution is optimal, as it produces maximal vasoconstriction with minimal epinephrine-related side-effects.

Epinephrine-containing solutions can severely compromise the local wound defense mechanisms by their vasoconstricting effects, and therefore should not be used in heavily contaminated wounds. Their use is also contraindicated in areas such as fingers and toes, which are supplied by terminal, segmental blood vessels. Epinephrine should also be avoided in patients with heart and peripheral vascular disease.

Signs of toxicity, which are remarkably similar among the different local anesthetic solutions, are always dose-related and include numbness, tingling, diplopia, mental confusion, and convulsions.

Allergy to the ester-linked local anesthetics (e.g., procaine, cocaine) is well documented, and cross-sensitivity exists between the ester-linked moieties. Allergy to the amide-linked local anesthetics (e.g., lidocaine, bupivacaine, mepivacaine) is virtually nonexistent, and most reported reactions are vasovagal in nature. No cross-sensitivity exists between the amide-linked and ester-linked local anesthetic agents.

Limiting the total dose of local anesthetic administered is the surest way to avoid systemic toxicity. The vasoconstrictive effect of epinephrine decreases the rate of anesthetic clearance from the wound, thus adding to the safety margin (Table 1). Should a toxic reaction occur, however, the surgeon must be prepared to oxygenate the patient and administer intravenous diazepam to increase the seizure threshold to the local anesthetic, and place the patient in the Trendelenburg position to ensure adequate cortical blood flow.

Certain wounds are particularly adapted to regional anesthetic techniques. Such techniques allow wider exploration and manipulation of deeper tissues than would be possible with local blocks. Regional techniques also avoid distortion of local tissues and allow precise alignment of injured parts. Regional anesthesia is especially applicable in extremity injuries (e.g., axillary block; isolated ulnar, median, or radial nerve blocks; digital nerve blocks, sciatic or femoral nerve blocks; spinal or epidural anesthesia; Bier blocks). Trigeminal nerve blocks are useful in providing segmental facial anesthesia. Details regarding specific anesthetic techniques are provided in the chapter on *Anesthetic Management*.

Lidocaine, and most other local anesthetics do not provide satisfactory local anesthesia in areas of established infection. Biochemical and physical mechanisms have been postulated for this clinical finding. Local anesthetics, which are weak bases, are inactivated by the acidic environment (e.g., increased lactic acid production) found in areas of infection. In addition, diffusion of local anesthetic

TABLE 1 Suggested Maximum Dosages of Local Anesthetics

Agent		mg/kg	Total Dose in Average 70 kg Patient
Lidocaine	with epinephrine	7	500 mg
	without epinephrine	4	300 mg
Procaine	with epinephrine	14	1,000 mg
	without epinephrine	8	
Cocaine		1	

solution is hampered by loculations and other physical barriers present in infected wounds. If the wound cannot be adequately examined or treatment rendered with either local or regional nerve block techniques, general anesthesia may be indicated. After adequate anesthesia has been achieved, the wound may be examined and definitive management rendered.

WOUND PREPARATION

Hair Removal

Shaving the operative area with a clean disposable razor is frequently recommended. This may be particularly useful in dense hair-bearing areas. However, clinical data suggest that preoperative shaving is associated with increased wound infection rates. Depilatory use does not enhance the wound's susceptibility to infection. Although shaving may facilitate wound management, it may invite bacterial proliferation and wound infection if the infundibulum of the hair follicle is injured. This can be avoided by clipping the hair 1 or 2 mm above the skin or by using depilatory agents. Care should be taken to remove all shaved hair from the wound, as any hair left behind in the closed wound will act as a foreign body, inviting infection and compromising the wound healing process.

Hair definitely should not be shaved if the laceration traverses the eyebrow or other hair-bearing area. The juncture between the hair-bearing and non-hair-bearing skin presents a critical landmark which will allow accurate alignment of wound edges, thereby avoiding a step-off deformity, particularly in the brow line.

Skin Degerming

Although it is possible to sterilize surgical instruments, one cannot completely sterilize the skin of either the surgeon or the patient without damaging or destroying it. However, skin degerming techniques, have been developed to decrease bacterial counts on the surgeon's hands, within the wound, and on the surrounding skin. A distinction must be made between techniques employed to decrease the resident bacteria on intact skin and those designed to decrease the bacterial contamination of the open wound. One must avoid placing anything into the wound that may cause further tissue injury or impede wound defense mechanisms. In the final analysis, one should avoid placing anything into the wound that one would not place into the conjunctival sac of the eye.

Initial cleansing of the skin surrounding the wound should be carried out by the physician or a member of the operating team employing soap, a nonirritating solution, or a fat solvent. Ionic soap and detergents are satisfactory skin cleansers, but are extremely irritating to the open wound and, if allowed to bathe the wound, actually increases the potential for wound infection. After application to intact skin, the surgical scrub solutions should be removed by thorough rinsing with water. Such cleansing removes transient microflora, gross contaminants, and coagulated blood from the skin surrounding the wound.

A degerming agent should next be applied to the intact skin surrounding the wound. Commonly used solutions include iodine and iodine compounds, hexachlorophine, and alcohol solutions. Povidone-iodine (Betadine), which is nonirritating to intact skin and has a rapid onset of action and a broad antimicrobial spectrum, is the most commonly used skin disinfectant. Such solutions reduce the number of resident and contaminating bacteria on the intact skin surface. The iodine in these compounds is bound to a nonsurfactant moiety (polyvinylpyrrolidine)—large molecules which, if absorbed through the wound, are retained by the body owing to the kidneys' inability to excrete them. In addition, if povidone-iodine gains access to an open wound, free iodine can be absorbed, leading to disturbingly high serum levels. When placed in an open wound, antiseptic solutions destroy not only bacteria, but also cells responsible for local defense and tissue repair, and may actually increase the incidence of wound infection. Therefore, such solutions should not be used in open wounds.

Necrotic tissue, exogenous debris, and bacteria promote the development of wound sepsis. A simple wash of the open wound with physiologic saline solution or a balanced salt solution may mechanically remove up to 90 percent of contaminating bacteria. However, normal saline (pH 5.0) may be irritating to the wound, particularly to the intima of blood vessels; lactated Ringer's solution (pH 6.7) is preferable to saline. Antibiotics may be added to the irrigating solution for heavily contaminated wounds.

The efficacy of wound irrigation is related to irrigation pressure. In heavily contaminated wounds, simple irrigation with an Asepto syringe does not adequately reduce the bacterial concentration. Pulsatile pressure delivered at 7 to 10 p.s.i., however, effectively removes debris, including bacteria, from the wound without disseminating microorganisms into the tissues. Irrigation with a 35-ml syringe through a 19-gauge needle produces irrigation pressures of 7 p.s.i., a useful technique in an emergency room setting. Higher irrigation pressures are to be avoided, as tissue damage and increased potential for wound infection may result.

Mechanical cleansing of the wound by direct scrubbing techniques is effective for removal of particulate contamination and bacteria, but may further injure local tissues. If mechanical scrubbing is required, a highly porous sponge will minimize tissue trauma. Brushes and low-porosity sponges are apt to inflict further tissue injury in an open wound, but may be required to remove imbedded debris to avoid the persistence of abrasion tattoos. Soaps, detergents, and surgical scrub brushes should not be used in open wounds, as they inflict further tissue injury and decrease the wound's resistance to infection.

Surgical Debridement

Although conservative debridement is recommended for most wounds, it must be adequate. Necrotic wound edges must be debrided, regardless of the location or former importance of the devitalized tissue. Surgical debridement may also be required to remove severely contaminated tissues or wound edges that are so irregular as to make wound closure impractical. Closely parallel lacerations may be converted to a single wound by excising the intervening skin bridge.

The simplest method of debridement is total excision of the wound, creating a surgically clean one, but this should be limited to wounds that do not involve specialized structures. Complete excision of the wound is possible only in regions containing an abundance of soft tissues, such as the thigh or buttocks. Selective debridement of all grossly nonviable tissue is essential in wounds containing vital structures. Under special circumstances, tendons, fascia, or dura of questionable viability may be retained, but must be protected from further injury through desiccation. These structures may survive as free grafts if appropriate wound coverage is provided.

Guidelines for determining tissue viability must be based on careful examination of the wound and sound clinical judgment. A completely reliable test to predict tissue viability has not been perfected, although inspection of the wound with Wood's lamp for fluorescence following an intravenous fluorescein injection does provide a reflection of tissue perfusion at that moment. Especially with burn, crush, and blast injuries, the exact extent of tissue damage may be difficult to determine during the initial evaluation. The diffuseness of the tissue damage makes precise initial surgical debridement impossible. In such circumstances, grossly devitalized tissue should be debrided, but tissue of questionable viability may be initially preserved. The demarcated necrotic tissue can be debrided at a "second look" procedure in 24 to 48 hours.

Avulsed or amputated tissue will become necrotic unless the part can be converted to a graft or the blood supply re-established. Unless cellular destruction has occurred, avulsed skin can frequently be debrided, defatted, and reapplied successfully as a free graft. Composite tissues rarely survive as free grafts, and microvascular revascularization should be considered if feasible.

Hemostasis

Thorough wound debridement and prevention of fluid collections are primary goals of good wound management. A blood clot acts as a foreign body and provides an excellent culture medium for bacteria within the wound. Hematoma is a common cause of skin graft loss, and its presence beneath a skin flap may compromise the flap's viability. Therefore, every effort must be made to obtain meticulous hemostasis before closing the wound. Even small clots within the deep recesses of a wound may lead to fibrosis and palpable thickening in the postoperative period.

Spontaneous hemostasis may occur in an acute wound owing to vasospasm, fibrin deposition, and platelet plugging. If a known vessel traverses the wounded area, it should be examined for injury, regardless of the presence or absence of bleeding at the time of exploration.

Hemostasis can be achieved by the application of pressure or biologic solutions (e.g., crystalline collagen, thrombin solution) to the wound or by direct manipulation of injured vessels. Vessels may be suture ligated, clipped, or electrocoagulated. Vessels larger than 2 mm in diameter should be precisely clamped with as little adjacent tissue as possible and clipped or tied with the finest appropriate ligature to avoid necrosis of a large mass of tissue distal to the tie. Metal and synthetic absorbable (polydioxanone) ligature clips are commercially available. However, sutures and clips are foreign bodies and increase the wound's susceptibility to infection. Braided, nonabsorbable sutures have the highest propensity for infection in contaminated wounds and should be avoided. Quantitative bacterial studies have demonstrated that a single, buried silk suture enhances the possibility of infection by a factor of 10,000 times. Monofilament synthetic sutures are least reactive, but their low friction coefficient makes them unsuitable as ligatures, except in the repair of large vessels. For these reasons, absorbable sutures (e.g., polyglycolic acid, polyglactin, catgut) are recommended for use as suture ligatures in acute wounds.

Smaller vessels may be electrocoagulated. Vessels must be precisely clamped and the minimal amount of electrical energy necessary to provide hemostasis employed. Indiscriminate electrocoagulation results in significant amounts of charred, necrotic tissue within the wound, which increase the wound's susceptibility to infection.

Antibiotics

The reward for meticulous wound debridement and physiologic closure is timely healing without suppuration and rapid restoration of function. Fortunately, most civilian wounds are not heavily contaminated and contain less than 10^2 bacteria per gram of tissue at the time of presentation in the emergency room. Quantitative bacterial studies demonstrate that the critical factor in predicting wound sepsis is the number rather than the type of bacteria remaining in the wound at the time of closure. Infection predictably occurs if wounds containing more than 10^5 bacteria per gram of tissue are closed without adjunctive measures. The most important factor in preventing wound infection is adequate surgical debridement. If the likelihood of wound infection remains high, antibiotic prophylaxis is indicated.

Prophylactic antibiotics markedly decrease the risk of postoperative sepsis if the antibiotic can be delivered before the bacteria arrive in the tissues. Understandably, it is unlikely that the patient will have adequate antibiotic tissue levels at the time of acute injury, but if indicated, antibiotics should be administered promptly in the emergency room following wound evaluation and after culture specimens have been obtained. The effectiveness of antibiotics in preventing subsequent wound infection is greatly reduced by any delay in starting therapy. Prophylactic antibiotics have a negligible, if any, beneficial effect if initial administration is delayed 4 hours following injury and bacterial contamination. In elective situations, prophylactic antibiotics should be administered during induction of anesthesia.

It has already been mentioned that wound quantitative bacterial counts give an accurate prediction of subseuqent potential for wound infection. Properly managed wounds containing less than 10^5 bacteria per gram of tissue at the time of closure heal per primum without infection. Insight into the magnitude of bacterial contamination is provided by knowledge of the mechanism of injury and by the clinical appearance of the wound, but a more definitive assessment of the degree of contamination can be obtained by quantitative microbiologic assays. The "rapid slide technique" can provide the surgeon with this crucial information within 20 minutes (Table 2).

Clean acute lacerations rarely present with bacterial counts greater than 10^5 bacteria per gram of tissue. Following proper irrigation and debridement, such wounds can usually be closed primarily without risk of infection and do not require prophylactic antibiotic therapy. Wounds resulting from crush or blast injuries, on the other hand, frequently contain large quantities of devitalized tissue, foreign debris, bacteria, and blood clots. The level of bacterial contamination should be determined following irrigation and debridement. If counts greater than 10^5 organisms per gram of tissue persist, but the extent of tissue injury does not contraindicate wound closure, prohylactic antibiotics may allow uncomplicated primary wound closure and healing. A Gram stain from the wound helps to determine the appropriate antibiotics. However, antibiotics are effec-

TABLE 2 The "Rapid Slide" Bacterial Quantitative Assay

1. Clean the surface of the wound biopsy area with 70 percent isopropyl alcohol.
2. Obtain the biopsy specimen with a 3- or 4-mm dermal punch or with a scalpel. No anesthesia is required for an open wound.
3. After the tissue is weighed, flamed, and diluted 1:10 with thioglycollate (1 ml/g), it is homogenized.
4. Spread exactly 0.02 ml of the suspension with a 20-lambda Sahli-pipette on a glass slide. The inoculum is confined to an area 15 mm in diameter.
5. Oven-dry the slide for 15 minutes at 75° C.
6. Stain the slide using either a Gram stain or the Brown and Brenn modification for tissue staining, to accentuate the gram-negative organisms.
7. Read the smear under 1.9 mm (magnification × 97) objective and examine all fields for the presence of bacteria.
8. The presence of even a single organism is evidence that the tissue contains a level of bacterial growth greater than 10^5 bacteria per gram of tissue.

tive in preventing wound infection only if the bacterial levels are less than 10^9 organisms per gram of tissue. If closed, wounds containing greater than 10^9 bacteria per gram of tissue following debridement suppurate regardless of the presence or absence of prophylactic antibiotics. Such grossly contaminated wounds (including those contaminated by feces, pus, or heterosaliva) should not be closed primarily. In such circumstances, the wound should be debrided and topical antimicrobials (e.g., silver sulfadiazine) added to the wound management regimen until bacterial counts drop below 10^5 bacteria per gram of tissue to allow delayed primary closure.

Previous comments have been limited to the treatment of acute wounds. However, the same basic principles apply to the management of chronic wounds. All chronic wounds (e.g., pressure sores, full-thickness burns, leg ulcers) contain granulation tissue—by definition, granulation tissue contains bacteria. Successful closure of chronic wounds is also predicated on the surgeon's ability to control the bacterial contamination. Regardless of the method employed for wound closure, suppuration results if the final bacterial counts exceed 10^5 per gram of tissue and prophylactic antibiotics are withheld. Clinical evaluation of granulation tissue provides a notoriously inaccurate estimate of the degree of contamination; as in the management of acute wounds, the surgeon should validate his clinical impressions by obtaining a quantitative bacterial assay.

Intravenous antibiotics do not reach adequate levels in granulation tissue to have an effect on bacterial concentrations quantitatively, but may affect them qualitatively, leading to a more virulent, antibiotic-resistant organism. Intravenous antibiotics are not indicated in the treatment of chronic soft tissue wounds except to treat surrounding cellulitis. Reduction of excessive bacterial flora can be accomplished by meticulous attention to surgical techniques and by the judicious application of topical antimicrobials.

Any wound may provide the portal of entry for *Clostridium tetani*. Nail puncture wounds, splinter injuries, burns, and other traumatic wounds require tetanus prophylaxis (Table 3).

WOUND CLOSURE

Timing of Closure

Time elapsed since injury does not by itself represent a significant determinant for wound closure. The decision to close a wound is predicated on many factors, the most important of which is the level of contamination. The primary goal is to reduce the bacterial inoculum below the critical level of 10^5 organisms per gram of tissue prior to wound closure. However, a laboratory test must not replace sound clinical judgment. When faced with less than ideal circumstances

TABLE 3 Tetanus Prophylaxis

| Type of Wound | Patient Not Immunized or Partially Immunized | Patient Completely Immunized Time Since Last Booster Dose | |
		5 to 10 yrs.	10 yrs. †
Clean minor	Begin or complete immunization per schedule; tetanus toxoid 0.5 ml	None	Tetanus toxoid 0.5 ml
Tetanus prone	Human tetanus immune globulin, 250–500 units; tetanus toxoid, 0.5 ml, complete immunization per schedule; antibiotic therapy as indicated	Tetanus toxoid 0.5 ml; antibiotic therapy if indicated	Tetanus toxoid 0.5 ml; human tetanus immune globulin, 250–500 units; antibiotic therapy if indicated

(e.g., retained foreign body, necrotic tissue following debridement) or diminished wound defense mechanism (associated with systemic illness, malnutrition, impaired local blood supply, and so on), primary wound closure may produce disastrous results, regardless of the initial quantitative bacterial counts.

The timing of wound closure represents a compromise between the likelihood of infection and the ability to provide favorable conditions for closure. If appropriate, primary wound closure is clearly advantageous over other methods. An open wound invites fibrous tissue proliferation and contraction, both of which detract from final function and appearance. The wound should not be closed indiscriminately, as infection will defeat any possible gains from primary closure.

If left open, contaminated wounds gradually gain resistance to infection over a 4-day period. After initial debridement, the open wound may be dressed with sterile, fine-mesh gauze. A moist or greasy dressing prevents wound desiccation. The presence of wound debris, drainage, or fever dictates the frequency of dressing changes. On the fourth day, a quantitative bacterial assay helps to determine the appropriateness of wound closure. Following further debridement and antibiotic coverage as necessary, the wound may be closed using sterile technique. If the wound is not located in a critical area and if it is small, it may be preferable to allow healing by second intention.

The most aesthetically pleasing scars and the most satisfactory return of function usually result from healing by first intention. Anything that interferes with primary healing may result in additional scarring and a less acceptable result. Proper wound debridement, closure, and postoperative management are prerequisites for satisfactory primary healing. Initial wound care has a significant influence on subsequent healing; surgical technique remains the most important determinant of successful wound closure. This includes gentle manipulation of injured tissues, precise sharp debridement, prudent use of electrocautery, avoidance of excessive or strangulating sutures, prevention of tissue desiccation, and diligent postoperative management.

Methods of Closure

Once the decision to close the wound has been made, the surgeon must choose an appropriate method. The decision requires an understanding of the objectives of repair as well as the materials necessary to effect such a repair. The ultimate goal of any closure is to achieve precise tensionless alignment of the injured parts without further injury to adjacent structures. This allows prompt restoration of function and cosmetic appearance.

The surgical technique chosen to effect closure must be individualized for each wound. Generally, the simplest method compatible with a satisfactory outcome is selected. This concept has been described as the ''reconstructive ladder'' approach to wound closure. Whenever possible, as with simple lacerations, the wound should be closed by primary approximation. Following complex wounds associated with tissue loss, it may become impossible to close the wound edges directly by approximation without undue tension. If an adequate soft tissue base is present, a skin graft may suffice for wound closure. In more complex wounds containing exposed bones, tendons, nerves, vessels, dura, or other vital structures, one must progress up the ''reconstructive ladder' and design a flap to provide an appropriate solution for closure of the defect. Local flaps are generally technically simpler to use than distant flaps and are thus preferable whenever appropriate circumstances exist. In certain clinical situations or in certain anatomic locations (e.g., large complex wounds involving the distal leg or ankle region), a distant flap may provide the only practical wound coverage. Free tissue transfers are reserved for these most complex wounds.

The choice of appropriate material for wound closure is based on its biologic and mechanical properties as well as characteristics of the tissues being approximated. Composition of the material, strength, knot efficiency, tissue response, and wound location should all be considered. The surgeon's armamentarium includes a variety of suture materials, stainless steel staples, and surgical tapes. To a degree, however, the choice of material for surgical closure is less important than the surgical technique. Each suture must be properly placed and tied without excessive tension to minimize ischemia of the wound edges. The least reactive and the smallest size and amount of suture material that will adequately effect tissue approximation, particularly in contaminated wounds, should be employed.

The necessity to close individual layers of the wound is based on knowledge of local wound stresses, presence of dead space, and the necessity for accurate approximation of tissues. Dense connective tissues (e.g., dermis, fascia, ligaments, tendons) represent the strength layers of any wound closure. These tissues heal slowly, however, and the suture material chosen to approximate them should be capable of maintaining its strength until satisfactory union has occurred. Ideally, such a suture should incite a minimal amount of local tissue reaction. Synthetic, monofilament, nonabsorbable sutures are best suited for this purpose.

Muscle and adipose tissues do not hold sutures well. Closure of these layers is occasionally necessary in order to obliterate dead space. In the laboratory model, dead space resulting from tissue loss has been shown to increase the likelihood of infection. However, obliteration of dead space with sutures, enhances the possibility of infection because the sutures act as foreign bodies in the wound. Suturing of the dead space is particularly contraindicated in the closure of contaminated wounds. When necessary, the dead space should be obliterated with a minimal number of loosely tied absorbable sutures.

Skin closure may be performed in layers or by full-thickness percutaneous sutures. Surgical tapes or staples may also be considered. The choice of method depends on the location of the wound, its direction, and local stress factors. Wounds that are oriented in the direction of skin wrinkles are subjected to less tension during healing, and consequently produce a more favorable scar. Examples include transverse lacerations involving the forehead or neck. Wounds that cross the lines of maximal stress are subjected to increased tension during healing and have a propensity to widen and hypertrophy with time. Examples include lacerations over the deltoid region or the cheek. In most situations, the acute wound should be debrided and closed without any attempt at reorientation of the direction of the scar. The scar should be allowed to mature before considering scar revision.

The degree of wound gaping prior to epidermal reapproximation reflects the potential width of the scar. Particularly in areas of high skin tension, layered wound closure is indicated to minimize the final width of the scar. The dermis should be anatomically realigned with interrupted inverted sutures. A few well-placed 5-0 or 6-0 clear nylon sutures provide adequate reapproximation of the dermal layer until the wound has healed and the scar matured. However, dermal nylon sutures may remain palpable or visible through the skin. Absorbable sutures are more frequently employed for dermal closure. Catgut sutures, which are made from animal protein (available either in the plain or chromic form), are frequently employed for dermal closure. However, catgut sutures display erratic behavior in loss of strength, absorption, and tissue reaction. For these reasons, many surgeons prefer to use synthetic absorbable suture (e.g., polyglycolic acid, polyglactin) for dermal reapproximation. Even though these sutures do have longer holding power than catgut, they too lose their holding power before wound maturation is complete. Recent studies with polydioxanone monofilament absorbable sutures have demonstrated prolonged breaking strength retention, a reliable absorption profile, and minimal tissue reaction. Experience with polydioxanone is still limited, but perhaps this suture will prove to be the most appropriate material for dermal approximation. Following closure of the dermis, the strength layer of the wound, the epidermal layer can be adjusted with fine, nonabsorbable, monofilament sutures—chosen for their low tissue reactivity—or surgical tape. If sutures are employed, they should be replaced before the fifth postoperative day with surgical tape to avoid unsightly crosshatching of the final wound. This method of wound closure is designed to provide the least noticeable scar and is most appropriate for facial lacerations.

Percutaneous sutures that incorporate both the epidermis and dermis and a small amount of underlying subcutaneous tissue are frequently employed to close wounds elsewhere in the body. Such sutures are usually removed 7 to 14 days later. Without dermal support during the subsequent maturation phase, the scar tends to widen and hypertrophy. Here too, however, a layered closure and early replacement of the superficial sutures by surgical tape may minimize the subsequent scar.

Factors in obtaining a satisfactory scar include eversion of the wound edges to effect precise epidermal coaptation and proper suture tension to minimize ischemia of the wound margins. In order to obtain everted wound edges, the sutures must be placed so that the depth of each bite exceeds its width. It has been clearly shown that the size of suture material employed is not so important as the tightness of the closure or the length of time that the sutures are left in situ. Sutures should be removed before the seventh day to avoid epithelization of the suture tracts with a resultant objectionable (railroad) appearance of the scar. Monofilament, synthetic nonabsorbable sutures (e.g., nylon, polypropylene) are most frequently employed for percutaneous skin closure. Silk sutures, which are natural fibers, are significantly more reactive and have been shown to increase the incidence of wound infection. Silk should not be used in acute wounds, except occasionally for closure of intraoral mucosal laceration.

Stainless steel sutures, skin clips, and staples have been employed for years because of their presumed inertness. However, studies have suggested slightly increased infection rates, probably owing to the mechanical irritation because of their rigidity. This fact will be of little, if any, clinical significance if the staples are removed before the seventh postoperative day. A number of prepackaged skin staplers are now available. Most staplers are designed to produce an everted skin closure and can do so quickly. The main advantage of staplers is a significant reduction in wound closure time, particularly with extensive lacerations or in such specialized situations as securing multiple skin grafts.

Surgical tapes have the advantage of not requiring anesthesia to minimize painful stimuli during wound closure. Such techniques are particularly attractive in the care of the pediatric population. Taped wounds also have the least propensity for infection. In certain situations, one may close the deeper layers of the wound (including the dermis) with sutures and close the epidermal layer with tape—thus avoiding the need to later remove skin sutures. Microporous, rayon reinforced wound tapes are widely used. Adherence is enhanced if all moisture is removed and the skin defatted with acetone before tapes are applied. Tincture of benzoin may initially enhance tape adherence but it is quickly solubilized by skin oils and loses its adherence capabilities, thus contraindicating its use. However, wound tapes do have significant disadvantages. It is difficult to obtain precise anatomic approximation of the skin edges with surgical tapes, particularly with irregular lacerations. It is impossible to obtain an everted closure solely with tape. Moreover, tape only approximates the superficial portion of the wound and leaves deeper layers vulnerable to biomechanical stresses, which may result in widening and a more prominent scar.

Wound Drains

Justification for drains has been stated to include obliteration of dead space and egress of material foreign or harmful to a particular location. Drains are rarely indicated in the closure of acute superficial wounds. Percutaneous drains constitute foreign bodies, enhance tissue necrosis, and serve as conduits for bacterial contamination. Contrary to popular opinion, drains do not prevent the formation of hematomas or seromas. If good surgical technique has been employed, it is unnecessary to drain most superficial wounds in the acute situation. If bleeding cannot be controlled at the time of operation, delayed primary wound closure should be considered. However, drains may be an important adjunctive measure in the treatment of superficial abscesses. The specific indications for drainage of body cavities and organs are discussed in separate chapters.

POSTOPERATIVE WOUND CARE

The surgeon's responsibilities do not end with wound closure. The surgeon must provide maximal support of the patient and a suitable environment for satisfactory wound healing, and he must direct the patient's rehabilitation.

Although wound healing may be considered a local phenomenon, the ideal milieu for the wound can only be provided by total patient care. Attention must be paid to associated injuries. In addition, nutrition, blood volume, and oxygenation must be maintained. A social worker may provide valuable assistance to a patient with a physically disabling injury. Likewise, a psychiatirst may help a patient to cope with an altered body image following a disfiguring injury.

The sutured wound should be protected from the environment with a dressing impervious to exogenous microbial contamination. Experimental studies have demonstrated that closed wounds can be infected by surface bacterial contamination within the first 2 or 3 days. Following this period, sutured wounds gain considerable resistance to infection, and dressings no longer serve a protective role. Taped wounds demonstrated superior resistance to infection, becoming resistant to surface contamination within 2 hours following wound closure.

A dressing may serve a number of functions that may contribute to healing. Ideally, a dressing should provide an atmosphere conducive to satisfactory wound healing. The dressing should keep the wound surface free of excess fluids to minimize maceration and bacterial proliferation while avoiding desiccation. The main functions of a dressing may be listed as follows: protection, immobilization, compression, absorption, debridement, medication, and cosmesis. As the wound heals, its needs may change and necessitate a different type of dressing.

Most dressings consist of a contact layer, an absorptive layer, and an outer wrap. Dry gauze is frequently applied to a freshly closed wound. Such a dressing adheres to the epithelium and vascular tissue of the wound and may result in interference with wound healing during dressing changes. Preferably, the contact layer should consist of nonadherent plastic-coated material or gauze impregnated with a bland ointment. Plastic-coated dressings (e.g., Telfa) or gauze impregnated with bismuth ointment (e.g., Xeroform) or petrolatum provides a satisfactory contact layer. This contact layer should be applied as a single sheet to allow continued egress of wound fluid through the contact layer. Fluffed gauze sponges, mechanics' waste, and bulk cotton may be added as an absorptive layer, to allow the dressing to conform to a desired shape, and to provide immobilization of the wounded part. Nonstretchable, firm, roller gauze bandage and adhesive tape complete the typical dressing, thus providing a compact and stable immobilizing influence. A plaster or aluminum splint may be added to the dressing to enhance immobilization.

Occlusive tapes limit vapor transmission, promoting tissue maceration and bacterial growth. Porous paper tapes are preferable as they allow moisture to be transmitted through the interstices of the tape, with resultant dry skin beneath the tape, which inhibits bacterial proliferation.

Immobilization may avert further tissue damage. Immobilization of the site of injury is essential in the management of contaminated wounds because lymphatic flow is thus reduced n the immobilized part, thereby minimizing the spread of wound microflora. Immobilization places the wound at rest, thus decreasing pain and metabolic demands of the tissues. In addition, immobilization may protect the newly formed capillaries from disruption, thus avoiding small clots and allowing the wound to heal more expeditiously. When combined with elevation and pressure, the transudation of fluid is minimized. Immobilization may be aided by bulky dressings, skin tapes, or splints. The length of immobilization varies according to the demands of local tissues and the status of the wound. However, prolonged immobilization may defeat its possible advantages.

One cannot overemphasize the advantage of elevating the injured part to minimize edema with its resultant deleterious effects. This is particularly applicable to extremity injuries. Edema, which has been stated to be "the mother of scar," slows down the machinery of repair and increases fibrous tissue proliferation. Elevation of the wounded part above the level of the heart is the simplest method of limiting the amount of edema. In certain situations, compression of the wound with bulky dressings may subserve the benefits of elevation. However, one must not apply tourniquet-like constriction to proximal parts or distal venous and lymphatic congestion could result. In extremity injuries, compression dressings should extend from the most distal point proximally, but access to the toes or fingertips should be maintained to allow assessment of the neurovascular status. Maximal wound edema occurs within the first 48 hours and gradually resolves over the next week. It may be necessary to adjust an extremity dressing during periods of fluctuating tissue edema.

A clean wound should have very little drainage and require few dressing changes. Unless clinical signs dictate otherwise, the initial dressing should be left intact over most sutured wounds for the first 48 hours. As mentioned previously, sealed wounds will be highly resistant to surface bacterial contamination by this time, and further dressings may be unnecessary. In most clinical situations, the patient with a well-healing wound may shower by the third day. However, wounds that continue to drain serous fluid require continued protection with an appropriate dressing.

Certain wounds are not amenable to the satisfactory application of a dressing. It is frequently difficult to apply a conforming dressing to sutured facial lacerations. Meticulous suture line care may provide a reasonable alternative. This involves frequent cleansing with saline or dilute hydrogen peroxide solution to remove adherent coagulum, thus decreasing the likelihood of stitch abscess formation. Following cleansing, a thin layer of antibiotic ointment should be applied to the suture line.

Dressings may also be used to debride an open wound. The traditional wet-to-dry method utilizes avulsion of adherent tissues to provide the debridement. This method is effective if performed properly, but one must remember that the dressing does not discriminate between viable and nonviable tissues and tissue injury results with each dressing change. Moistening the dressing prior to removal defeats the purpose of such a dressing. A wet-to-dry dressing should not be employed in wounds containing viable periosteum, perichondrium, paratenon, or perineurium because such tissues desiccate during the "dry" phase, resulting in further tissue damage.

Enzymatic debridement provides an alternative to the wet-to-dry dressing. An enzyme produced by *B. subtilis* (Travase) is effective in removing particulate necrotic debris and coagulum without producing significant injury to viable tissues.

Medicated dressings are occasionally indicated. Topical antimicrobial agents, particularly silver sulfadiazine (Silvadene) and mafenide (Sulfamylon) are frequently employed to control surface contaminants in chronic granulating wounds. These agents are also useful in the management of partial-thickness injuries or wounds containing marginally viable tissues to decrease the potential for bacterial invasion with subsequent conversion to a full-thickness injury and necrosis. However, topical agents retard wound epithelization and should be discontinued as soon as their objectives have been reached (mainly bacterial counts less than 10^5 organisms per gram of tissue).

A surgeon should not discount the importance of a neat dressing. To the patient or casual observer, the sight of a wound may be abhorrent and incite fear or anxiety. A carefully applied dressing reassures the patient that the best possible wound care has been provided.

Rehabilitation may require the assistance of a physical or occupational therapist. The surgeon's responsibility to the patient does not end until the scar has matured and the patient has returned to the mainstream of life.

NEUROLOGIC INJURY

TRIAGE OF HEAD-INJURED PATIENTS

THOMAS A. GENNARELLI, M.D.

The seriousness of head injuries is readily apparent, but recent studies concerning the frequency of occurrence of such injuries and their associated morbidity and mortality serve to solidify these clinical impressions. At least 2 million people incur head injuries each year in the United States, and more than 400,000 patients with head injuries are admitted to hospitals in the United States every year, approximately half of whom are involved in motor vehicle-related injuries. Deaths resulting from head injury are frequent, totalling 40,000 to 60,000 per year and numbering 24 to 36 per 100,000 population. Head injuries account for 1 to 3 percent of all deaths from all causes, 25 percent of all trauma deaths, and 50 to 60 percent of all deaths due to motor vehicle trauma. Furthermore, approximately half of the 3.5 million days of hospitalization per year from motor vehicle trauma represent hospital stays of head-injured patients, and half of the 35,700 man-years of work time that is lost by regular wage earners because of motor vehicle injuries each year can be attributed to head injury. The cost of head injuries therefore represents a substantial portion of the 83 billion dollar cost of trauma.

It is well appreciated that severe head injury is associated with high mortality and high morbidity. In a recent multicenter study, the cumulative mortality of seven head injury centers in the United States was 41 percent. Only 26 percent of these severely injured patients had good recovery; 16 percent were moderately disabled, and 17 percent were either severely disabled or vegetative. It is perhaps less well appreciated that minor head injuries may also be associated with important sequelae. A recent report has documented a high degree of morbidity in patients who were unconscious for less than 20 minutes and who were hospitalized for 48 hours or less. Three months after injury, one-third of the patients who were gainfully employed prior to injury were still out of work. The majority complained of headache and memory problems, and a large number of these patients showed a variety of objective neuropsychologic dysfunctions on formal testing. Considering the additional number of patients who are rendered unconscious or suffer post-traumatic amnesia, estimated at 1.9 million per year, it is apparent that head injury is a major public health problem, considerably larger than we had been led to believe in the past. The solution to this problem lies in (1) the application of preventive measures to mitigate the occurrence and severity of these injuries, (2) a coordinated effort to provide optimal, early, and definitive care for these patients, and (3) a program for appropriate rehabilitation and follow-up.

TYPES OF HEAD INJURY

In general terms, it is convenient to view head injuries as consisting of three distinct varieties. A knowledge of the different pathogenesis and pathophysiology of these varieties allows a more appropriate specific management of such injuries (Table 1).

Skull Injuries

Skull fractures can occur without damage to the brain and is itself not an important cause of neurologic death or disability. Skull fractures can be classified in many ways. For example, they are considered open fractures if the dura is torn and closed fractures if it is not. More conventionally, fractures are catego-

TABLE 1 Classification of Head Injuries

Skull injuries
  Vault fracture
    Linear
    Depressed
  Basilar fracture

Focal Injuries
  Epidural hematoma
  Subdural hematoma
  Contusion
  Intracerebral hematoma

Diffuse brain injuries
  Mild concussion
  Classic cerebral concussion
  Prolonged coma
    Mild DAI
    Moderate DAI
    Severe DAI

rized into those of the vault and those of the base. Basilar skull fractures can present with CSF otorrhea or rhinorrhea, subconjunctival and periorbital hemorrhage (raccoon eyes), or hemotympanum, and usually are not visible on conventional skull films. Injuries to the neural substance of the brain are the primary cause of neurologic dysfunction and can readily be divided into two categories, focal and diffuse.

Focal Injuries

Focal brain injuries are those in which the lesion is large enough to be visualized with the naked eye. The entities causing focal brain injury include contusions, subdural hematoma, epidural hematoma, and intracerebral hematoma. These lesions cause neurologic problems both by virtue of the local brain damage and by causing masses within the cranium, which lead to brain shift, herniation, and ultimately brain stem compression. Brain stem compression is the cause of coma in patients with focal injury. These injuries constitute approximately 50 percent of all cases of head injury in patients admitted to the hospital and are responsible for approximately 66 percent of deaths due to head injury.

Diffuse Injuries

Diffuse brain injuries are associated with more widespread or global disruption of neurologic function and are not usually associated with macroscopically visible brain lesions. Rather, they can cause widespread disruption of both the function and the structure of the brain. When sufficiently severe, the diffuse brain injuries produce coma, not by a compressive effect on the brain stem, but by direct damage to the brain stem or cerebrum. Since diffuse brain injuries, for the most part, are not associated with visible macroscopic lesions, they have historically been lumped together to mean all injuries not associated with focal lesions. Recent evidence suggests that the diffuse brain injuries represent trauma to innumerable axons of the brain. In the milder injuries, this diffuse axonal injury (DAI) is purely functional in nature, but as the severity of injury increases, the amount of DAI increases and physical disruption of axons occurs. The severe diffuse axonal injury is associated with larger amounts of axonal tearing and has a poor prognosis. Several categories of diffuse brain injury are now recognized and will be discussed.

Mild Concussion.   Several concussion syndromes exist that involve temporary disturbances of neurologic function (such as memory) without loss of consciousness.

Classic Cerebral Concussion.   Classic cerebral concussion is a temporary, reversible neurologic deficiency associated with temporary (less than 6 hours) loss of consciousness.

Diffuse Injury. Prolonged traumatic coma that lasts longer than 6 hours and is not due to mass lesions (that is, brain stem compression) is usually associated with axonal damage, and this entity has recently been termed diffuse axonal injury (DAI). Previously, these injuries have been known by many names (e.g., diffuse injury, brain stem contusion, shearing injury), but the term "diffuse axonal injury" more realistically reflects their pathogenesis. These injuries form a continuum of increasingly severe injury and therefore there is no absolute boundary between them. However, the following three distinctions can be made for clinical convenience:

1. *Mild DAI.* A coma that lasts 6 to 24 hours, mild DAI is next to classic concussion in severity, but may be associated with long-standing or permanent neurologic or cognitive deficits.
2. *Moderate DAI.* This is defined as a coma that lasts more than 24 hours and is associated with little or no evidence of brain stem dysfunction. More severe than mild DAI, moderate DAI is associated with mortality of 20 percent and significant morbidity in survivors.
3. *Severe DAI.* Severe DAI is characterized by regularly occurring signs of brain stem dysfunction in patients who are comatose longer than 24 hours (with no mass lesion). This entity has substantial mortality (57%) and morbidity and is associated with widespread damage to axons of the cerebrum and the brain stem.

The diffuse brain injuries account for 40 percent of severely head-injured patients, and although they constitute only 33 percent of head injury deaths, they are the most serious cause of persisting neurologic disability in survivors.

ASSESSMENT OF SEVERITY OF INJURY

Early care of the patient with head injury begins with assessment of the severity of injury and protection of the brain from further insult until definitive diagnosis and definitive therapy can be achieved. Both early and definitive care are aimed at recognizing and treating one of the two fundamentally different types of head injury: focal or diffuse. The ultimate outcome from head injury depends on which type of injury is present, how severe that injury is, and how aggressively it is managed.

The severity of brain injury can be established in less than one minute by evaluating (1) level of consciousness, (2) pupillary function, and (3) lateralized weakness of the extremities. Abnormality of all three is highly suggestive of a focal mass lesion that requires surgery, whereas only the former may be abnormal in diffuse brain injury.

Level of consciousness is best assessed by the Glasgow Coma Scale (GCS), a system that evaluates eye opening and best motor and verbal response. The score is determined by adding the best response in each category and ranges from 3 to 15 (Table 2). Because of its reproducibility, a difference of 2 on the GCS signals a change in neurologic status; a decrease of 3 is worrisome, usually indicating an enlarging hematoma, and demands prompt treatment. It should be noted that coma is defined according to the elements of the GCS as follows: no eye opening, not following commands, no word verbalizations.

The GCS is intended as a global measure of brain dysfunction and in itself contains considerable prognostic information. There is a progressive decrease in mortality as the initial GCS increases from the most severe injury (GCS 3). It is important that injury severity assessment be performed promptly and sequentially after injury to determine the degree of improvement or deterioration that has occurred. Two factors that adversely affect the severity assessment and do not reflect brain injury are the drug use and existing hypotension. The former involves principally alcohol and barbiturates, which are neurologic depressants and decrease the GCS; therefore, a true assessment of the injury component can be made only when the patient is free of these agents. Similarly, hypotension or shock, which frequently accompanies severe multiple system injury, causes decreased cerebral perfusion and loss of consciousness unrelated to brain injury. Therefore, assessment of the level of consciousness by GCS cannot be made until the systolic blood pressure is over 80.

Pupillary function is assessed by the size, equality, and response to bright light. With or without ocular injury, pupillary asymmetry greater than 1 mm must be attributed to intracranial injury until proved otherwise. With few exceptions, the larger pupil is on the side of the mass lesion. Diffuse brain injuries can also cause pupillary asymmetry, but these are usually mild and not associated with the "blown" pupil of third nerve compression attributable to transtentorial herniation. In patients who have a high GCS (moderate-to-mild injury severity), pupillary asymmetry may begin before the level of consciousness decreases, and thus before the GCS falls. Unilateral or bilateral pupillary areflexia is generally a highly unfavorable prognostic sign in adults with severe head injury, but need not be so in children. In addition to obvious ocular injuries, pupillary asymmetry and areflexia may be due to vitreous hemorrhage as the result of increased intracranial pressure, to direct vitreal and retinal injury, or to intracranial injury

TABLE 2 Glasgow Coma Scale

Eye Opening		Best Motor Response		Best Verbal Response	
Spontaneous	4	Follows command	6	Oriented	5
To voice	3	Localizes	5	Disoriented	4
To pain	2	Flexion withdrawal	4	Inappropriate words	3
None	1	Abnormal flexion	3	Sounds only	2
		Extension	2	None	1
		None	1		

or transection of the optic nerves associated with basilar skull fracture.

Lateralized extremity weakness is determined by testing motor power in patients who are able to cooperate or by observing asymmetry of movement in response to painful stimulus. As injury severity worsens, lateralized weakness is more difficult to appreciate, and so small differences may be much more important. Thus, with patients in coma, attention must be paid to the rapidity and amount of movement that occurs in response to painful stimuli. A greater latency before movement begins or less vigorous movement is indicative of lateralized extremity weakness. Although lateralized weakness can occur with diffuse brain injuries, it is much more likely to be a sign of focal swelling within that hemisphere or an intra-axial lesion such as an intracerebral hematoma.

The purpose of assessing injury severity is to triage patients. Patients should be considered to have serious injuries by the following criteria:

1. A GCS of 10 or less (8 usually indicates coma and less than 8 always means coma).
2. A decrease in the GCS by 3 or more irrespective of the initial GCS.
3. Pupillary inequality greater than 1 mm irrespective of the GCS.
4. Lateralized extremity weakness irrespective of the GCS.
5. Markedly depressed skull fractures.
6. Open cranial wounds with CSF leakage (including otorrhea and rhinorrhea) or with brain exposed.

Other injuries that do not meet these criteria may become serious injuries if an expanding intracranial mass develops. Therefore, caution is advised in the developing of criteria for discharge from the emergency department after head injury. Most neurosurgeons prefer hospital admission and observation for all patients with skull fracture and for any patient with a GCS less than 15. Most of these admissions are brief, but serve to extend the observation period for patients who have more slowly developing intracranial hematomas.

PATIENT FLOW TRIAGE SYSTEM

Based on the variables in the assessment of injury severity just discussed, it is possible to develop a systematic approach to the triage of head injury patients. Figures 1 and 2 outline such a system. It must be understood that the scheme presented here is a guideline; owing to the complexity and multiplicity of brain injuries, it is not and cannot be either foolproof or all-inclusive.

The first, and most important, triage tool is a determination of the level of consciousness based on the GCS. All patients who score less than 9 are severely ill and require immediate attention. This is also true of some patients with GCS scores of 9 or more, and they must not be neglected just because they are not currently comatose. In fact, some would argue that more attention should

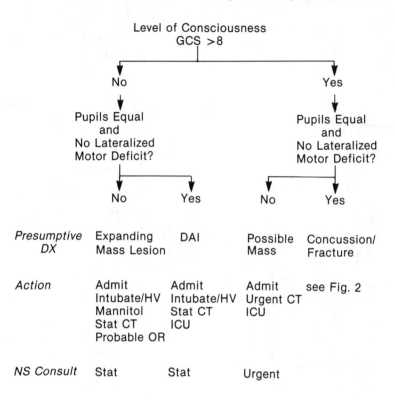

Figure 1 This flow chart outlines a systematic approach to the triage of patients with head injury.

be given to patients with GCS scores of 9 or more, since their chances of survival (salvage) are potentially better.

In a patient with a score less than 9, it must immediately be determined whether the pupils are unequal or whether there is better movement (or less abnormal movement) on one side; in either case, it must be presumed that an expanding mass lesion is present (epidural, subdural, or intracerebral hematoma or large contusion). Since these lesions are potentially correctable by surgical decompression, a rapid definitive diagnosis must be made by CT scan. Before the patient is transported to the CT scanner, hyperventilation (HV) should be started via an endotracheal tube and a bolus of mannitol (1 g per kilogram) should be given to medically decompress the brain.

A comatose patient with equal pupils and equal extremity movements may

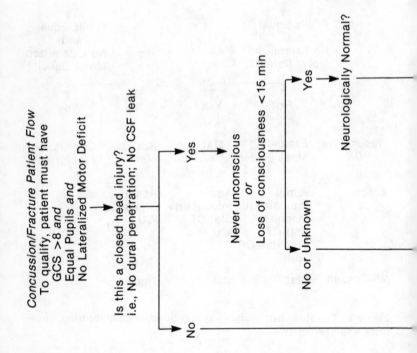

Concussion/Fracture Patient Flow
To qualify, patient must have
GCS >8 *and*
Equal Pupils *and*
No Lateralized Motor Deficit

Is this a closed head injury?
i.e., No dural penetration; No CSF leak

No

Yes

Never unconscious
or
Loss of consciousness <15 min

No or Unknown

Yes

Neurologically Normal?

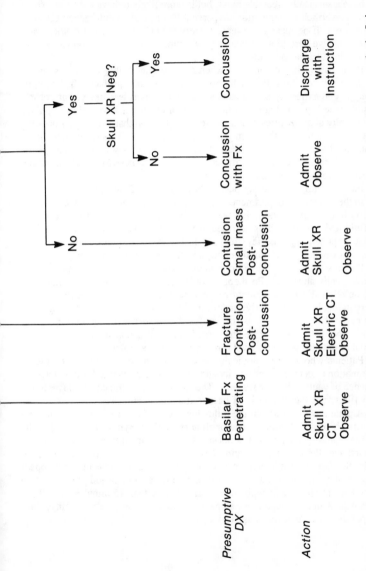

Figure 2 This flow chart outlines a systematic approach to the patients with a concussion or fracture, or both. It is a continuation of the flow chart in Figure 1.

still have a surgically treatable mass, but is more likely to have a diffuse axonal injury. Nevertheless, intubation, hyperventilation, and an emergency CT scan are required. If no mass is present, surgery is not indicated, but medical care in the intensive care unit is necessary to optimize cerebral metabolism and to monitor intracranial pressure.

If the patient is not comatose when first examined (that is, has a score of 9 or more), he or she still may harbor a serious cranial problem. If the pupils are equal and extremity movements are similar, this is less likely, but not impossible (see Fig. 2). Patients who are not in coma but have either pupillary or extremity abnormalities usually have a focal lesion that is not (yet) of sufficient size to compress the brain stem and cause coma. All such patients must be admitted and undergo CT scans. Elective surgery may be necessary if the CT scan demonstrates a mass that is questionable; otherwise, medication and expectant close observation are the rule.

Patients who seem less seriously injured (see Fig. 2) must be evaluated further in the emergency department. Wounds must be carefully inspected for dural penetration, for indriven foreign bodies of bone fragments, and for cerebrospinal fluid leakage, as well as otorrhea or rhinorrhea. These injuries, as well as obviously penetrating injuries (such as gunshot wounds), require admission, diagnostic evaluation, and possible surgical repair of the open injury.

Patients who do not have open injuries and are not in coma may still be neurologically abnormal. Postconcussion confusion may persist for some time and, on clinical grounds, cannot reliably be distinguished from early signs of an expanding lesion. Similarly, under no circumstance should an intoxicated patient be discharged when he is still confused or disoriented "because he's still drunk." No patient should be discharged until his mental status is completely normal or until his preinjury level is reached if prior neurologic disability existed.

Patients who are neurologically normal must have a complete neurologic examination to determine normality and can then be discharged if they have no evidence of vault or basilar fracture. The former is determined by conventional skull films, but the diagnosis of basilar fracture is clinical.

A patient who has any of the following is considered to have a basilar fracture: cerebrospinal fluid otorrhea or rhinorrhea; hemotympanum; blood in the external auditory meatus that is not due to direct ear injury; subconjunctival hemorrhage, the posterior margin of which cannot be seen; raccoon eyes; or the Battle sign. It must be appreciated that the latter three signs may not appear for several hours following injury. Admission for a short period of observation is prudent for all patients with coma lasting longer than 15 minutes, for all patients with skull fracture, and for all patients with a neurologic abnormality, since the possibility of delayed mass lesions exists.

THE HEAD

HENRY M. BARTKOWSKI, M.D., Ph.D.
LAWRENCE H. PITTS, M.D.

Head injuries account for approximately half of trauma fatalities and result in more than five million days of hospitalization and 30 million days of work lost annually in the United States. The yearly incidence of significant head injury is projected to be about 200 cases per 100,000 population for all regions of the United States. Although prevention of head injury ultimately will reduce morbidity and mortality most effectively, we currently must direct our attention toward aggressive management of craniocerebral trauma after impact. Primary mechanical brain damage that occurs at the moment of injury cannot be repaired by therapeutic intervention; thus, current management of head injury is an attempt to prevent secondary insults to the traumatized brain.

During initial treatment of head injury, restoration of normal cardiopulmonary function is of paramount importance. Resuscitation must be accomplished promptly in the emergency room. Unconscious patients should be intubated immediately for airway protection as aspiration can cause sudden pulmonary compromise leading to hypoxia and hypercapnia that cause additional insult to the brain. Even without evidence of aspiration, between 30 and 50 percent of patients with traumatic coma are hypoxic when first treated, and endotracheal intubation allows mechanical ventilation with increased arterial Po_2 and increased Pco_2. Head injury alone does not produce shock except in the terminal phases of brain death when medullary failure leads to cessation of respiration and to agonal hypotension. The significance of shock cannot be overemphasized. Patients presenting with severe head injury and hypotension suffer a 90 percent mortality while patients with a similar degree of head injury who are not in shock have a 50 percent mortality. Hypotension must be assumed to be due to hypovolemia and its cause sought from bleeding into the chest, abdomen, or extremities.

In order to reverse possible hypoglycemia or narcotic overdose, which may contribute to neurologic depression, we routinely administer 50 cc of 50 percent dextrose and 0.8 mg of naloxone to comatose patients after obtaining blood and urine specimens for routine and toxicologic studies.

PHYSICAL EXAMINATION

The initial physical examination must include sufficient observations to determine an accurate baseline evaluation, recorded in a manner that will allow clinical changes to be readily appreciated by subsequent examiners. Vital signs are, of course, essential. Abnormalities of pulse and blood pressure may reflect a primary cardiac event as the etiology of the patient's disorder. On the other hand, it is well established that hypertension with bradycardia, the Cushing reflex, is a sign of increased intracranial pressure and signifies an intracranial mass lesion until proved otherwise. Associated injuries must be identified and therapy instituted because such injuries may lead to airway compromise, blood gas abnormalities, or shock, all of which will compound neurologic damage (Table 1). A cervical spine injury should be assumed to exist, and the head and neck kept in a neutral position until a lateral cervical spine film excludes spinal instability.

The scalp must be inspected carefully for lacerations or puncture wounds. Small puncture wounds may be the only outward sign of penetrating injuries. They may occur anywhere on the scalp and commonly may be missed by the examiner if located in the dependent occipital area. Depressed fractures may or may not be identified by digital palpation of the scalp or exploration of a laceration. As in the case of puncture wounds, depressed fractures may involve any portion of the calvarium. In the case of an open brain injury, no further inspection is warranted; these wounds must be debrided and closed in the operating room.

Basilar skull fractures are diagnosed on the basis of physical findings. Circumscribed unilateral or bilateral periorbital ecchymoses (raccoon eyes) are indications of intraorbital bleeding from fractures of the floor of the frontal fossa. Blood in the external canal indicates a basilar fracture through the lateral portion of the temporal bone. A temporal bone fracture medial to the tympanic membrane results in a hemotympanum. Ecchymosis overlying the mastoid (Battle's sign) represents blood dissecting to the skin from a mastoid fracture; it usually is delayed for 12 to 24 hours after initial injury. Leakage of cerebrospinal fluid via the nose (rhinorrhea) or the ear (otorrhea) is a manifestation of meningeal disruption at the site of a basilar fracture and carries the risk of meningitis. Damage to the seventh or eighth cranial nerves may accompany temporal bone fractures. Facial palsy of immediate onset represents direct facial nerve injury at the site of temporal bone fracture and requires early diagnostic evaluation and possible early surgical repair. Delayed onset facial palsies usually resolve spontaneously without surgical intervention. Tearing and stretching injuries to the auditory and vestibular nerves severely disrupt hearing and balance and are irreparable by any currently available surgical or medical treatment.

TABLE 1 Multisystem Injuries Associated with Major Head Injury

Head injury and facial injury	14%
Head injury and chest injury	16%
Head injury and extremity injury	20%
Head injury and abdominal injury	21%
Head injury and at least one other injury	39%

EMERGENCY NEUROLOGIC EXAMINATION

The initial neurologic examination must be rapid and complete; immediate therapeutic and diagnostic actions hinge on the findings. The examination must determine the level of consciousness, brain stem or spinal cord dysfunction, and the presence of peripheral nerve injury. Level of consciousness has been described poorly by a variety of imprecise words such as lethargy, stupor, or obtundation, words that vaguely describe changes in neurologic function in different patients or in the same patient at different times. An alternative to these terms has been the Glasgow Coma Scale (Table 2). This system records the patient's response to verbal and painful stimuli and has been widely adopted at trauma centers. It is a valuable tool for following a patient's improvement or deterioration, is highly reliable, and is accompanied by remarkably little variation among examiners.

The integrity of midbrain, pontine, and medullary function is determined by cranial nerve examination. The pupillary light reflex allows evaluation of the optic and oculomotor nerves. A pupil that is dilated and unresponsive after injury indicates ipsilateral transtentorial herniation from an expanding mass lesion. The oculocephalic reflex (doll's eyes maneuver) consists of conjugate eye deviation contralateral to the direction of head rotation. The reflex evaluates connections between the vestibular aparatus, pontine gaze centers, and sixth and third nerve nuclei in the pons and midbrain. The head should be turned to elicit the response *only* if a cervical fracture has been excluded by appropriate cervical spine x-ray studies. In the event of a cervical fracture, the pontine gaze center and its connection to the third and sixth cranial nerves can be evaluated by the oculovestibular reflex (caloric testing). The expected response to cold water irrigation of the auditory canal in a comatose patient is conjugate deviation of the eyes toward the irrigated ear. Supraorbital pressure can be used to elicit a facial grimace to test seventh nerve function in a comatose patient. Cough and gag reflex can be used to evaluate lower cranial nerve and medullary function.

TABLE 2   Glasgow Coma Scale

Class	Eye Opening	Best Motor Response	Best Verbal Response
4	Spontaneously	6 Follows commands	5 Oriented
3	To voice	5 Localize painful stimulus	4 Confused
2	To pain	4 Complex arm movement	3 Inappropriate words
1	None	3 Reflex flexor posturing	2 Incomprehensible sounds
		3 Reflex extensor posturing	1 None
		1 Flaccid	

DIAGNOSTIC PROCEDURES

In the emergency room, when a comatose patient is being initially evaluated, a chest film and a lateral cervical spine film should be obtained immediately to rule out pneumothorax, hemothorax, or other pulmonary lesions that may lead to hypoxia or hypercapnia and to rule out a cervical spine fracture, respectively. Skull films should be obtained for any penetrating injury or if a depressed fracture is suspected on physical examination. Computerized tomographic (CT) scanning has largely replaced skull roentgenography, arteriography, and ventriculography in the diagnosis of skull fracture and traumatic intracranial lesions. Radioisotope scanning has no role in the early phases of head trauma.

CLASSIFICATION

Head injured patients can be placed into four groups, depending on the severity of injury.

Brain Stem Dysfunction

Patients with signs of brain stem dysfunction require immediate aggressive investigation and treatment. Transtentorial herniation is accompanied by the triad of ipsilateral sluggish pupillary constriction to light, depressed consciousness, and contralateral or ipsilateral hemiparesis. This complex requires immediate treatment consisting of:

1. Emergency endotracheal intubation to optimize arterial oxygenation, allow hyperventilation, and protect the airway against obstruction from blood, vomitus, or pharyngeal soft tissue.
2. Maintenance of normal blood pressure by intravenous fluid resuscitation and placement of the patient in Trendelenburg position, since lowering of systemic pressure in the face of elevated intracranial pressure (ICP) can cause inadequate cerebral perfusion and cerebral ischemia.
3. Use of hyperosmotic agents such as mannitol (1.5 g per kilogram) infused rapidly intravenously.
4. Immediate transport to the operating room for placement of an emergency temporal burr hole on the side of the dilated pupil. If an extracerebral hematoma is found, a craniotomy is performed to evacuate the clot. If a hematoma is not found by burr hole exploration, the patient is taken for an immediate CT scan (if available, otherwise cerebral angiography) to diagnose intraparenchymal lesions including hemorrhage and focal edema. It is essential to relieve brain stem compression as quickly as possible to prevent irreversible ischemic damage.

5. Based on a clinical trial in our institution, corticosteroids are ineffective in improving outcome from severe head injury. The efficacy of barbiturates in improving outcome has not been adequately established, and their use is accompanied by substantial cardiovascular side effects; thus they cannot be recommended for widespread use until appropriate trials are completed.

Focal Neurologic Deficit

Patients with focal neurologic deficits (e.g., hemiparesis, dysphasia) in the absence of brain stem compression (e.g., pupillary dilatation, abnormal eye movements) should be evaluated by CT scanning if available, or by cerebral angiography. If the patient has a decreasing level of consciousness while the study is being performed, mannitol should be given (1.5 g per kilogram infused rapidly intravenously), followed by surgery if indicated by the diagnostic study. If CT scanning reveals a mass lesion, immediate decompression is performed via craniotomy. Speed is the most important factor in treating a mass lesion; the sooner the brain is decompressed the better the outcome.

Depressed Consciousness: No Focal Deficit

In patients with a depressed level of consciousness, but no focal deficit, careful serial observation may be employed to determine whether the patient will improve neurologically without specific intervention. If the patient fails to display neurologic improvement within a few hours or shows any deterioration, a CT scan or cerebral angiogram should be performed. If a mass lesion, infarct, or edema is not found, a thorough metabolic work-up should be done to determine the cause of altered consciousness.

No Apparent Neurologic Deficit

Patients who are neurologically intact following head injury are unlikely to develop delayed complications. Even patients with classic "lucid intervals" before deterioration usually have significant headache or some degree of lethary when seen after injury. Short periods of retrograde or antegrade amnesia are of no prognostic importance; however, prolonged amnesia manifest by continuing confusion and inability to answer simple questions is a significant neurologic deficit and requires close observation. Nausea and vomiting are common after head injury in children and generally of no prognostic value. However, severe vomiting may necessitate hospitalization for treatment of dehydration. The child is intravenously hydrated at two-thirds maintenance intake so as to avoid over-hydration and worsening of any brain edema that may be present.

Patients who have skull fractures and in whom there was a loss of consciousness for greater than several minutes should be hospitalized for close observation for a 24-hour period, since the patient initially may be lucid but then deteriorate as with an epidural hematoma. If the circumstances surrounding the head injury are unclear, and problems such as seizures or syncopal episodes may have precipitated the injury, admission should be considered to evaluate these possibilities. If the patient can be observed by reliable and intelligent family members or friends, he or she may be observed at home with careful instructions given for recognition of signs of possible deterioration and for obtaining additional medical consultation or care if necessary.

Compound depressed fractures require immediate operation to prevent development of intracranial infection. These fractures are debrided and the bone fragments are washed in an antibiotic solution (such as bacitracin, 50,000 units in 500 ml of normal saline) and reserved for immediate replacement. Dural and brain lacerations are debrided and the dura repaired either primarily or by the use of pericranial or fascia lata grafts. Large dural lacerations overlying basilar fractures may be repaired by onlay grafts of temporalis fascia, fascia lata, or pericranium.

Intracranial pressure is monitored in all postoperative and comatose nonoperative patients via a catheter placed into the lateral ventricle, if possible, or into the subdural space. Alternatively, a threaded bolt can be placed through a small drill hole in the skull, under which the dura has been opened. An intraventricular catheter gives the most accurate readings and can be used as a therapeutic measure by the withdrawal of intraventricular fluid to reduce intracranial pressure.

The catheter system is filled with an antibiotic solution such as tobramycin or gentamicin, 10 mg in 20 ml of normal saline. This same solution is used to fill the transducer. Epidural fiberoptic intracranial pressure monitors are being used more widely and offer a satisfactory alternative to the fluid-filled systems. They do not permit withdrawal of cerebrospinal fluid for control of intracranial pressure, which is possible with intraventricular catheters. Intracranial pressures up to 20 mm Hg are considered to be within normal limits; above that level the pressure is considered to be abnormal and appropriate treatment is indicated to reduce the pressure.

POSTOPERATIVE CARE

Supportive care following the initial resuscitation and/or surgical intervention is a critical phase in the management of head injury that is optimally provided in an intensive care unit. The skills of the anesthesiologists and medical and surgical subspecialists can be added to those of intensive care nurses and respiratory therapists to keep the patient as stable as possible during the post-traumatic period.

When it occurs, intracranial hypertension is most pronounced in the first 2 to 3 days after trauma. Exceptions to this rule include such patients as those with diffuse cerebral swelling, in whom the ICP may remain elevated for 10 to 14 days. Patients with ICP above 20 torr show a significantly higher morbidity and mortality than those whose ICP can be controlled below this level. Death almost uniformly results with uncontrolled intracranial hypertension above 40 torr. It is imperative to obtain adequate control of intracranial hypertension by using a combination of the following:

1. *Surgical decompression.* Removal of even relatively small quantities of hematoma or necrotic brain may markedly lower ICP and prevent herniation.
2. *Head elevation.* Enhances venous drainage and lowers venous pressure.
3. *Ventricular fluid drainage.* Can immediately lower ICP. In the case of diffuse cerebral swelling it is of limited value because little cerebrospinal fluid (CSF) is available for removal.
4. *Hyperventilation (PCO_2 25 to 30 torr).* Cerebral vessels constrict in response to hypocapnia. It is best used for short periods, being allowed to return to mildly hypocarbic levels (PCO_2 30 to 35 torr) as other methods of controlling intracranial hypertension are employed.
5. *Hyperosmotic therapy.* Mannitol may be administered in doses of 0.5 g per kilogram every 3 hours. Its use is best guided by actual ICP monitoring. Mannitol should not be used when serum osmolality exceeds 330 milliosmoles since serum osmolality above this level can cause cerebral dysfunction.
6. *Diuretics.* Furosemide (Lasix) may decrease elevated ICP both by dehydration secondary to diuresis and by inhibiting production of CSF by the choroid plexus. Diuretics may be used alone or in conjunction with hyperosmotic therapy. A common dose is 0.3 mg per kilogram every 4 to 6 hours.
7. *Maintain normothermia or moderate hypothermia (35° to 37°C).* Lowers cerebral metabolism and may reduce elevated ICP. Attempts to lower body temperature may be accompanied by generalized shivering, and this increased muscular activity can elevate ICP by thoracic contraction and elevation of central venous pressures.
8. *Barbiturate coma.* Its efficacy in head injury has not been clearly established and requires further evaluation.

Anticonvulsants are routinely used in patients with coma-producing head injuries. The presence of intracranial hematomas, depressed fractures, or post-traumatic amnesia lasting longer than 24 hours increases the likelihood of early seizures. Relatively few seizures occur after the first year following injury, and these late seizures are not diminished in frequency by the early use of anticonvulsant therapy. Diphenylhydantoin or phenobarbital should be used during the first 12 months after head injury and then are gradually discontinued over several months if the patient has remained seizure-free. We recommend 300 mg of Dilantin daily or 30 to 45 mg of phenobarbital three times a day as maintenance dosage. Anticonvulsant therapy can be restarted in the small population of patients who develop late seizures.

Late sequelae of head injury include the postconcussion syndrome and cerebrospinal fluid leaks. The former, which consists of headache, dizziness, and memory deficits, has no specific therapy, but usually resolves within weeks to months. Late CSF leaks may occur following basilar skull fracture. These usually do not subside spontaneously or with conservative treatment and generally require surgical repair.

SPINE AND SPINAL CORD

FRANKLIN C. WAGNER Jr., M.D.

Injuries to the spine and the spinal cord can be deceptive; they may not always be clinically apparent when masked by other injuries. Furthermore, even though the spine, spinal cord, and nerve roots are anatomically closely related, the spinal cord may escape damage when the spine and the surrounding soft tissues are injured. Nonetheless, the potential for a spinal cord injury in such a case does exist.

For these reasons, the index of suspicion for spine and spinal cord injury should be especially high when the patient is unconscious as a result of a head injury, when the patient has been injured above the clavicle, and when the patient has been injured in a high-speed motor vehicle accident. The spine in these patients should be immobilized and any unnecessary movement or manipulation avoided until spinal injury can be excluded.

SPINAL INJURIES

One or a combination of mechanisms may produce a spinal injury. These mechanisms include axial loading, distraction, extension, flexion, and rotation. Understanding a spinal fracture in terms of these mechanisms lessens the likelihood of enhancing them and, thereby, the possibility of increasing the damage when treating the fracture.

Axial loading at the level of the first cervical vertebral (C1) may result in a blowout of the ring, the so-called Jefferson fracture. This fracture is unstable, and in one-third of cases, it is associated with a fracture of the second cervical vertebra (C2).

Three types of fractures that may involve the odontoid process (dens) of C2 are as follows: type I, which occurs above the base of the odontoid and is most often stable; type II which occurs at the base of the odontoid and usually is unstable; and type III, which involves the body of C2 and may be stable.

Extension and distraction or extension and axial compression may damage the posterior elements of C2. This results in the unstable "hangman's fracture."

The cervical spine, between and including C3 and C7, is mobile compared to the thoracic spine, which is fixed by the rib cage. Therefore, the C3 through C7 vertebrae may be injured by excessive flexion, extension, axial loading, and rotation.

Fractures involving the thoracic spine, especially from T2 through T10, are most likely caused by hyperflexion. The resulting wedge compression of one or more vertebrae is usually stabilized by the relative rigidity of the rib cage.

Internal stabilization may be required to prevent further deformity should the angulation exceed 30 degrees.

Thoracolumbar fractures result most often from a combination of hyperflexion and rotation. Because of the number of vertebral elements damaged, fractures at this level of the spine are extremely unstable. Lumbar spine fractures usually result from hyperflexion. If the disruption of the posterior elements is severe, internal stabilization is required.

SPINAL CORD INJURIES

Numerous methods of classifying patients with spinal cord injuries have been utilized. These methods have included classifications based on the amount of retained function and classifications in which patients have been grouped into different syndromes according to their neurologic findings. The most important prognostic consideration is whether the patient has a complete or an incomplete lesion.

The patient with an incomplete lesion is more likely to regain a significant percentage of his lost neurologic function than is the patient with a complete lesion. On examination, the patient with an incomplete lesion is found to have some preserved sensory and/or motor function below the level of his injury; the patient with a complete lesion has none.

The "level" of the spinal cord injury is the most distal segment of the spinal cord with fully intact sensation and movement. This method of determining the level of injury has been adopted because retained but impaired sensation and movement for at least three levels below this point may indicate damage to the nerve roots rather than the spinal cord.

Functional Assessment

Certain anatomic features of the spinal cord influence the examination of the patient with spinal cord injury. The cervical spinal cord segments, C5 through T1, are represented in the upper extremities, but have little or no representation on the trunk. Therefore, if the arms are not examined and superficial pain is tested by pinpricks on the trunk where the C4 dermatome is immediately cephalad to the T2 dermatome, the examiner may form an incorrect impression of the patient's sensory level. The nerve fibers that convey the sensation of touch are most widely distributed in the white matter of the spinal cord. Consequently, if the examiner does not ask the patient to distinguish between sharp and dull sensation when testing with a pin, the preservation of touch may be mistaken for the presence of superficial pain. The fibers subserving superficial pain in the sacral area are located in the periphery of the cervical spinal cord and may escape injury when the more central portion of the cord is damaged. The presence of sacral sparing, however, may indicate that the sensorimotor paralysis is not complete.

After birth, the spine grows more rapidly than the spinal cord so that the cord appears to ascend within the spinal canal. Consequently, the spinal cord terminates in the majority of adults at the lower (lumbar) end of the vertebral body of L1. The sacral segments of the spinal cord, S1 through S5, which compose the conus medullaris, are located approximately at the level of the L1 vertebra, while the spinal cord segments L1 through L5 correspond with T10 through T12. The nerve roots emerge from the spinal cord at the appropriate segments and make up the cauda equina as they travel caudally in the spinal canal before leaving the canal beneath the pedicles of the corresponding vertebrae, i.e., the L5 nerve beneath the pedicle of the L5 vertebra. An injury, therefore, at the thoracolumbar junction may damage both the spinal cord and the cauda equina, and the level of the spinal cord injury may not correspond to the level of the spinal fracture-dislocation.

Assessment of Spinal Films. A systematic method of reviewing spinal films lessens the likelihood of overlooking abnormalities. In the cervical spine, all seven cervical vertebrae must be visualized. Since the seventh cervical vertebra is frequently obscured on the lateral view by the shadow of the shoulder, it may be necessary to pull the patient's arms down and thereby depress the shoulders or, alternatively, obtain a swimmer's view.

Spinal Alignment. Once adequate x-ray studies have been obtained, the alignment of the spine may be assessed. In all regions this may be done by determining the smoothness of the two curves formed by the anterior and posterior aspects of the vertebral bodies. Two additional curves are visualized in the cervical spine on the lateral view. These are formed by joining the points where the laminae fuse with the bases of the spinous processes, thereby delimiting the posterior aspect of the spinal canal, and by connecting the tips of the spinous processes.

Certain measurements may indicate malalignment of the vertebrae and possible spinal cord compression. A displacement of one vertebral body on another exceeding 3 mm suggests a dislocation. An angulation between adjacent vertebral bodies of more than 11 degrees indicates malalignment. A reduction of the anteroposterior diameter of the cervical spinal canal, formed anteriorly by the posterior aspect of the vertebral bodies and posteriorly by the junction of the laminae and spinous processes, to 13 mm or less may indicate spinal cord compression.

Spinal Vertebrae. Following the assessment of spinal alignment, the integrity of the bones may be inspected. The contour, height, and presence of lucencies in the bodies, pedicles, facets, laminae, transverse processes, and spinous processes should be noted.

A reduction in the anterior height of the vertebral body of more than 3 mm, compared to the posterior height, suggests a compression fracture. An oblique lucency through the vertebral body may mean a tear-drop fracture, and the lack of parallel facets may indicate a lateral compression fracture. An avulsion fracture produces a lucency through the spinous process. A distance greater than 3 mm between the posterior aspect of C1 and the anterior odontoid process is consistent with a dislocation, whereas a lucency through the odontoid process of C2 indicates a fracture.

Soft Tissue Spaces. Changes in the soft tissue spaces surrounding the spine point to a spinal injury. Hemorrhage accompanying such an injury commonly results in a widening of the prevertebral space of more than 5 mm. A fracture may obliterate the prevertebral fat strip at the same level. A torn interspinous ligament is likely to widen the space between spinous processes and be associated with an anterior spinal fracture.

PREHOSPITAL AND EMERGENCY ROOM EVALUATION

The prehospital emergency medical system should have trained personnel who are familiar with spinal injuries and can safely and expeditiously evacuate patients with known or suspected spinal injuries to hospitals with neurotrauma care capabilities. During the rapid transport of such patients, the cervical spine should be immobilized with a semirigid collar, and the remainder of the spine should be supported on a long spine board. If necessary, the airway should be maintained with either a nasal or an oral airway.

When the patient arrives in the emergency room, immobilization should be maintained until a portable lateral film of the suspected spinal injury is obtained. The results determine whether further immobilization is required. Although not essential at this point, a full series of spinal films, including anteroposterior and lateral projections and an open mouth view of the odontoid process of C2, should be obtained before definitive treatment is undertaken, since unsuspected fractures at different levels are not uncommon.

Once a spinal fracture or fracture-dislocation has been identified, it is appropriate to obtain a computerized tomographic (CT) scan of the involved area. The axial views, along with the sagittal reconstructions, provided by this scan give additional information about the type of fracture-dislocation and the degree to which the spinal canal may be comprised.

Initial Management

When fracture-dislocation of the cervical spine is confirmed, the fracture should be further immobilized, and closed reduction of the dislocation should be undertaken by means of skeletal traction. As progressively greater weights are added, it is imperative to check the patient frequently, both neurologically and radiologically, in order to prevent the hazard of distraction and further injury to the spinal cord.

The amount of time allotted to achieving a closed reduction is determined by the patient's neurologic status. If weights have been incrementally applied to a maximum of 50 to 70 pounds over a 1- to 2-hour period without effect, it is unlikely that additional weights or time will accomplish a reduction. In the patient with an incomplete lesion, an open reduction is then considered. When the patient has a complete lesion, more time is devoted to accomplishing a closed reduction and achieving adequate alignment so that proper bone and soft tissue healing occurs.

Although positioning and manipulation may accomplish a closed reduction of a fracture-dislocation of the thoracic or lumbar spine, the necessary forces are less easily controlled than in reduction of the cervical spine. For this reason, an open reduction may be contemplated sooner with a fracture-dislocation involving the thoracic or lumbar spine, especially in the patient with an incomplete lesion.

In patients with incomplete lesions in whom closed reduction has been accomplished with no neurologic improvement, additional diagnostic imaging may be considered. Metrizamide myelography, followed by computerized tomography, may demonstrate post-traumatic swelling or compression of the spinal cord such as is produced by an acutely herniated disc.

Surgery

When there is persistent compression by bone after a closed reduction has been attempted or by soft tissue as shown by myelography even though a closed reduction has been achieved, the surgical approach to the spinal canal may be anterior, anterolateral, posterolateral, or posterior. Which approach is employed should be determined by the location of the displaced bone or soft tissue, the extent of the compression, and how the damaged spine may be effectively stabilized should that be required.

PERIPHERAL NERVE

LAWRENCE H. PITTS, M.D.

Peripheral nerve trauma is a relatively uncommon, but very important, cause of significant posttraumatic disability. To enhance the patient's functional recovery, careful evaluation and a thoughtful treatment plan must be initiated soon after injury.

Nerve injuries are most readily characterized as sharp or blunt although there are situations, such as gunshot wounds or injuries adjacent to bony fractures, in which the two types of lesions are combined. Because the therapy is so different, it is important to consider the implications of these two distinct types of nerve trauma.

Sharp lacerations of peripheral nerves, such as those inflicted by knives or glass, sharply divide the nerve with relatively little damage to nerve or its blood supply other than immediately at the site of laceration. These injuries often are accompanied by significant injury to nearby arteries whose lacerations may represent a true surgical emergency, depending on the vessel size. These wounds usually are promptly explored and the vessels repaired, with care to avoid further injury to surrounding nerves. If possible, local hematomas should be evacuated to prevent pressure injury to nerves. Proper exposure of the injured nerves often require somewhat larger exposure than that required for vessel repair. If the cleanly cut nerve ends can be identified, they can be reapproximated in the operating room. The operating microscope is used to identify and realign matching fascicles or small epineural vessels on the nerve surface for optimal repair. The nerve ends are anastomosed, using fine monofilament sutures to approximate the epineurium. Sharp lacerations of the nerve are relatively less common than blunt injuries.

Blunt injuries to peripheral nerve or brachial or sacral plexus can arise from direct blows, fractures, nerve stretch, compression neuropathies, and gunshot wounds among other causes. The force of the injury is dissipated over a segment of nerve, the extent of which is ill defined in the acute phase. Because the extent of injury generally cannot be appreciated even by direct inspection of the nerve, these injuries are treated expectantly, repair being delayed for weeks or months (to be discussed).

The appropriateness of waiting for spontaneous recovery of peripheral nerve function is based on an understanding of the degree of neural injury and its anatomic basis (Table 1).

From the anatomic definition of degree of injury, expected times of recovery can be determined. Primary injuries, i.e., blockage of electrical conduction only, should recover completely within 3 to 4 weeks. Secondary injuries require axonal regeneration from the site of injury to the target sensory organ or muscle, the amount of regeneration required being approximately 1 mm per day or

TABLE 1 Anatomic Basis of Degree of Neural Injury

Degree of Injury	Anatomic Basis
First degree	Conduction block, no anatomic disruption
Second degree	Axonal loss, intact neurilemmal sheath
Third degree	Loss of axon and myelin sheath
Fourth degree	Fascicular disruption with epineurial loss
Fifth degree	Nerve disruption with perineurial loss

1 inch per month; thus the time from injury to recovery can be estimated. Since the neurilemmal sheaths are intact in secondary injuries, myelinated axons will regenerate and travel to their appropriate organ, giving complete recovery if the end-organ has not atrophied during the time of regeneration.

Considerable recovery of third-degree injuries can be anticipated although, with loss of myelin sheaths, some aberrant regeneration occurs along with some degree of local scarring at the injury site and less than total recovery. Recovery is much less complete in fourth-degree injuries with loss of fascicles and considerably greater neuroma formation at the injury site. There is no regeneration in fifth degree injuries without surgical repair and subsequent nerve regeneration. Generally, there is a mixture of injury degrees in nerves that have not been transected.

It is clear then that initial clinical evaluation of a peripheral nerve injury may not allow accurate prediction of outcome. If the wound is such that complete nerve transection is certain, attempted operative repair is the only course available for re-establishing future nerve function. In cases of lesser injury, however, one cannot make an accurate prognosis within 4 to 6 weeks of injury. Therefore, with blunt injuries, nerve repairs are not appropriate soon after injury, and must be delayed until it becomes possible to assess early spontaneous recovery. If the nerve is known to be completely transected, earlier repair is indicated (to be discussed).

EMERGENCY CARE OF PERIPHERAL NERVE INJURIES

Many peripheral nerves, particularly those in the brachial plexus and upper arm, are associated with major vascular structures whose care takes precedence over nerve repair. External hemorrhage must be controlled promptly and its source recognized and corrected. This often requires temporary hemostasis with definitive exploration for vascular injury done promptly in the operating room. Fractures can occur concomitantly with nerve damage and may themselves be the source of neurotrauma, so that fracture realignment is important in the care of peripheral nerve injury. Since delayed wound infections around injured nerves severely jeopardize their recovery, it is imperative that early and careful wound debridement and cleaning be carried out in cases of penetrating wounds and peripheral nerve trauma. Such debridement may require exploration in the operating room for optimum results.

After hemostasis and initial wound dressing are accomplished, an examination of the extremity is necessary to delineate possible vascular interruption (cool, pulseless limbs), fractures, and specific neurologic deficits. The details of neurologic examination are beyond the scope of this chapter, but motor, sensory, and reflex function should be assessed carefully, with special attention to both radicular innervation and innervation by specific peripheral nerves. If there is *any* residual neural function in the affected nerve or nerve root, the lesion is incomplete with a vastly better recovery potential than when there is no demonstrable function on examination. Since dermatomes vary slightly from patient to patient, the examination must be done carefully to identify complete injuries when they are present. Detailed documentation of the examination is important since this provides a critical baseline against which to judge future improvement or deterioration.

If operative intervention is not indicated, careful follow-up is required by physicians with an interest in peripheral nerve dysfunction to document recovery or recommend therapy in the absence of recovery. For penetrating injuries, follow-up wound care is important to ensure freedom from, or prompt treatment of, infection should it occur. The emergency room physician should make certain that the patient has an appropriate plan for follow-up care.

EARLY OPERATIVE INTERVENTION

Hemostasis and restitution of extremity blood flow is the most important initial care of many penetrating wounds causing nerve injury. Adequate exposure must be obtained for vascular repair along with appropriate debridement of contaminated penetrating wounds. If the injury is caused by penetration with an extremely sharp object, and if neural transection is identified during wound exposure, and if the wound is unlikely to become infected, a primary repair of the nerve is appropriate. This requires an experienced microsurgeon and availability of appropriate instruments and operating microscope, so that a fine epineurial repair can be done soon after injury. Since such clean nerve lacerations are distinctly uncommon, and since most nerve injuries have a blunt component, primary repair is unusual after peripheral nerve injury. If the nerve has been bluntly transected, it is impossible to determine soon after injury how far proximal and distal to the injury site there will be nerve death and subsequent scarring. If inadequate neural debridement is effected and damaged nerve ends joined, a significant neuroma will form with unacceptable anastomotic results. A more appropriate course is to identify the transected neural elements and, by means of a nonabsorbable wire or nylon suture, to suture them to surrounding tissue so that the ends remain adjacent. Such partial approximation of the nerve ends minimizes nerve retraction and gap width so that subsequent neural repair may be possible with an end-to-end anastomosis rather than cable grafting.

After initial wound management, early postoperative care must ensure adequate limb perfusion and recognition and treatment of compartment syndromes to prevent subsequent nerve ischemia and injury. It is important to recognize and treat wound infections, which can further injure the damaged nerve and cause a poor recovery after treatment of the nerve injury.

Most peripheral nerve injuries result from nonpenetrating blunt injuries, or the penetrating injury has a blunt component precluding early definitive repair. Many such nerve injuries are in continuity, and the degree of recovery cannot be ascertained for one or more months following surgery. Commonly, blunt nerve injuries are followed expectantly for 3 to 4 months, both to assess the possibility of spontaneous recovery of first-degree injuries and to allow the beginning of nerve regeneration in second- and third-degree injuries. If improvement cannot be demonstrated within 3 to 4 months of injury, the patient should be evaluated by a surgeon with special expertise in peripheral nerve injury repair. Late operative exploration may be necessary to optimize the eventual outcome after nerve trauma. The documentation on sequential examinations of the peripheral migration of a Tinel's sign (local nerve tenderness to percussion) would indicate that some spontaneous recovery is occurring and might warrant further expectant therapy in anticipation of spontaneous improvement in neurologic function. The absence of a distally moving Tinel's sign increases the likelihood that operative exploration and repair would be superior to further expectant therapy.

Since most neural injuries are in continuity, it is not possible to determine the degree of nerve injury by visual inspection. Intraoperative electrophysiologic monitoring, including peripheral nerve stimulation and action potential recording, must be available intraoperatively to determine whether there is electrical continuity across the injury site. If there clearly is conduction across the injury site, further expectant therapy may be indicated. If there is no conduction across the injury site, nerve transection and anastomosis should be done. If the length of injured nerve and gap width are too great, cable graft repair using sural nerve is appropriate. Some nerve mobilization can be accomplished by joint flexion and soft tissue dissection along the nerve. However, the surgeon must exercise extreme care not to devascularize the nerve or perform an end-to-end anastomosis under tension since such repairs usually result in neuroma formation and ineffective nerve regeneration across the repair site. If adequate nerve mobilization cannot be achieved to allow a repair without tension, one or more segments of sural or other sensory nerve can be used to bridge the injury gap. Whenever possible, an attempt should be made to rejoin fascicles above and below the injury site; it is frequently difficult to determine proper matching of the fascicles if the gap is wide. For optimal repair, a skilled, experienced surgeon must have available appropriate microsurgical instruments and the operating microscope in addition to electrophysiologic monitoring equipment. If these resources are unavailable, the patient should be referred to an appropriate facility where they are available.

POSTOPERATIVE CARE

Wound infections must be recognized and treated promptly. If specific extremity positioning, such as joint flexion, was necessary to achieve a tension-free end-to-end anastomosis, the extremity must be splinted in that position until soft tissue healing is strong enough to allow gradual extension of the affected joints, usually beginning 4 to 6 weeks after repair. Within 2 to 3 months of surgery, gentle, progressive active and passive range-of-motion exercises should be initiated under the guidance of a physical therapist to maximize joint mobility and tendon flexibility in the limb in anticipation of reinnervation of limb motor and sensory function. The patient requires periodic follow-up appointments with the operating surgeon to carefully guide this recovery phase.

OUTCOME AFTER PERIPHERAL NERVE SURGERY

Improvement after peripheral nerve repair is closely dependent on the patient's age. Children can have dramatic recovery of motor and sensory function after transection and repair, with and without cable grafting. Since regeneration after cable grafting requires neural growth across two suture lines, these repairs are less satisfactory than end-to-end anastomoses, although cable grafting is superior to repairs done under tension. In general, it is realistic to anticipate useful motor and sensory recovery across one joint, but useful regeneration of function across two joints is uncommon. Return of protective sensation can be an extremely valuable result after peripheral nerve surgery even if functional motor recovery does not occur, although substantial motor recovery certainly occurs in some cases.

MAXILLOFACIAL TRAUMA

MAXILLOFACIAL TRAUMA

ROBERT L. WALTON, M.D.
JURIS BUNKIS, M.D.
GREGORY L. BORAH, M.D., D.M.D.

Injuries of the maxillofacial region are common, particularly in urban areas, where victims of automobile collisions and physical assaults constitute a large proportion of the emergency room traffic. The severity of injury is not often reflected in initial appearances. Copious bleeding, early swelling, and associated neurologic disturbances frequently make accurate clinical assessment difficult, if not impossible. Early management, therefore, is often limited to control of life-threatening emergencies and other time-dependent problems such as compromised vision.

This chapter constitutes a summary of the techniques we have found useful in the management of acute injuries of the maxillofacial complex. Although this chapter focuses primarily on the management of facial fractures, we have included special sections addressing facial nerve, parotid, and laryngeal injuries.

GENERAL CONSIDERATIONS

The timing of therapy depends on numerous variables of which age, associated injuries, and antecedent medical problems play a pivotal role in the decision-making process. Obviously, each patient must be individualized. Our philosophy has been to effect wound closure and fracture reduction as early as possible. From a wound healing point of view, this approach makes good sense, yet the factors governing this act defy generalization. In the heat of the resuscitation/stabilization battle, there is little chance or sense in pursuing a precise, comprehensive therapeutic assault. For facial fractures, a "grace period" of about 10 days (except for mandibular fractures) allows time for an organized "team" assessment and operative plan. Massive soft tissue swelling is perhaps a relative contraindication to early operative reduction of facial fractures. If surgery is delayed, every effort to hasten the dissolution of swelling should be implemented. This includes debridement and simple closure of open wounds, elevation of the head, and immobilization of the fracture. The latter may require the simple implementation of a liquid diet (usually through a straw), a Barton bandage, or gross wire fixation of the dentition. Contamination of mandibular fractures through the oral cavity usually is not a major consideration unless operative reduction is delayed beyond 2 to 3 days or there is a significant amount of periodontal disease or dental caries. In these situations, we prefer to irrigate the oral cavity with a Cleocin solution, 300 mg per 100 cc water, every 6 hours. This method has significantly decreased the incidence of infections in our patients.

In patients with severe midfacial and/or mandibular trauma, presenting with acute upper airway obstruction, a cricothyroidotomy is preferred over direct oral or nasotracheal intubation because it is quick, carries minimal risk, and avoids unnecessary manipulation of the injured parts. Furthermore, it is difficult to perform a precise midfacial fracture reduction encumbered by the tether of a nasotracheal tube. In the same context, oral tracheal tubes are not employed in fractures of the mandible or maxilla. Moreover, both of the latter techniques are uncomfortable for the patient. The cricothyroidotomy is left in place until after the operative management of the facial fractures, when the patient has recovered sufficiently to maintain an adequate airway. The airway can be maintained safely via the cricothyroidotomy. Rarely is it necessary to convert a cricothyroidotomy to a tracheostomy if the injury has been confined to the maxillofacial region. A primary tracheostomy is performed in the operating room for those maxillofacial injuries associated with laryngeal or hypopharyngeal obstruction, intracranial injury, chest or high spinal cord injury, or anticipation of prolonged postoperative airway problems. If the airway is not acutely compromised, nasal or oral tracheal intubation is preferable prior to tracheostomy, provided this can be accomplished by direct visualization of the hypopharyngeal structures; otherwise a cricothyroidotomy is performed first.

A thorough physical examination is performed prior to any diagnostic studies. Evaluation of the cervical spine is a first-line priority which precedes any detailed facial study. Most facial fractures can be diagnosed easily with a minimum of x-ray studies. A stereo Water's roentgenogram is perhaps the single most informative view in the standard "facial series." Specialized views of the mandible (posterior-anterior, lateral oblique, or Panorex) are often necessary in evaluating fractures of the subcondylar regions or assessment of dentition in the fracture line. If available, the computerized tomogram (CT) is an extremely accurate tool in the radiologic examination of the facial skeleton. This method exposes the patient to less radiation than does standard tomography and allows visualization of areas that cannot easily be examined by conventional techniques. Over the past 2 years, we have exclusively employed the CT examination for all complex upper and midfacial fractures.

SOFT TISSUE INJURIES

The basic precepts of wound management will be dealt with in another chapter. Suffice it to state that the maxillofacial region constitutes a complex anatomy with specialized structures that serve innumerable important functions. For this reason, extensive debridement of the facial wound should be avoided. The rich vascular supply to this region allows salvage of tissues that otherwise might be discarded. In heavily contaminated wounds, minimal debridement and delayed closure are perhaps the most appropriate therapy. Specialized injuries of the face, such as those involving the facial nerve, the parotid gland and its duct, and the larynx, will be addressed.

Facial Nerve Injuries

Any wound that lies in the anatomic distribution of the facial nerve must be carefully assessed for injury to the nerve. In the conscious, cooperative patient, a thorough motor test is appropriate. Because of the extensive interneural communication of the buccal and zygomatic branches of the facial nerve, a simple laceration of one or several branches may not produce any significant loss of motor function. Nerve lacerations medial to the pupil are not repaired because it is at this level that the nerve arborizes extensively and enters the facial musculature. In the unconscious patient or the uncooperative patient, all wounds suspect for facial nerve injury are explored in the operating suite. If major life-threatening injuries are present, the facial wound is simply closed with skin tapes or monofilament suture and explored at a later date. Early exploration and repair is mandatory for an optimum result. In all cases, the operating microscope is employed utilizing magnifications of 16 to 25 power. A nerve stimulator is used to help identify the cut distal end of the nerve—this is only effective during the first 4 days following nerve injury owing to the loss of conductivity of the distal nerve end, which accompanies neuronal degeneration, another key consideration for early primary repair. To the inexperienced surgeon, locating the divided ends of the facial nerve is no easy task. Here, a keen familiarity with local anatomy is paramount to success.

First the wound is gently irrigated to remove all clots and debris. Next the superficial myoaponeurotic system (SMAS) is identified. This lies just below the superficial fat as a fine fibrous layer which is continuous with the platysma inferiorly and the superficial temporal fascia superiorly. Just beneath this layer lies the plane of the facial nerve. Utilizing ocular loupes ($2.5\times$ to $4.0\times$ magnification), the wound is then explored to identify the nerves. Not all nerves are of the motor type—many sensory nerves lie in this area as well. The nerve stimulator (set at 0.5 mv) will help to identify the motor branches. After a distal branch is identified, it is tagged with a 6–0 monofilament suture, and its corresponding proximal counterpart is located. In this fashion, the entire wound is explored. After all the nerves have been identified and tagged, the deeper layers of the wound are closed. Next, using the operative microscope and microsurgical technique, the cut nerve ends are coapted with two 10–0 sutures placed through the epineurium. If a clean division of the nerve is present, simple cleaning of the fibrous tissue 1 to 2 mm from the nerve end is all that is necessary. Irregular or jagged lacerations are prepared by sharp amputation with a broken razor blade. Care is taken to avoid any unnecessary manipulation of the cut nerve end. Extremely small branches or branches that lie together easily, without tension, are repaired with a single epineural suture. Lacerations involving the main trunk of the facial nerve are repaired with fine epineural suture after precise fascicular alignment of the proximal and distal ends.

If segments of the nerve (greater than 1 cm) are missing, primary nerve grafts are employed if the condition of the wound, as well as the patient, permit. The greater auricular nerve is an excellent source of autogenous tissue for grafting the facial nerve and its branches. Other cutaneous sensory nerves, such as the antebrachial cutaneous and sural nerves, are also employed, but are less desirable because of their size discrepancy and distant donor site location. If for some reason a primary neurorrhaphy or graft cannot be performed, the proximal and distal nerve ends are tagged with 6–0 monofilament suture. The suture is placed through the entire thickness of the nerve end and 5 mm long tails are left for later identification. Reexploration of these wounds has shown that, even with tagging, the nerve ends are extremely difficult to identify owing to their diminished size and local scarring.

After the nerve repair has been completed, the skin is closed in layers and reinforced with skin tapes. Skin tapes placed directly over the wound closure site help to splint the area of nerve repair and minimize vascular oozing and possible disruption of the repair. This splinting is maintained for 3 weeks.

Even in the best of circumstances, the amount of recovery from a total facial nerve laceration is less than 50 percent of the original function. Dyskinesis (mass action) is a frequent complication of facial nerve repair, particularly if the level of injury is at a major division or of the nerve trunk itself. Lacerations of the marginal mandibular branches are notorious for poor recovery.

Parotid Injuries

The majority of parotid injuries are characterized by a penetrating wound that lacerates the capsule and separates the parenchyma or parotid ducts. Because of the intimate association of the parotid gland and Stenson's duct with the buccal branch of the facial nerve, injury to one structure should be suspect for injury to the other.

Simple lacerations of the parotid capsule are managed by closure with an absorbable suture. Division of some of the minor collecting ducts from the parenchyma requires no specific therapeutic intervention except for the usual wound debridement and closure. Salivary leakage from these severed ducts is contained by the wound and usually ceases as the wound heals. Occasionally, a sialocele forms and is resolved by serial aspirations.

Transection of Stenson's duct requires surgical intervention; otherwise, a salivary fistula may result. The wound is explored and enlarged if additional exposure is needed. The distal duct is located by passing a Silastic catheter through its mucosal orifice. The injecting of methylene blue or other dye through this duct for purposes of localization is to be avoided because it is rarely necessary and the dye causes staining of the surrounding tissues, which further complicates the anatomy. The proximal duct end is more difficult to find. It is helpful to dry the wound with a sponge blotter and then gently compress the parotid parenchyma. The proximal duct is usually found at the site of salivary pooling. Once identified, the duct is cannulated in-continuity and the two segments are repaired. A single-layered repair is employed, avoiding the ductal mucosa. Direct repair of the epithelial mucosa of this duct is complicated by the formation of an obstructing intraluminal mass—the result of a retained nidus of suture material.

The Silastic cannula is secured to the buccal mucosa with a nonabsorbable suture and then removed after 7 to 10 days. It is not necessary to drain these wounds.

Injuries that result in loss of the anterior portion of the parotid duct and its orifice are managed by rerouting the proximal duct through the buccinator muscle and suturing the duct end to the edges of a buccal mucosal slit. The duct is kept cannulated for 10 to 14 days to allow maturation of the new orifice.

Complete loss of the extraparenchymal portion of Stenson's duct represents a major therapeutic challenge. In most cases, primary reconstruction is impractical and carries the risk of further soft tissue injury. In these cases, it is perhaps wise to accept a controlled parotid fistula. This is easily created by cannulating the remnant parenchymal portion of the duct and directing the salivary flow to the oral cavity. Delayed reconstruction is then performed weeks or months later.

Ligation of the parotid duct has been avocated as an alternative method of management, but carries a substantial risk for the production of a parotid fistula. If significant parenchymal and/or ductal injury precludes salvage or reconstruction, it is probably best to excise the entire gland. Radiation therapy will eliminate salivary secretion by destroying the glandular components of the parotid. This method, while effective, results in extensive soft tissue fibrosis, pigmentation of the skin, and unknown potential future sequelae. It should be reserved for those isolated cases that cannot easily be managed by surgical excision.

Blunt trauma to the parotid causes parenchymal injury, hematoma, or both. The parotid becomes massively swollen, tender, and susceptible to infection. In most cases, bleeding within the parotid capsule is diffuse and subsequently resorbed by the parenchyma. For these cases, supportive measures such as iced compresses, broad-spectrum antibiotic prophylaxis, analgesics, and a bland diet result in rapid resolution of the problem. Massive hematomas should be drained immediately. Needle aspiration is rarely effective and thus a direct incision and evacuation of the clot is preferred. These wounds are then drained to allow egress of the necrotic glandular debris. Salivary fistulas occasionally result from this procedure, but rarely are permanent unless the major ductal system has been injured.

Parotid abscesses can complicate blunt trauma to the gland. These are managed by simple drainage and antibiotic therapy. Care must be exercised, however, to avoid injury to the facial nerve branches.

Laryngeal Trauma

Blunt or penetrating trauma of the larynx requires immediate attention to the airway. Blind or hastily placed endotracheal tubes carry the risk of extending the injury, and attempts at their placement may be unsuccessful. If the airway is acutely compromised, an emergent tracheostomy is performed. This should be conducted expeditiously under good illumination and adequate instrumentation. Gaping wounds of the larynx can be intubated directly until the patient's condition is stabilized and he or she can be transported to the operating theater for formal tracheostomy. Blunt injuries to the larynx must be observed carefully if minimal or no airway obstruction is encountered at the initial examination. Edema or hemorrhage into the neck over the ensuing 48 hours may subsequently obstruct the traumatized air passage, necessitating tracheostomy. Similarly, progressive subcutaneous emphysema requires direct management.

Contusions of the anterior neck may not result in fracture of the cartilaginous skeleton of the larynx or acute compromise of the airway. These patients are placed at bed rest with the neck stabilized and the head of the bed elevated at least 30°. Humidified oxygen by face mask keeps the traumatized airway moist and reduces the patient's tidal volume. Swallowing is painful and is often accompanied by pharyngeal spasm and/or aspiration. For this reason, no oral feedings are instituted for at least 48 hours. The patient is supported with intravenous fluids and, ideally, hyperalimentation. Antibiotic therapy is instituted as a prophylaxis and continued for approximately 72 hours. Analgesics and sedatives are kept to a minimum to avoid depression of the respiration and possible precipitation of an airway obstruction. These patients generally do well with conservative therapy, though some may experience lingering voice changes or difficulties with swallowing.

Blunt trauma causing acute airway obstruction signifies fracture and collapse of the laryngeal skeleton. The larynx must be explored and repaired to establish a functional organ. After tracheostomy, the larynx is explored through a transverse anterior neck incision, exposing the anatomy from the hyoid bone to the trachea. The strap muscles are separated in the midline and retracted laterally. These can be detached from the hyoid superiorly for greater exposure. The larynx is next examined, and specific consideration is given to the anatomic relationships between the hyoid and cricoid cartilages and the stability of each. Fracture, collapse, or separation of either is an indication to perform a laryngotomy. Simple, relatively stable fractures of the thyroid cartilage are repaired with fine monofilament or wire sutures placed through small drill holes on each side. One should avoid placing these sutures through the laryngeal mucosa—a possible advantage in preventing suture granulomas.

The laryngotomy is performed through a midline incision, which first divides the thyroid cartilage. An oscillating saw or knife is used to make a vertical incision, which extends down to, but not through, the laryngeal mucosa. Occasionally, the thyroid cartilage is vertically fractured, making this incision unnecessary. In any event, the mucosa behind the thyroid cartilage is carefully dissected for approximately 5 mm on each side of the midline. Next, a vertical incision is made through the cricothyroid membrane in the midline and is carried up to the anterior commissure of the glottis. The anterior commissure is divided exactly at its apex, and the incision is then directed laterally just below the epiglottic cartilage. Care must be exercised to avoid injury to the internal branch of the superior laryngeal nerve during this dissection. Illumination of the operating field is facilitated by a fiberoptic headlight or a disposable, gooseneck light placed from above into the larynx.

The lumen of the larynx is then carefully explored. The mucosa may be hemorrhagic and edematous, and there may be lacerations. The articulations of the cricoid, thyroid, and arytenoid cartilages are examined. Any dislocations should be manually repositioned and secured by simple sutures through the appropriate ligaments. It is particularly important to repair the avulsed ligaments with fine absorbable sutures (5-0 or 6-0), incorporating just enough tissue to allow stability. A major problem lies in the post-traumatic fibrosis of the cricoarytenoid joint, which severely impairs vocalization. This can be minimized by fine surgical techniques.

Mucosal lacerations are trimmed and carefully closed with absorbable sutures. In these types of injury, mucosal loss is rare. However, if any defects remain they can be closed by local mucosal advancement or the placement of a mucosal graft (preferably from the cheek). It is not desirable to create flaps from the adjacent laryngeal mucosa because these tend to distort the laryngeal lumen, and their viability may be compromised as a consequence of the original trauma. Split-thickness mucosal grafts are excellent for this purpose. The graft is tailored to match the mucosal defect and then secured to the bed and adjacent mucosa with fine catgut. We have not found it necessary to stent these grafts, unless a particularly large area is being resurfaced. Stents are foreign bodies, quite irritating, and can themselves contribute to laryngeal fibrosis. If a stent is used, it is secured to the anterior larynx with pull-out sutures, so that the larynx and stent move in unison.

The laryngotomy is closed in layers, using fine interrupted catgut sutures for the mucosa. The cricothyroid ligament and extramucosal soft tissues are repaired with synthetic absorbable suture material. The thyroid cartilage is then reapproximated with 5–0 stainless steel wire. Horizontal mattress sutures placed through small drill holes across the isthmus of the thyroid cartilage work well in securing the two halves. Care must be taken to avoid twisting the wires too tightly because they can cut through the cartilage. The remaining cartilage fractures are then repaired.

The avulsed or detached laryngeal muscles and ligaments are then repositioned and secured to the laryngeal framework with absorbable sutures. If severe disruption of the laryngeal anatomy has occurred, the repaired larynx can be suspended from the hyoid bone to help stabilize the parts and to remove tension from the repair. Two absorbable sutures are anchored laterally to the hyoid and then affixed to either the cricoid cartilage or the first tracheal ring. The tension is set firmly, causing the larynx to "rest" in the neck untethered.

The skin is closed over drains placed alongside the larynx. The tracheostomy is kept in place for 7 to 10 days or until it can be plugged and removed without compromising the airway.

Penetrating trauma of the larynx is managed in the same way as described for severe blunt trauma except that the laryngotomy may have to be modified somewhat to suit the anatomy of the laryngeal wound. In addition, these wounds should be suspect for nerve, vascular, or esophageal injury. Division of the superior laryngeal or recurrent laryngeal nerves should be managed by precise repair utilizing microsurgical technique and magnification. With these injuries, careful postoperative care must be administered to prevent aspiration and/or airway obstruction.

In the extreme case, despite diligent care, laryngeal function rarely returns to normal. At minimum, permanent voice changes are encountered. The sequelae of fibrosis, joint immobility, airway compromise, and skeletal distortion give cause for further attempts at reconstruction.

FACIAL FRACTURES

Nasal Fractures

Nasal bone fractures are the most frequently encountered fractures of the facial skeleton. Bleeding from the nose is the most common presenting sign and, in some patients, may be copious (particularly in hypertensives). The thin membrane bones of the nose shatter in unpredictable fashion when broken. However, most fractures are minimally displaced and thus represent a minor therapeutic problem. Roentgenograms of nasal fractures are not particularly useful from a therapeutic point of view and so are not generally obtained. The key points in assessing these injuries are the alignment of the nasal pyramid and septum, the symmetry of the nasal profile, and the presence of a septal hematoma.

If the condition of the patient permits, the head is elevated and ice packs are placed over the root of the nose. The patient is sedated with diazepam (5 to 10 mg IM) and generally given an analgesic/antiemetic (Demerol, Thorazine) parenterally. If massive swelling is present, a simple intranasal examination is all that is performed initially, allowing 3 to 4 days for the swelling to subside before instituting definitive therapy. A thorough intranasal examination is performed at the time of reduction. This requires excellent lighting—preferably a head lamp or reflector. Instrument requirements are minimal and consist of a rubber-shod elevator, a long-bladed nasal speculum, alligator forceps, Asch nasal forceps, a needle-point cautery, and suction. Topical and local infiltration anesthesia is most commonly employed. Cocaine hydrochloride is an excellent topical anesthetic for use intranasally. Its vasoconstrictive effects are indispensable in shrinking the edematous nasal/septal mucosa. Prior to administering this drug, a careful history should be obtained regarding possible allergies or sensitivities. The surgeon should also be familiar with the systemic effects of cocaine and the signs of toxicity (headache, anxiety, chills, tachycardia, irregular respirations, nausea, numbness or tingling of the extremities). Overdoses of this drug should be rapidly treated by discontinuance of the drug followed by intravenous administration of a short-acting barbiturate. Instrumentation for artificial respiration should also be available should respiratory arrest occur.

With regard to dosage, 5 to 10 cc of a 5 percent solution of cocaine hydrochloride is enough to moisten six small cotton pledgets, which are placed intranasally. This dosage rarely causes toxic reactions in an adult patient. Into each naris, one cotton pledget is introduced and the septum and lateral nasal walls are swabbed throughout. One pledget is then directed posteriorly along the nasal floor below the inferior turbinate to a depth of 4 to 6 cm. A second pledget is introduced and the swabbing repeated. This pledget is directed posterosuperiorly below the middle turbinate until resistance is encountered (site of sphenopalatine ganglion). A third pledget is impacted high in the nasal vault at the root of the nose. The pledgets are left in position for 10 to 15 minutes. During this time, one can perform local and regional percutaneous infiltration of Xylocaine (2%) with epinephrine (1:200,000) solution. A total of 6 to 10 cc is sufficient for blocks of the infraorbital and infratrochlear nerves, as well as local infiltration along the nasal-malar groove, dorsum, tip, and nasal spine. The anesthetic is used sparingly to avoid soft tissue distortion.

The nasal vaults and septum are examined with a speculum. Septal hematomas are evacuated through a vertical mucosal incision and the cavity is examined for bleeding points, which are cauterized. It usually is not necessary to suture these incisions. Septal fractures and dislocations are then reduced with an elevator or the Asche forceps and held in this position with bilateral nasal packs. Comminuted fractures of the nasal septum, if unstable, require stent fixation. For these purposes, sterilized x-ray celluloid is excellent stent material. A stent is simply tailored with scissors to conform to the septal anatomy. Greasy medicated gauze is applied over each side of the reduced nasal septum and is backed with the celluloid stent material. The stent-septum-stent sandwich is then fixed with through-and-through sutures of 3–0 Prolene. Care must be taken to avoid excessive tension in the sutures to prevent septal necrosis or ulceration. The stents are left in place for 2 weeks and removed.

In most instances, displaced fractures of the nasal bones can be reduced by direct intranasal manipulation with an elevator or by simple external molding with the thumb and forefinger. A dislocated nasal septum is often reduced by these maneuvers as well. After reduction, the intranasal structures are re-examined. Any small irregularities are then reduced and molded with the Asche forceps. The end point for reduction is primarily visual—a straight nose, symmetry of the nasal walls, and a midline septum.

Some greenstick fractures of the nose are stable on reduction and require no additional support. Comminuted, unstable fractures of the bony, cartilaginous nasal pyramid are best managed by intranasal packing and external splinting. We prefer a petrolatum-impregnated intranasal pack placed according to the method described by Kazanjian and Converse (layered gauze strips carefully packed into the nasal cavity). It is often helpful to insert a small rubber or Silastic tube along the nasal floor to serve as an airway as well as a pressure equalizer in the nasopharynx. These tubes make the patient more comfortable by preventing the "plugged-ear" sensation that accompanies swallowing.

The nasal packs are left in place for 4 to 5 days, which is usually enough time for the fractures to become "sticky" enough to not require support. The presence of an intranasal pack causes mucosal irritation and copious rhinorrhea. This nuisance can be reduced by administering a decongestant such as pseudoephedrine.

There are different types of external nasal splints, all of which have their particular advantages and disadvantages. We prefer the following method: after reduction of the nasal fracture and intranasal packing, the nasal dorsum is cleaned with an alcohol solution. Microporous half-inch tape is applied in overlapping, transversely oriented strips from the nasal root to the tip. This is backed in similar fashion with half-inch cloth adhesive tape. Next, plaster strips are cut and applied over the taped area in "sloppy-wet" fashion until a 3- or 4-ply thickness is achieved. The plaster is then smoothed gently with the finger, congealing all the layers, and the excess water is blotted with a dry sponge. Care is taken to avoid getting any of the plaster into the eyes. After the custom splint is dry, it is secured by cross-taping to the cheeks. A small 2 × 2 gauze nasal drip pad is placed and held into position with a rubber band. This pad is changed when soiled by nasal discharge. The external nasal splint is removed in 5 to 7 days.

Nasal Fractures in Children

Nasal and septal fractures in children are at risk for producing growth disturbances and thus require special consideration. Any injury causing nasal bleeding in a child should be interpreted as a possible nasal/septal fracture. Examination and therapy are best performed under general anesthesia. Cocaine nasal packs are employed to shrink the edematous mucosa. Particular attention is directed to injuries of the nasal septum. Septal hematomas are devastating in this age group and require immediate drainage. If associated with a septal fracture, the hematoma may be bilateral. In these cases, a small portion of the cartilage should be removed, and the opposite hematoma evacuated through the same mucosal incision.

Naso-orbital Fractures

Severe blows to the nasal bridge may result in a communition of the supporting bony structure of the intercanthal region. These injuries are complex and represent the most difficult to manage of the maxillofacial region. There is often associated neurologic trauma resulting from telescoping of the nasal pyramid posteriorly and superiorly through the cribriform plate. Neurosurgical intervention may be indicated if signs of frontal lobe injury, intracranial bleeding, or extensive dural lacerations are present. CSF rhinorrhea is a common finding and, in the absence of neurologic signs, is not a contraindication for surgical reduction of the fractures. There is no evidence that a broad-spectrum antibiotic is effective as a prophylaxis against meningitis. CT scan imagery of the upper midface is the best noninvasive diagnostic tool for evaluation of these injuries. If a neurosurgical emergency exists on presentation a definitive, combined intracranial and extracranial approach is effected. Otherwise, the patient is stabilized and the surgical repair is performed at a convenient time when the swelling has subsided (Table 1).

Goals of Therapy

The goals of management lie in restoration of the anatomic continuity of the fractured parts, drainage of the affected paranasal sinuses and lacrimal apparatus, and soft tissue repair. The thin, eggshell bones of the medial orbital wall, the honeycomb ethmoidal labyrinth, and the floor of the frontal sinus shatter unpredictably as the nasal root is imploded by the point of impact. A precise anatomic reduction of these fragments is neither possible nor practical. The key here is to re-establish correct relationships of the nasal pyramid to the frontal root and base of the skull and to realign the major pillars of the orbital-nasal complex (e.g., supraorbital rims to frontal bone and its nasal process, nasal bone to frontal bone and frontal process of maxilla, frontal process of maxilla to maxilla and zygoma). The position of the medial canthal tendon is altered in these injuries, producing a traumatic telecanthus deformity (pseudohypertelorism). Usually, the tendon attachment to a fragment of the medial orbital wall is preserved. This

TABLE 1 Facial Fractures: Composite of Clinical Radiographic Findings, Surgical Approaches, and Complications for Specific Facial Fractures

Fracture	Clinical Presentation	Radiographic	Surgical Approach	Complications
Naso-orbital	Symptoms: pain, visual abnormalities. Signs: massive periorbital and upper facial edema and ecchymosis, epistaxis, traumatic telecanthus, foreshortening of nose with telescoping. Associated intracranial injuries.	Views: CT scan. Findings: disruption of interorbital space and comminution of nasal pyramid. Frontal, zygomatic, orbital maxillary fractures common.	ORIF via coronal "Meisterschmitt" approach or direct "open sky" approach through wound. Severe comminution may require outrigger suspension to head frame, frontal sinus repair, drainage, canthal tendon alignment, and fixation	Residual upper mid-face deformity ("dish face"). Telecanthus. Frontal sinus/nasolacrimal system pathology with mucocele, mucopyocele, dacryocystitis.
Zygoma Arch	Symptoms: pain lateral cheek, inability to close jaw. Signs: swelling, crepitus over arch, obvious asymmetry.	Views: Water's submentovertex. Findings: depression of arch, comminution.	"Greenstick fractures": closed reduction via brow or temporal approach. Comminuted: reduction and stabilization by circumosseus wiring to external rigid stent. Unstable: ORIF by direct coronal approach.	Contour irregularities of arch area, flattening of arch.
Body "tripod fracture"	Symptoms: pain, trismus, diplopia, numb upper lip, lower lid bilateral nasal area. Signs: swelling, ecchymosis of malar and periorbital areas. Palpable infraorbital rim "step-off". Entrapment of extraocular muscles with disconjugate gaze. Scleral ecchymosis, displacement lateral canthal ligament.	Views: Water's submentovertex, CT scan. Findings: clouding, air/fluid level maxillary sinus, separation of zygomaticomaxillary, zygomaticofrontal, and zygomaticotemporal suture lines.	Non- or minimally displaced: conservative. Displaced/comminuted: ORIF via brow and infraciliary approach. Entrapment: orbital floor exploration and reconstruction via infraciliary approach. Caldwell-Luc with sinus stent. Complex comminuted: outrigger suspension.	Residual malar deformity, enophthalmos, diplopia, infraorbital nerve anesthesia, chronic maxillary sinusitis.
Orbital floor	Symptoms: diplopia, orbital pain.	Views: Water's, CT scan, tomograms.	No entrapment, enophthalmos, or adnexal herniation:	Enophthalmos, diplopia. Recurrent orbital

TABLE 1 Facial Fractures: Composite of Clinical Radiographic Findings, Surgical Approaches, and Complications for Specific Facial Fractures—Continued

Fracture	Clinical Presentation	Radiographic	Surgical Approach	Complications
	Signs: periorbital edema, ecchymosis, enophthalmos, extraocular muscle entrapment, disconjugate gaze. Hyphema, subluxation of lens, retinal detachment, rupture of globe with direct eye trauma.	Findings: air/fluid level maxillary sinus, herniated adnexa and/or orbital floor fragments in maxillary sinus.	conservative therapy. Entrapments, enophthalmos or herniated adnexa; orbital floor exploration via infraciliary approach, reconstruction (cartilage, bone or alloplastic material). Antrostomy with sinus stent.	cellulitis with implant (alloplastic) extrusion.
Mandible Condyle	Symptoms: pain at fracture site, referred pain to ear. Signs: crepitus, excessive salivation, swelling of condylar region, deviation of jaw toward fracture, cross-bite or open-bite deformity.	Views: AP, oblique, Water's, Panorex. Findings: nondisplaced, or displaced anteriorly and medially.	Non- or minimal displacement: IMF. Displaced ORIF via submandibular or transoral route.	Ankylosis of TMJ. Chronic TMJ
Angle	Symptoms: pain at fracture site, inability to close mouth. Signs: swelling at angle of jaw, ecchymosis, crepitus, malocclusion.	Views: Panorex, mandibular series. Findings: nondisplaced (favorable) or posterior fragment displaced upward and medially (nonfavorable).	Favorable: IMF Nonfavorable: ORIF via intraoral or submandibular route.	Nonunion, malunion osteomyelitis.
Body	Symptoms: pain at fracture site, limitation of movement. Signs: swelling, ecchymosis, crepitus, malocclusion.	Views: Panorex, mandibular series. Findings: nondisplaced (favorable), or post. fragment displaced upward and medially, anterior fragments rotated lingually (nonfavorable).	Favorable: IMF. Nonfavorable: ORIF, via extraoral approach. IMF with lingual splints.	Osteomyelitis, infection (tooth in fracture line.)
Symphysis	Symptoms: pain. Signs: malocclusion, frequent	Views: mandibular series, submentovertex.	ORIF via submental incision. IMF with lingual splints.	Residual malocclusion. loss of chin projection,

TABLE 1 Facial Fractures: Composite of Clinical Radiographic Findings, Surgical Approaches, and Complications for Specific Facial Fractures—Continued

Fracture	Clinical Presentation	Radiographic	Surgical Approach	Complications
	association with soft tissue wounds of lower lip, tongue.	Findings: nondisplaced or lingual rotation of anterior fragments, may be associated with angle or condyle fractures.		asymmetry. Osteomyelitis.
Maxilla LeFort I (transverse)	Symptoms: pain upper jaw, numb upper teeth. Signs: midfacial edema and ecchymosis, epistaxis, malocclusion, mobility of maxillary dentition.	Views: Water's, Panorex, CT scan. Findings: opaque maxillary sinus, displacement of fragments of alveolus if comminuted. Fracture through maxillary sinus and pterygoid plates.	Disimpaction, IMF with skull cap or internal fixation to pyriform margin.	Loss of teeth, infection, malocclusion.
LeFort II (pyramidal)	Symptoms: pain midface, numb upper lip, lower lid, lateral nasal area. Signs: midfacial edema and ecchymosis, epistaxis, malocclusion, mobility of midface, nasal flattening, anesthesia infraorbital nerve territory.	Views: Water's, CT scan. Findings: opaque maxillary sinuses, separation through frontal process, lacrimal bones, floor of orbits, zygomaticomaxillary suture line, lateral wall of maxillary sinus and pterygoid plates.	Disimpaction, IMF with suspension to internal wire fixation to solid structure above fracture (infraorbital rim, frontal bone). Direct transosseus wiring via infraciliary approach.	Nonunion, malunion, lacrimal system obstruction, infraorbital nerve anesthesia. diplopia, malocclusion.
LeFort III (craniofacial dysjunction)	Symptoms: pain face, difficulty breathing. Signs: "donkey-face" deformity. malocclusion, mobile face, marked facial edema and ecchymosis, epistaxis, CSF rhinorrhea.	Views: Water's, CT scan. Findings: separation of mid-third of face at zygomaticofrontal, zygomaticotemporal, and nasofrontal sutures, and across orbital floors. Opaque maxillary sinuses.	IMF and cranial suspension to wire fixation at frontal bones. Direct wiring via brow incisions, naso-orbital incisions.	Nonunion, malunion, malocclusion. lengthening of midface, lacrimal system obstruction.

allows for repositioning of the fragment back into its normal anatomic position, where it is secured to the stable nasal pillar and maxillary process as well as to the opposite tendon by a through-and-through wire. The positioning of these tendons correctly is difficult and prone to considerable error, which is not apparent at the time of reduction unless a wide exposure is achieved.

Surgical Exposures

Some surgeons prefer a direct approach through the nasal root via an "open-sky" technique. We occasionally use this approach if there is an open wound here which provides access or can be enlarged satisfactorily without producing an objectionable scar. The retraction of the soft tissue causes distortion of important landmarks, which are particularly important in gauging bone to soft tissue relationships. We prefer the Meisterschmitt or degloving exposure for these injuries. A coronal scalp incision is made from ear to ear, and the scalp is dissected forward below the galea to the supraorbital rims. The periosteum is incised high above the orbital rims, and a subperiosteal dissection is continued over the supraorbital rims and laterally below the temporalis muscle. The superior orbital neurovascular bundle may be dissected from its foramen with a fine osteotome to provide greater exposure. Centrally, a subperiosteal dissection is continued over the nasal bones to the upper lateral nasal cartilages. The medial orbital wall is exposed, and the lacrimal sac is dissected from its fossa, leaving the nasolacrimal duct intact. The anterior ethmoidal vessels are identified here and divided. The subperiosteal dissection is continued inferiorly, exposing the infraorbital rim and frontal process of the maxillary bone. If greater exposure of the maxilla and infraorbital rim is needed, a subciliary incision is made along the lower eyelid medially to the lacrimal punctum. The orbicularis muscle is divided, and the dissection is continued behind the muscle to the orbital rim.

This exposure gives excellent visualization of the entire naso-orbital complex. Reconstructive efforts can then be based upon the full "birds-eye" view of normal and abnormal anatomy.

Surgical Repair

First priorities are given to reconstruction of the stabilizing pillars of the naso-orbital region. Preoperative radiographic assessment will determine if this can be safely done without a craniotomy. Occasionally, neurosurgical exploration with exposure of the anterior cranial fossa is the most conservative and safest approach. This can easily be performed through a frontal craniotomy via a Meisterschmitt exposure. The nasal pyramid is disimpacted with an Asche forceps and is brought forward. The nasal bones are then secured to the stable frontal root with stainless steel wires (26-gauge). The nasal processes of the maxillary bone are wired to the maxilla and the nasal bones. If severe comminution of these bones is present, each piece is carefully positioned anatomically and wired at two points to neighboring pieces with No. 30 stainless steel wire. In this fashion, the puzzle is reconstructed, but no attempt is made to wire together the thin, delicate flakes of the lamina papyracea, lacrimal, or ethmoid bones. These pieces are usually attached to periosteum or mucosa, and upon reduction and fixation of the naso-orbital pillar, they generally lie in satisfactory position. If severe comminution is present with marked lateral displacement of the ethmoidal bones, reduction can be accomplished by direct gentle molding with an Asche or Walsham forceps. This "pinching" together of the nasal bridge is effective in maintaining the anterior projection of the fractured segments.

Medial Canthal Tendons

The medial canthal tendons are usually repositioned in the reconstruction of the naso-orbital pillar. This reduction can be reinforced internally or externally to maintain the projection of the nasal bridge and the security of the canthal fixation. Internal reinforcement is preferred when the lateral walls of the pyramid are not comminuted and, when reduced, maintain their anatomic position. In these cases, a No. 26 stainless wire is passed through two drill holes that traverse the nasal bridge just above the attachment of the canthal tendons. When tightened, this wire maintains a rigid fixation of the central structures.

Medial Orbital Walls

If the medial orbital walls are comminuted, a simple internal wire fixation is insufficient for support, but allows collapse of the surrounding fragments. These fractures are best stabilized by external splint fixation. After the nasal bridge, canthal tendons, and medial orbital wall fragments have been positioned and wired, through-and-through wires are placed across the nasal bridge just superior to the canthal tendon attachments. These wires are then brought through the nasal skin on each side and attached to contour pledgets fashioned from Alumifoam splints (foam side toward the skin). The splints aid in molding the fractured bridge framework as well as in maintaining the requisite anterior projection of the nasal pyramid. If the medial canthal tendons have been avulsed from their bony attachments, they are reattached by fixation to the reconstructed nasal bridge. It is important to delineate the exact point of fixation here to avoid postoperative discrepancies in palpebral orientation. A helpful solution is to gauge the fixation points of the *lateral* canthal tendons. A line (wire) connecting these two points will fall across the bridge at the correct point of fixation for the medial tendons. A small hole is drilled through the nasal bridge at this level. It is important to position this hole anterior to the lacrimal fossa or its remnant to ensure proper positioning of the canthal tendon. (The canthal tendon normally splits and attaches to the anterior and posterior rims of the fossa.) Next, the medial canthal tendons are wired to each other through the hole. A No. 30 stainless steel wire is excellent for these purposes.

Occasionally, severe comminution of the naso-orbital complex precludes adequate internal or splint stabilization. In these cases, outrigger fixation via a plaster head cap or cranial "halo" device is necessary. We prefer the halo device, which is fixed to the cranium. This is more precise and allows visualization of the scalp and frontal region, a feature that is particularly advantageous following craniotomy. Plaster head caps become loose with time and are a source of constant complaint. A wire is secured to a stable fragment or passed through the canthal block and attached to the outrigger device. The vector of traction is determined by the direction of collapse. If satisfactory reduction can be maintained by simple traction, the wire is secured to the outrigger appliance at the proper point. This is maintained for 2 weeks or until bony fixation is adequate. Combinations of internal wiring, external splint, or outrigger fixation may be necessary to achieve and maintain the desired reduction.

The Nose

After reduction and stabilization of the naso-orbital pillar and medial canthal tendon attachments, the nose is examined. Disruption of the bony-cartilaginous juncture of the nasal dorsum can cause severe deformities of the nasal profile and is also a harbinger of possible septal fractures or dislocation. A careful intranasal examination is performed, with topical cocaine hydrochloride used to shrink the edematous mucosa. Any septal fractures or dislocations are reduced (see *Nasal Fractures*). Septal hematomas are evacuated. The nose should not be packed in the presence of CSF rhinorrhea. If a combined intracranial, extracranial approach is used, and the dural defect repaired, a light nasal packing is inserted and removed in 3 to 4 days. The dorsal nasal cartilage is fixed to the nasal bones with fine wire sutures placed in horizontal mattress fashion through small drill holes. Absorbable sutures are insufficient to maintain reduction here and should not be used.

Sinuses

The next consideration is given to the drainage of the ethmoidal, sphenoidal, and frontal sinuses. If an adequate reduction is achieved, these sinuses will drain satisfactorily. In severe impaction-type injuries, the ostia of the frontal sinus may lose its continuity with the ethmoid. This may result in the formation of a frontal sinus mucocele or mucopyocele. The cause is obstruction of the nasofrontal duct. In these cases, drainage of the frontal sinus must be effected. Access to the frontal sinus can often be achieved through a fracture of its floor or anterior wall or through craniotomy; otherwise a 5-mm sinusotomy is performed anteriorly and a drainage tract is established by probe exploration through the nasofrontal duct. The probe is directed to beneath the anterior portion of the middle turbinate. This tract is maintained by stenting with a 12 F Silastic catheter, which is brought out through the naris and sutured to the nasal floor. The tube is left in this position for 3 to 4 weeks. It is irrigated daily with a sterile saline solution. Both frontal sinuses should be drained. In some cases in which wide exposure of one sinus is present through a fracture segment, the intersinus septum can be burred away, creating a common sinus for unilateral drainage.

Lacrimal Apparatus

The lacrimal apparatus must be inspected for injury. Common sites of disruption occur in the lacrimal sac and the nasolacrimal duct. Canalicular injuries should be suspected if the medial canthal tendon has been avulsed from its bony attachments. If no injuries are detected by gross visualization, it is helpful to cannulate the lacrimal punctum on the upper or lower eyelid and inject 2 to 3 cc of saline solution into the lacrimal system. If saline returns via the noncannulated punctum and into the nose beneath the inferior turbinate, this is good evidence that the lacrimal system is patent and all components communicate with each other. If the saline leaks into the wound, careful inspection of the canaliculi and lacrimal sac is necessary to determine the site of injury. We repair lacerated canaliculi with fine 9–0 monofilament nonabsorbable sutures over a Silastic stent using operative magnification. Lacrimal sac injuries are first probed to determine patency of the nasolacrimal duct. If resistance to probing is encountered, adjacent fracture segments in line with the nasolacrimal duct are manipulated until the probe can be easily passed into the nose below the inferior turbinate. The duct is stented with a Silastic catheter gauged to fit snugly, but not tightly. The catheter is sutured to the nasal floor and left in place for 3 weeks. The lacrimal sac is then closed in one layer with fine interrupted 8–0 monofilament sutures.

In severe crushing or avulsion type midfacial injuries, the lacrimal collecting system may be so traumatized that repair is impossible. In these cases, it is best to close the wound and perform a dacryocystorhinostomy or other drainage procedure at a later time. In some cases, a primary dacryocystorhinostomy is performed if the nasal wall has not been comminuted and is stable.

Primary Bone Grafting

Injuries resulting in the loss of bony support of the medial orbital wall, nasal bridge, orbital rim, or floor are treated by primary reconstruction using bone grafts. This technique is preferred over a staged reconstruction because it achieves the desired goal in one operation and is unencumbered by the formation of difficult scar tissue. A corticalcancellous bone graft is harvested from the iliac crest and tailored according to the demands for reconstruction. Onlay grafts are generally employed for isolated reconstruction of an orbital wall, floor, or rim. In massive injuries with loss of the entire nasal root and medial orbital walls, a "butterfly" graft is employed with the body serving as the nasal root and dorsum, and the folded wings as the medial orbital walls. In these cases, remnants of the ethmoid sinus are removed with a rongeur. The frontal sinuses are drained, and a nasal lining is constructed using septal and lateral mucosal flaps. The grafts are fixed to the adjacent stable bony structures with interosseous wire. These wounds are not usually drained, although every effort is made to obtain absolute hemostasis prior to closure. Broad-spectrum antibiotics are administered preoperatively, intraoperatively, and postoperatively for 48 hours unless CSF rhinorrhea persists, in which case they are continued until the problem is resolved.

The coronal scalp incision is closed in layers and an occlusive bulky head dressing is applied. Postoperatively, the patient is kept at bedrest with the head elevated 30 degrees. Dressings over the face, and particularly the eyes, are avoided. Vision and neurologic status checks are performed at intervals of 4 to 6 hours. Swelling, which is usually extensive, begins receding by the third day. Most patients tolerate liquids without difficulty by the second postoperative day. The diet is advanced as conditions permit. Analgesics are given parenterally in frequent small doses (morphine is preferred). Severe postoperative pain is uncommon and, if persistent, signals a potential complication.

Frontal Sinus Fractures

A blow of significant magnitude is required to fracture the frontal bone, especially the supraorbital rims. These injuries are frequently associated with intracranial injury and are often managed at the time of craniotomy. Simple, nondisplaced fractures of the frontal sinus require no intervention. Broad-spectrum prophylactic antibiotic therapy is occasionally instituted.

Comminuted outer table frontal sinus fractures are explored through the adjoining forehead laceration or via a coronal scalp exposure. The sinus cavity is examined and the nasofrontal duct is probed to ensure patency. The fracture fragments are carefully reduced and secured with interosseous wires if the reduction is unstable. Even in severely comminuted fractures, the anterior wall can be reconstructed safely provided sinus drainage is ensured and a rigid interosseous fixation achieved. It is not necessary to "obliterate" the frontal sinus in these injuries; there is no biologic basis for filling the sinus cavity with devascularized fat or muscle.

Inner table fractures of the frontal sinus are associated with dural and brain injuries and frequently require craniotomy. The bone of the inner table is relatively thin and shatters on impact, at times making reconstruction impossible. If the fragments can be reduced to reconstruct a continuous inner table, this method is preferred. At times, painstaking effort must be made to precisely fit the individual fracture pieces into their proper position. Fine No. 28 stainless steel wire is employed for these purposes. When the inner table is fractured beyond repair, the segments are completely removed and the edges of the sinus cavity are smoothed of any irregularities. The sinus is stripped of its mucosa to the nasofrontal duct. Careful submucosal dissection of the orifice of the duct is performed so that a sleeve of duct mucosa is mobilized. This is doubly ligated with fine (5–0) synthetic absorbable suture and trimmed of any excess mucosa. The stump is then cauterized. Any remnants of suspected mucosa in the sinus cavity are likewise cauterized. A plug of corticalcancellous bone harvested from the craniotomy site or outer table is tapped into the orifice of the nasofrontal duct after the edges of the duct have been freshened with a burr. The outer table is reconstructed as previously outlined. Initially the sinus cavity fills with serum, CSF, and clot, but gradually becomes occupied by the frontal portion of the brain. If both walls of the sinus have been destroyed, the preferred procedure is "cranialization" combined with a primary bone graft reconstruction of the outer table.

Supraorbital rim fractures occasionally involve the frontal sinus. The key here is assurance of patency of the nasofrontal duct by stenting or a "window" procedure through the intersinus septum for drainage through the opposite side. Bony defects are reconstructed primarily with corticalcancellous iliac crest or split rib bone grafts. Alloplastic materials such as Methylmethacrylate, Silastic, and Teflon have been utilized for reconstruction of the frontal region in acute trauma. Their advantage lies in ease of reconstruction, avoidance of a donor site, and availability. We prefer autogenous material if the patient's general condition permits and if no penetrating intra-abdominal injury is present. Autogenous bone is better tolerated by the patient, is permanent, and when healed is a less susceptible nidus for bacterial infection.

Fractures of the Zygoma and Orbit

Lateral or oblique blows to the midface are absorbed by the malar region. Although the zygoma itself is uncommonly fractured, its attachments to the maxilla, frontal, and temporal bones are vulnerable to disruption. If the zygoma is displaced, disruption of the orbital floor and lateral wall is encountered. Direct forward blows to the orbit are absorbed by the orbital rims. The eye and ocular adnexa are compressed in the orbital vault, causing the weakest part, the floor, to fracture. There is probably a component of both mechanisms in a large percentage of malar complex fractures. In assessing these injuries, primary attention is given to the eye and its function. The maxillary sinus, which is involved in all fractures of this sort, is considered not only as a route of operative access, but also as a source of complication if inappropriately managed (see Table 1).

Indications for Surgery

Surgical management of these fractures is performed as early as possible, particularly when entrapment of the extraocular muscles or massive disruption of the orbital floor is present. Delay of surgical intervention in these cases not only continues the inevitable inflammatory process, but also invites progressive ischemia of fat and muscle leading to fibrosis, diminished extraocular muscle function, and enophthalmos. Undisplaced fractures do not require surgical treatment. Our indications for surgery are as follows: (1) clinical or roentgenographic displacement of the zygoma or orbital floor, (2) documented enophthalmos, and (3) early diplopia with a positive forced duction test.

The goals of surgical therapy are basically twofold: restoration of normal function and appearance. Release of entrapped or herniated orbital contents, precise reduction of displaced fractures, primary reconstruction of bony and soft tissue defects, and sinus drainage procedures constitute the therapeutic sequences employed to achieve these goals.

Isolated Zygomatic Arch Features

Isolated zygomatic arch fractures are usually of the "greenstick" variety and are easily managed via the Gillies' approach through a temporal incision. Local anesthesia with general standby may be employed for the majority of these cases. Occasionally, muscle relaxation may be required for reduction of the fracture. A vertical incision is made within the hairbearing scalp directly over the temporalis muscle. A blunt elevator is slipped below the temporalis fascia to the undersurface of the zygomatic arch. The depression of the arch is palpated and slight counterpressure is applied here to "control" the reduction. The fracture is then elevated, using the forefinger as a fulcrum for the elevator. These fractures can be heard or felt to "click" back into normal position. After reduction the fracture is palpated for stability; if it is stable, a protective splint fashioned from a finger splint is molded to arch over the fracture site. It is taped to the forehead and mandibular angle and left in place for 10 days. A soft diet is recommended during this time as it is possible, with forceful chewing, to dislodge the fracture segments.

Unstable or Comminuted Zygomatic Arch Fractures

Unstable or comminuted zygomatic arch fractures require internal or external fixation. Numerous adjunctive techniques have been employed based on the temporal fossa "packing" principle. Balloon catheters, vaginal gauze, and rubber drains have all been employed as packs placed beneath the zygomatic arch to maintain an anatomic reduction. This technique is not favored because it is imprecise, creates an "open fracture" situation with the risk of infection, and is bothersome for the patient. Open reduction of the unstable arch is a more direct approach and can be accomplished through a coronal incision or an incision placed over the arch in a wrinkle line. Both approaches require general anesthesia, expose the patient to the risk of injury to the facial nerve, and are time-consuming. We have occasionally performed an open reduction of a comminuted zygomatic arch in conjuncton with another procedure involving fractures of the frontal/orbital complex. The coronal "degloving" approach gives a wide exposure of the entire arch, making open reduction quite easy. A simple method of external fixation is achieved by placing a percutaneous wire suture around the depressed arch and securing this to a stable arch splint (contoured finger splint), which is taped to the forehead and cheek or mastoid eminence. In severe comminution, two or more wires can be used to obtain and maintain an accurate reduction. Postreduction roentgenograms are taken to check the fracture alignment; adjustments of the wire tension can be made if any displacement is encountered. The splint is left in position for 10 to 12 days and then removed.

"Tripod" Fractures of the Zygoma

Classic "tripod" fractures of the zygoma are managed by open reduction when displaced. If there is clinical or roentgenographic evidence of orbital content herniation into the maxillary sinus, entrapment of the extraocular muscles, or marked disruption of the orbital floor, exploration of the orbital floor is performed. For minimally displaced fractures, a brow incision is made to expose the zygomaticofrontal suture line and this access is used to reduce the fracture with a blunt elevator through the temporal fossa. Careful palpation of the arch and infraorbital rim during this reduction determines its end point. If the fracture remains stable, the brow incision is simply closed. The Gillies' temporal incision is not a good approach for these fractures because the unstable fracture requires a brow incision anyway.

Unstable and Severely Displaced Fractures

If the fracture is unstable or if severe displacement or comminution is present, a brow and lower eyelid exposure is performed. The zygomaticofrontal suture line is cleaned of its periosteum and a figure-of-8 No. 26 interosseous wire is placed either anteriorly or posteriorly through fine drill holes. The wire is not twisted. Next, the orbital rim and floor are exposed via an infraciliary transmuscular incision. The line of incision on the lower eyelid is marked as it is for a belpharoplasty—2 to 3 mm below the lash line, extending laterally in a wrinkle crease, but not beyond the orbital margin (scar becomes apparent here). The skin and subcutaneous tissues are infiltrated with a solution of 1 percent Xylocaine with epinephrine (1:200,000), and 7 to 10 minutes are allowed for the full vasoconstrictive effect. The incision is begun laterally and is extended medially to the lateral lash margin. Next, the underlying orbicularis muscle is divided and precise hemostasis effected with the electrocautery. Using blunt-tipped tissue-cutting scissors, a tunnel is dissected behind the orbicularis to the lacrimal punctum. The scissors are used to cut the skin and muscle along the inscribed line. Two fine sutures are placed through the upper cut edge of the lid incision and connected to clamps for upward retraction of the eyelid; this protects the cornea and tenses the tissues to allow easier dissection. The composite skin-muscle flap of the lower eyelid is dissected to the orbital rim. Care is taken to keep the dissection just behind the muscle in the fine fibroareolar tissue in front of the orbital septum. This plane is relatively bloodless, though small bleeders are encountered medially and laterally. Precise hemostasis is obtained at all times with a fine needle-point electrocautery. Alternative exposures to this region include the transconjunctival and the infraorbital rim approaches. The transconjunctival approach carries the risk of corneal abrasion and does not provide adequate exposure if interosseous wire fixation is required. Its benefits lie in ease of dissection and a concealed surgical scar. The infraorbital rim approach is relatively bloody, carries the risk of injury to the infraorbital nerve, and creates a conspicuous scar on the face. Its advantages lie in its direct approach to the inferior orbital rim and floor and the avoidance of ectropion formation in the lower eyelid. The infraciliary lower eyelid approach is believed to represent a compromise between these two approaches and incorporates some of the advantages inherent in each. Ectropion of the lower eyelid has occurred with this approach, but in most cases is a temporary phenomenon that resolves by gentle massaging of the eyelid. For the most part, ectropion can be avoided by employing fine surgical technique and obtaining absolue hemostasis prior to wound closure.

The inferior orbital rim is exposed medially beyond the zygomaticomaxillary suture line (fracture line) and laterally to the point of ascendancy of the lateral orbital rim. If the medial portion of the inferior orbital rim is fractured, the dissection is continued along the rim until a stable buttress is encountered. Occasionally, a counter-incision placed anterior to the lacrimal fossa in the nasomalar crease facilitates this exposure. After the entire orbital rim defect has been exposed, a periosteal incision is made along the lower margin, and a subperiosteal dissection of the rim and lateral orbital floor is performed. Usually, the lateral orbital floor or a portion of it is intact, allowing the dissection to commence in ''known'' territory. The subperiosteal dissection is continued posteriorly to the inferior orbital fissure and medially to the rim of the fracture. At the zygomaticomaxillary juncture, the infraorbital nerve and artery are encountered. Care is exercised here to avoid injury to these structures. The dissection is continued medially to expose the stable components of the orbital rim and medial orbital floor. After the medial and lateral dissections are complete, there is usually encountered a tether or actual herniation of the periorbital soft tissues through the fracture line in the orbital floor. It is important *not* to forcefully attempt to retract this tissue from its impingement for fear of causing permanent nerve, muscle, or fat injury. In these cases, distraction of the fractured zygoma will allow atraumatic manipulation and reduction of these tissues. For these purposes, it has been found advantageous to secure a traction wire on the zygomatic portion of the orbital rim (through a small drill hole) and to use this anchor to help distract the zygoma while manipulating its reduction via the brow approach. The wire anchor helps in directing the reduction to the appropriate position after the orbital contents have been freed.

When extracting the herniated or entrapped tissues, it is important to employ a gentle technique and to make every attempt to visualize the anatomy clearly. Usually, the contents are easily freed by distraction. Occasionally, in delayed cases, swelling, inflammation, and early fibrosis are encountered. The herniated tissues must then be gently dissected or "teased" from their abnormal position. After the soft tissues have been freed, the zygoma is reduced and secured by interosseous wiring of the zygomaticomaxillary suture line and tightening of the previously placed zygomaticofrontal wire. A two-point stabilization is adequte for most fractures of this type.

After the zygoma has been reduced, the orbital floor is carefully examined. In most cases, there is adequate bony support to prevent herniation. If the orbital floor is comminuted and the fractures are unstable or a defect is present which allows collapse of the orbital soft tissues, a reconstruction is performed. First, all of the loose fragments are removed and foreign body fragments are extracted from the maxillary sinus as these may provide a nidus for infection. The resultant orbital floor defect is closed with a bone graft harvested from the anterior wall of the maxillary sinus, the vomer, with nasal septal cartilage, or with an auricular cartilage graft. We prefer autogenous material for reconstruction of the orbital floor because it is better tolerated by the patient and has been associated with fewer complications. Certainly, a good number of antral bone grafts placed in the orbital floor are resorbed and replaced by fibrous tissue, but this is of little clinical significance because the remnant fibrous sling is stable and provides excellent support of the orbital contents. It is difficult to rationalize the biologic sense of placing an alloplastic material (Silicone, Teflon) in a potentially contaminated site comprising the roof of a paranasal sinus cavity. The orbital floor graft is placed over the defect or wedged between the adjoining sides of the floor remnants. The rim periosteum is closed to help stabilize the graft. Prior to wound closure, the operative site is carefully explored for bleeding points and these are cauterized. The brow and lower eyelid incisions are closed in layers.

Postoperatively, the zygoma is protected by an external splint or cup. Careful assessment of the vision is performed in the recovery room. The head is elevated to reduce swelling, and the patient is advised to avoid bending over or blowing the nose for 6 weeks following operation. Prophylactic antibiotics are administered in the perioperative period if a graft was employed and discontinued 48 hours after surgery. These patients frequently experience photophobia and require sunglasses for as long as 6 weeks following discharge from the hospital.

Comminuted Fractures of the Zygoma

Comminuted orbital rim and zygomatic body fractures are managed by piecemeal reduction and interosseous wire fixation of all the fragments. Periosteal attachments are preserved if they do not interfere with the drilling and wiring of the fragments. Care must be exercised when dissecting laterally over the zygomatic body to avoid injury to the zygomaticofacial sensory nerve, which exits the main body 1 to 2 cm inferior and lateral to the orbital margin. Injury to this nerve can be a source of annoying pain and discomfort to the patient.

After the rim and zygomatic body have been reconstructed and fixed to the rigid medial and lateral components, the complex often is unstable and prone to collapse—a common cause of postoperative malar deformity. In these cases, outrigger stabilization becomes necessary. One or two points along the orbital rim and/or zygoma are chosen for support. Stainless steel wires (No. 30) are passed through small drill holes at these points and brought out through the lower eyelid flap. At the completion of the procedure, the wires are connected to an outrigger appliance (preferably a skeletal head frame). Postoperative roentgenograms are used to gauge the external reduction. We do not use elastics for traction in these cases because there is a tendency for overcorrection leading to an exaggerated projection of the malar eminence or orbital rim, which is difficult to correct once the bones become rigid.

Primary Bone Grafting in Zygomatic Fractures

Primary bone grafting is employed for acute fractures of the zygoma and orbit when there is severe comminution and/or loss of bone. Prerequisites include a stable patient and adequate soft tissue coverage. The inferior orbital rim and floor are reconstructed with contoured iliac crest bone grafts. Split-rib grafts are an alternative source of graft material; they work well in children, but have a high resorption rate in the adult. Interestingly, grafts placed in children enlarge with the normal growth of the surrounding facial skeleton. In some, however, graft enlargement is not proportional, and a hypoplastic skeletal deformity may develop; the factors governing these phenomena are not completely understood. Alloplastic materials are occasionally employed as an alternative. As stated previously, they are not considered equivalent substitutes for autogenous material, particularly when utilized around the paranasal sinuses. Here, deficiencies in soft tissue coverage give rise to implant migration and sinus tract formation. We do not use alloplastic materials in children. Contour defects of the malar eminence, zygomatic arch, or orbital rim in adults, however, are ideally suited for these grafts.

Orbital Blow-out Fractures

Blow-out fractures of the orbital floor are managed in the same way as those associated with zygomatic fractures. The key exception here is the lack of distraction capability in the zygomatic fragment. If the herniated/entrapped contents cannot be easily reduced without injury, the floor fracture is widened, bit by bit, by shaving the fracture edges with a No. 15 scalpel blade until the mass is easily delivered. The orbital floor defect can be repaired with a bone or cartilage graft, as previously described. A Caldwell-Luc antrostomy is occasionally employed to facilitate the reduction of difficult trap-door fractures or large comminuted fractures of the orbital floor. A 4- to 6-cm incision is made just below the apex of the labial gingival sulcus, and a subperiosteal dissection of the anterior wall of the maxilla is performed. A large antral window is made with a fine diamond-tipped burr, and the sinus cavity is entered. (The antral bone graft thus harvested is saved and used for reconstruction of the orbital floor.) After the old blood and mucus are evacuated, the sinus cavity is explored. All loose fragments and sharp spicules of attached bony floor are removed to exlude possible foreign bodies in the sinus and prevent injury to the adnexal structures during reduction. An elevator is used to gently elevate the bone and soft tissues back into the orbital cavity. Care is taken to avoid stabbing the herniated adnexa with the instrument. Usually, a piece of attached orbital floor can be found which will serve as a platform for the elevator as the reduction progresses. After reduction of the fracture has been accomplished by this method, the floor is rarely stable unless a single large piece remains intact and can be wedged into position. If there is no significant bony defect in the orbital floor, the reduced fragments can be supported from below with a maxillary sinus pack. Numerous materials have been employed for this purpose and all have their advantages and disadvantages. Nonadherent inert materials work best. Gauze packings are malodorous and adhere to the bony fragments. Balloon catheters are easy to insert, but often do not elevate the orbital floor at the correct point. They may also cause pressure necrosis of the sinus mucosa. Custom low-pressure balloon catheters work well, but are expensive and frequently unavailable. We prefer a long half-inch Penrose drain. The drain is easily inserted and removed. It is nonadherent, maintains a good reduction of the orbital floor, and is well tolerated by the patient.

A medial wall antrostomy is made below the inferior turbinate, and the drain is passed from the maxillary sinus window into the nose and secured to the membranous septum with a silk suture. The sinus is then carefully packed in layers until the orbital floor fractures are in good position and stable. Excess drain is cut off, and the remaining end is notched with a "V" to ensure completeness of removal. The vestibular incision is closed in layers with absorbable sutures. The antral pack is left in this position for 10 to 14 days and then removed.

Antral packing is occasionally used for severely comminuted fractures of the zygoma and maxilla. We do not employ this technique, preferring direct wiring instead. When used, however, a balloon catheter, placed through a medial wall maxillary sinus antrostomy, has the requisite rigidity to immobilize the surrounding fragments. Unfortunately, this method remains somewhat imprecise.

Fractures of the Mandible

The mandible is unique among facial features owing to its functional detachment from the facial skeleton. Strong muscular forces applied to the mandible influence the direction and severity of displacement of its fractures. Unlike fractures of other facial bones, the mandibular fracture must be held in reduction by stronger methods of fixation and for longer periods of time. This key observation determines the ultimate mode of management. Timing of therapy is dependent on the relative severity of associated injuries and their importance in the overall status of the patient. Early therapy is preferred, especially in children, in whom fracture consolidation occurs rapidly (7 to 10 days). All mandibular fractures involving the teeth are considered open fractures because of the nature of the periodontal attachment, even if a laceration is not evident. Antibiotic prophylaxis is considered wise practice in such cases. Penicillin or erythromycin, given either intravenously or by mouth, is most appropriate in this situation. If fracture management is delayed beyond 48 hours, we generally prescribe clindamycin (300 mg per 100 cc saline every 6 hours) mouthwashes as an additional measure, particularly when significant periodontal disease or dental caries are present. The bathing of the fracture site with saliva and oral cavity bacteria causes massive contamination, which, if allowed to persist, can lead to nonunion or osteomyelitis of the fracture site.

The mainstay of mandibular fracture management is based on the concept of intermaxillary fixation. In general, this represents the most conservative treatment that will effectively reduce and stabilize the fracture. Other methods of mandibular fixation include interarch dental fixation, interosseous fixation, and external fixation. These methods may be employed in addition to intermaxillary fixation for specific fractures.

In managing these injuries, attention must be directed to the presence or absence of serviceable teeth on either side of the fracture. Fractures of the mandible may be favorable or unfavorable, depending on their direction or bevel and the influence of the muscles of mastication on specific parts. A keen understanding of these relationships is necessary before embarking on any therapeutic plan. Inasmuch as the goal of therapy is the re-establishment of normal or pre-injury mandibular function, the teeth serve as both the diagnostic and therapeutic means to this end (see Table 1).

Intermaxillary Fixation

A metal brace affixed to the dental arch with circumdental wires is the most common method of intermaxillary fixation in both closed and open procedures. Two types of arch bars are commonly employed. A pliable Niro type arch bar is easily adapted to irregularities in arch form and allows for close contouring of the bar to individual variations. However, it is not as stiff as the Jelenko type arch bar, which is rigid. The Jelenko is somewhat more difficult to conform to the arch, but allows for rigid stabilization, particularly in areas where there is hypermobile teeth. Generally 24 or 26 gauge stainless steel circumdental wire is best used for posterior teeth and 28 gauge wire is applied to the anterior teeth. Application of arch bars exerts a mild orthodontic force on individual teeth so care is taken, in regions such as the anterior segments, to minimize this force. The arch bars are applied to the upper and lower teeth and the jaws are brought into occlusion. Elastics placed between the arch bars guide and hold the segments in position with the maxillary dentition. The elastics are intially employed to effect a "gradual" reduction over several days. This is an excellent means of overcoming muscle spasm, which might be present initially. Once reduction is achieved, the elastics are replaced by wires. To be successful, intermaxillary fixation requires a reasonable complement of teeth. Large gaps of dentition, particularly around the fracture site(s), must be compensated by additional support (special splints or direct wiring). Arch bars alone do not afford sufficient stabilization for fractures of the mandibular body or symphyseal region or those fractures classified as "unfavorable." In addition, circumdental wiring tends to cause extrusion of the teeth—a point to consider in children or in adults with significant periodontal disease. A distinct advantage of arch bar intermaxillary fixation is that it can be done under local anesthesia with a minimum of instrumentation.

Lingual splints are useful adjuncts to arch bar fixation. They provide rigid stabilization, which checks unwanted rotational forces, and they also aid in preventing extrusion of the teeth. These are fashioned from dental models preoperatively or in situ at the time of operative reduction. The former method is preferable because it is more precise and saves operating time.

Other appliances used for intermaxillary fixation include interdental wiring (e.g., Stout, Risdon, Ivy loops), orthodontic bands, and acid-etch composite dental resins. Interdental wiring is occasionally useful as a temporizing measure to stabilize the fractured parts until the time is appropriate for a more definitive procedure. Although once used routinely in the management of mandibular fractures, this method has generally been replaced by direct arch bar fixation. However, it remains an excellent method of stabilization in the cooperative patient with a full complement of teeth. Orthodontic bands are effective in stabilizing the dentition. They are particularly useful in children because they do not cause extrusion of the dentition—a major problem when wiring primary teeth. However, their application is time-consuming and extremely expensive. Acid-etch composite dental resins represent a new generation of fixation devices. When applied properly, they provide excellent stabilization, do not cause extrusion of the teeth, and are not obstructive to the maintenance of daily oral hygiene. Their disadvantages lie primarily in their variable adhesiveness to the teeth—they are prone to fracture. These and similar appliances may soon supplant the standard circumdental wire.

Interosseous Fixation

Direct wiring of the fracture segments is indicated when intermaxillary fixation alone is insufficient in maintaining a proper alignment, as in cases of (1) fractures of the edentulous mandible, (2) displaced fractures in which one or more fragments do not contain teeth, (3) displaced fractures in children having deciduous dentition, and (4) fractures of both mandibular arches with a "floating" inter-arch segment.

The advantages of interosseous wire fixation of mandibular fractures are numerous. As with other fractures, direct exposure and wiring provide for a more precise, controlled means of reduction and stabilization. With internal support, the mandible can be released from intermaxillary fixation earlier (4 versus 6 weeks). The fixation provided is strong and is less susceptible to the forces of muscle pull. Disadvantages of this technique include the potential for operative injury to the facial or mandibular nerve, the creation of a facial scar, and possible infection. For the most part, these disadvantages can be minimized by careful operative technique and placement of incisions in the lines of minimum skin tension (wrinkle lines).

The placement of the interosseous wire should be planned so that the point of fixation is advantageous regarding the direction of muscle pull on the fragments. For example, an unfavorable fracture of the mandibular angle may open superiorly if a single wire is placed along the inferior border. In this case, a figure-of-8 wire or two wires may be necessary to effect a rigid stabilization.

When placing the drill holes, one must avoid injury to the dental roots and the mandibular nerve. If a high fixation is needed in the tooth-bearing position, wire fixation of the outer cortex will prevent injury to the cancellous components. In most cases, however, arch bar or lingual splint stabilization precludes the use of interosseous wiring in this area.

For most fractures of the mandible stabilized by interosseous wiring, we use a No. 24 or No. 26 stainless steel wire. It is important not to strip the periosteum extensively for fear of devascularizing the fracture segments. The fracture is reduced and held in reduction manually or with a bone clamp. Drill holes are made with a fine high speed drill, and the site is constantly irrigated with saline solution to avoid "burning" the bone. The wire is introduced, and both ends are pulled to engage the fragments. The ends are then twisted while maintaining moderate tension on the pull. The end point of twisting is based primarily on experience—we stop when the wire loop feels snug and elicits no play with movement. The wire breaks just after it loses its sheen at the apex of the twist. After the wire is secured, it is cut off about 10 to 15 mm from the apex indent while twisting it into one of the drill holes. When bringing the wire around the inferior border of the mandible, it is often helpful to notch the border with a burr and use this to seat the wire. This technique is helpful in preventing migration of the wire ligature and in preventing the palpable and sometimes painful wire lumps that can be felt through the skin. Every attempt must be made to close the periosteum over these repairs as well as to close the oral mucosa. These are contaminated wounds that contain a foreign body (wire). Synthetic absorbable sutures are preferred for the periosteal and/or fascial closures because of their decreased reactivity. Chromic gut (3–0) is used for the oral mucosa because it dissolves rapidly as the mucosa heals. (Synthetic absorbable sutures are not readily degraded in the oral cavity and often require removal.) We do not generally drain these wounds.

In most cases, the interosseous wire is left in position permanently; infection or irritation of the soft tissues is an indication for removal.

Other methods of interosseous fixation of the mandibular fracture include osteosynthesis compression plating, stapling, and K-wire fixation.

Compression plating of the mandibular fracture is a recent development borrowed from the orthopaedic experience. The method involves applying a special plate across the fracture site and securing the plate with screws into the outer cortex. This provides a rigid fixation of the fracture segments and requires less dissection than interosseous wiring. The technique is accurate and rather simple, though some experience is required to avoid errors in placement and drilling. Specially designed plates and screws constructed from stainless steel/molybdenum alloy are applied with a custom tool pack designed especially for this purpose. The hardware is expensive, and this remains the greatest disadvantage of this technique. In early cases, using the osteosynthesis plating, it was recommended that the hardware be removed 6 weeks following surgery. As more experience has been gained with the materials and technique, and as the plates have been magnified, these appliances may now be left in permanently. However, because of the relative bulk of the appliances, they are sometimes palpated easily in thin individuals, who may subsequently request their removal.

Large metallic staples have been employed for stabilizing fractured mandibles. The custom staples are tapped into small drill holes on each side of the fracture. These are sometimes used for the fixation of fractures of the edentulous mandible, particularly when there is a high degree of alveolar resorption and a rather fragile, thin mandibular remnant. The many problems associated with the use of these appliances include migration, breaking, splintering of the mandibular fragment during introduction, and extrusion. Their advantage lies in simplicity of application.

K-wire stabilization of mandibular fractures is occasionally employed either as a primary or a secondary means of fixation. It can also be used in temporary splinting of the fractured segments. Minimal periosteal dissection is required in the insertion of the K-wires—a potential advantage when treating comminuted fractures. K-wires are also helpful in maintaining correct spatial relationships of the fractured parts and are particularly useful when there are missing parts (i.e., as in blast injuries). They are best inserted with a power tool because of the density of the cortical bone of the mandible. Slower manually operated drills cause warping of the wire during insertion, with the production of large bone holes and a tendency for aberrant migration. Threaded K-wires are not recommended if the wire crosses through soft tissue (floor of the mouth) because the threads tend to grab the tissue and avulse resistant parts, such as nerves and blood vessels. A square "C-wire" is advantageous in some instances because it impacts the bone snugly and has less tendency for loosening and migration.

The disadvantages of K-wire insertion in the mandible are primarily that of infection, the potential for loosening and migration, and avulsion injury to soft tissue parts. Infection is related to the looseness of the K-wire and its proximity to the oral cavity. Loose wires should be removed. As a general rule, we avoid entering the oral cavity. In some instances, however, this is not practical. If the K-wire is rigid, bone infection is rare. In placing the K-wire, care should be taken to avoid major nerves and blood vessels. It is helpful to make a small incision (if the fracture has not been exposed) through the skin at the proposed entrance site and dissect bluntly to the bone, thus avoiding the soft tissue contacts with the wire as it engages and minimizing possible nerve or vessel injury.

External Fixation

Biphasic external fixation devices are excellent adjuncts to managing comminuted mandibular fractures, fractures complicated by missing parts, or fractures of the edentulous mandible. There are numerous methods for constructing a biphasic appliance. We prefer a simple but reliable technique, utilizing an endotracheal tube and threaded K-wires. The fracture segments are first reduced and brought into occlusion with the maxillary dentition. Arch bars, acrylic splints, dentures, or combinations of these are used to re-establish a correct dental alignment. Two K-wires, which pass through both cortical layers approximately 1 cm from the inferior margin are inserted into each mandibular fragment. In placing these wires, it is important to make adequate soft tissue incisions to avoid engagement of the surrounding soft tissues. The wires should also be oriented in a congruent horizontal plane. Next, an endotracheal tube is cut to match the appropriate arch span incorporating the protruding wires. The wires are cut approximately 4 cm above the skin level, and the shortened tube is impaled on the ends of the wires through small incisions placed on its facing surface. The positioned tube is filled with acrylic polymer injected through one end from a large truncated-tipped syringe. The polymer hardens after 10 minutes, creating a rigid external fixation device.

Biphasic appliances can be used in this fashion as an adjunct to interosseous fixation of the severely comminuted mandibular fracture or as an external "spacer" device for fractures complicated by missing parts. When properly secured, they can be employed for monomandibular fixation. Their disadvantages lie in the potential for infection, soft tissue injury during insertion and removal, and a rather imprecise means of fragment stabilization. These devices are not recommended in children because of possible injury to the unerupted tooth buds.

Craniomandibular fixation with a head frame or skull cap is not usually employed for isolated mandibular fractures. These methods are occasionally used in conjunction with other fractures of the facial skeleton and particularly those associated with subcondylar fractures of the mandible.

Teeth in the Line of Fracture

One is often confronted with the question whether to remove or retain a tooth in the line of fracture. There are many arguments for both sides of this controversy. Certainly, vital, firm, functional teeth in the line of fracture should not be removed. Conversely, one could not object strongly to the extraction of teeth with fractured roots, nonrestorable teeth, extremely loose teeth, or teeth with periapical or periodontal disease that are in the line of fracture. In many instances, teeth in the line of fracture aid in stabilization. Our philosophy in these cases is to remove all teeth in the line of fracture that might contribute to the development of infection. We do not consider any benefit gained from stabilization to outweigh the potential sequelae of infection.

Similar controversy exists regarding removal of impacted or partially erupted mandibular third molar teeth associated with the line of fracture. In these cases, we prefer to extract the tooth and secure the fragments with an interosseous wire through the buccal cortical plate. This approach has not, in our experience, caused any complication and indeed removes a lingering problem.

Treatment of Mandibular Fractures

The treatment of mandibular fractures can be divided into four major categories based on the anatomic region involved: (1) condylar fractures, (2) angles, ramus, and coronoid fractures, (3) body and alveolar ridge fractures, and (4) anterior fractures. There are numerous other classifications, but this method simplifies an otherwise complex arrangement. The following treatment plans take into account an understanding of the influence of the various muscle groups as they act on the fracture segments.

Condylar Fractures

Undisplaced or minimally displaced fractures of the condylar neck are treated conservatively by closed reduction and intermaxillary fixation for 3 weeks. In bilateral condylar fractures treated by closed reduction, intermaxillary fixation is continued for 4 weeks because of the tendency to develop an open-bite deformity.

Dislaced condylar fractures are best managed by open reduction and internal fixation in conjunction with intermaxillary fixation. Absolute indications for this approach include (1) displacement of the condyle into the middle cranial fossa, (2) lateral displacement of the condyle, (3) the presence of foreign body (e.g., bullet, shrapnel), (4) displaced condylar fractures in children, and (5) the inability to obtain proper occlusion by closed reduction. Open reduction and internal fixation should also be considered for displaced condylar fractures in patients having a social or medical problem that would preclude intermaxillary fixation (e.g., alcoholism, seizure disorder, neurologic problem).

The type of surgical approach used for these fractures depends primarily on the location of the fracture and the type of internal fixation to be employed. Two basic exposures are used: (1) the submandibular approach, and (2) the periauricular approach. The submandibular approach is most commonly used and gives adequate exposure for most condylar fractures except the very high neck fractures. An incision is made approximately 2 cm below the mandibular angle in a convenient neck crease. Care must be exercised to avoid injury to the marginal branch of the facial nerve, which is encountered just deep to the platysma anterior to the angle. Variations in the course of this nerve must be anticipated. In most cases, the inferior course of the nerve is not beyond 1.5 cm of the lower mandibular margin. The identified nerve is reflected superiorly and protected. At the level of the mandibular angle, the muscle insertions are divided, and a subperiosteal dissection of the lateral surface of the ascending ramus is performed to the fracture site. The distal fragment is retracted inferiorly to facilitate the exposure. The condylar fragment is usually displaced medially. Occasionally, it is helpful to bluntly dissect upward along the lingual surface of the ramus to engage the condylar fragment and guide it into position with digital manipulation. Care must be taken to avoid injury to the inferior alveolar nerve, which enters the mandible on the ramus at the lingula. Muscle relaxation is a helpful adjunct during this part of the procedure.

After the condylar fragments have been reduced, the fracture is stabilized with an interosseous wire, a wire loop, or by intramedullary pinning. We prefer the intramedullary pin technique because it is simple and temporary, and provides excellent stabilization during healing. A small burr hole is drilled on the lingual surface of the angle until cancellous bone is encountered. A square "C-wire" is inserted through the skin and drilled up the medullary canal of the ramus into the condylar fragment, stopping in the head of the condyle. Intraoperative roentgenograms are taken to check the pin and fragment positions. Retrograde pinning of the fracture is occasionally employed if aberrant pin migration is encountered with the antegrade method. The fracture site is exposed, and a percutaneous pin is directed through the open end of the distal fragment and captured as it exits the angle. The fracture is reduced and the pin drilled into the proximal fragment.

The pin is cut 2 to 3 cm from the skin surface and capped with a cork. It is removed after 3 weeks. Intermaxillary fixation is continued for 2 weeks and then a soft diet is begun.

Very high displaced neck fractures of the condyle cannot easily be reduced by the angle approach and are best managed by direct exposure and interosseous wiring. This may be accomplished through a postauricular incision, which divides the ear canal. The facial nerve and parotid gland are reflected to expose the lateral and posterior surfaces of the temporomandibular joint. A second approach is a preauricular Hockey stick incision, which also allows for reflection of the parotid gland and access to the joint from below the zygomatic arch. Care must be exercised to preserve, as much as possible, the soft tissue attachments to the condylar fragment; otherwise, aseptic necrosis of this structure will occur.

Bilateral subcondylar fractures are notorious for producing severe open-bite deformities if displaced and are managed according to the guidelines stated previously. One must restore at least one side to maintain proper posterior vertical height, which helps to prevent occlusal collapse and subsequent anterior open bite.

Subcondylar fractures in children carry the risk of growth arrest leading to abnormalities in jaw development and ankylosis of the temporomandibular joint. Most of these fractures are managed conservatively without intermaxillary fixation. A soft diet allows early mobilization of the condyle—a possible prophylaxis against ankylosis. In the same context, a displaced condylar fracture should be managed by open reduction, with special care to avoid unnecessary periosteal stripping. Jaw motion is begun at 2 weeks because these fractures heal rapidly.

Dislocation of the Temporomandibular Joint

In the absence of fracture, the condylar head is displaced anteriorly out of its fossa, tearing its capsule. The jaw becomes locked in an open-bite position, and there is considerable pain associated with muscle spasm.

Most of the dislocations spontaneously reduce by the simple injection of lidocaine solution (1%) into the joint capsule. If this is unsuccessful, a manipulative reduction is required. The patient must be cooperative. Although not mandatory, intravenous valium is often helpful as a sedative, as well as a muscle relaxant.

In our technique for reduction of dislocated temporomandibular joints, the operator's thumbs are placed just lateral to the occlusal plane of the molar teeth on the buccal gingival surface with the fingers grasping the mandible extraorally along the posterior ramus. Placement of the thumbs on the occlusal surface can lead to bite injury of the operator's thumb when the jaw snaps into position. Gradual firm pressure is exerted to push the posterior mandible downward while pulling the anterior mandible upward as the condyl is reduced. The jaw "clicks" into position, and the patient notices immediate relief. A general anesthetic may be required to overcome the muscle spasm in some cases.

Angle, Ramus, and Coronoid Fractures

By definition, these fractures do not contain tooth-bearing segments. Consequently, their stabilization depends on the indirect influence of intermaxillary fixation. Favorable fractures whose line of obliquity lies against the masticatory muscle pull are best managed by intermaxillary fixation if adequate upper and lower dentition is present. In the edentulous patient, dentures can be used to effect this stabilization. The dentures are secured to the mandible by circum-mandibular wiring and to the maxilla by suspension wires from the piriform aperture, nasal spine, infraorbital rim or zygoma. Intermaxillary fixation is generally concluded by the fourth week and followed by graded physiotherapy to improve opening and closing.

Open reduction of these fractures supplemented with intermaxillary fixation is reserved for those characterized by displacement, an unfavorably oriented fracture line, or bilateral fractures. The preferred surgical approach is through a submandibular or angle incision.

Fractures of the coronoid process generally do not require open reduction and can be managed adequately by intermaxillary fixation.

Body and Alveolar Ridge Fractures

These fractures are characterized by the inclusion of tooth-bearing segments. If stable teeth are present on both sides of the fracture and a complement of occluding maxillary dentition is present, intermaxillary fixation is the procedure of choice. Open reduction of these fractures is indicated if (1) teeth are present on only one side of the fracture and the fracture angle is unfavorable, (2) there are no stable occluding maxillary teeth in the presence of an unfavorable fracture, or if (3) the mandible is edentulous.

For body fractures, a submandibular approach gives the best exposure. One or two interosseous wires are affixed and the jaws are secured by intermaxillary arch bars or denture appliances. In children, open reduction and internal fixation of these fractures carries the hazard of injury to the unerupted tooth buds.

In these cases, one must make every effort to place the wires very low along the inferior mandibular margin. Osteosynthesis plates may also be employed to stabilize the reduced fracture fragments—their use may eliminate the need for intermaxillary fixation.

Alveolar ridge fractures do not generally require open reduction unless they are "flail" and attached to a substantial piece of bone. Loose nonviable teeth are removed along with the small detached remnants of the alveolar ridge. The remaining teeth and attached alveolus are reduced to the dental arch and secured to an arch bar. In these cases, we do not like to use circumdental wiring because it tends to extrude the teeth. Dental bands or acid-etched adhesive appliances are best employed for this purpose. Occasionally, special acrylic lingual or occlusal splints are used when the adjoining dentition is absent or there are associated anterior or body fractures of the mandible.

Avulsed Teeth

Successful replantation of avulsed teeth is dependent on the conditions under which the tooth has been stored and the time interval between injury and replantation. Replantation of the tooth within the first hour carries a success rate greater than 70 percent, whereas teeth that have been allowed to remain outside the alveolus for a period longer than 4 hours have a low success rate. The tooth should be kept moist if replantation cannot be performed immediately. The best storage medium is the saliva of the oral cavity, or the tooth can be placed in a sponge soaked with Ringer's lactate solution. The tooth socket should be thoroughly cleaned of blood clot at the time of replantation and irrigated copiously. The tooth should be placed out of occlusion so that it is not in contact with its opposing member in the other arch. The replanted tooth is best kept splinted by dental bonding or an acid-etched adhesive appliance if available; otherwise, a stiff Jelenko-type arch bar may be used to help hold the tooth in position. Replanted teeth should be splinted for a minimum of 4 weeks to allow for firm reattachment of the periodontal ligament.

Anterior Fractures

Symphyseal or parasymphyseal fractures require special attention because they cannot be maintained in adequate reduction by simple arch bar stabilization. The pull of the attached muscle groups causes the fragments to gape at their inferior margins, and the obliquity of the fracture line allows overriding of the fragments, producing a lingual tilt of one side. Rare midline fractures of the symphysis may not demonstrate these tendencies and are amenable to closed reduction.

Open reduction and intermaxillary fixation is the procedure of choice for the majority of these fractures. In the case of a symphyseal fracture associated with an angle or body fracture, a lingual splint is necessary to provide additional support for the intervening mandibular segment

Open reduction is performed by one of two approaches: the intraoral approach or the submental approach. We prefer the submental approach for comminuted fractures because minimal periosteal dissection is employed, thereby diminishing the chances of devascularizing a fracture segment. A 4- to 5-cm curvilinear incision is made under the chin, just inferior to the submental skin crease. The dissection is extended through the platysma to the fascia of the digastric muscles and then anteriorly to the inferior border of the mandible. At the fracture site(s), the periosteum is incised and elevated anteriorly and posteriorly just enough to allow placement of the drill holes along the inferior margin. The fracture is cleaned of debris and granulation tissue. If the fracture courses obliquely from anterior to posterior, a single hole is drilled through the overlapping segments and a wire is passed through the hole and secured tightly around the inferior margin. Perpendicular fractures are best stabilized by wiring through two adjoining holes or placement of a figure-of-8 ligature. The use of osteosynthesis plates as an alternative means of internal fixation has greatly simplified stabilization in these fractures. The periosteum is repaired with fine synthetic absorbable sutures, and the wound is closed in layered fashion. The gingival mucosa is usually disrupted in these cases, and this tissue should be debrided and closed when it is practical to do so. After the internal fixation is performed, the teeth are stabilized in proper occlusion by intermaxillary fixation. The additional support provided by a lingual splint is helpful in controlling the comminuted fracture and does not contribute to the extrusion of the incisor teeth (which in these cases may be loose, particularly those bordering the fracture). The advantages inherent to lingual splint stabilization have led us to use them more frequently for these fractures.

The intraoral approach is employed for simple fractures of the anterior mandible and fractures of the edentulous mandible. An incision is made in the labial gingival mucosa above the sulcus and a subperiosteal dissection is performed over the alveolar ridge of the mandible at the level of the fracture. A wire is placed through paired drill holes along the upper border and secured. This placement has the advantage of providing a fulcrum against the surrounding muscle pull, which tends to gape the fragments when the wire is placed along the lower border. Care must be taken to "seat" the wire or other appliance away from the alveolar crest to avoid denture erosion.

The intraoral "degloving" technique provides a very wide exposure of the anterior mandible, but necessitates rather extensive dissection. It is occasionlly used for simple anterior fractures of the dentulous mandible or for comminuted fractures if osteosynthesis plating is to be employed. (This does not require a posterior periosteal dissection.) Using this approach, we prefer a supraperiosteal dissection to the inferior border, where a 2- to 3-cm flap of periosteum is elevated, exposing the fracture site. The advantages of this technique lie in the wide exposure obtained and the avoidance of an external scar.

K-wires are occasionally employed for stabilization of these fractures. They are particularly useful in comminuted fractures when open reduction might jeopardize fragment viability. The fragments are manipulated into reduction and the K-wire is inserted percutaneously to engage the mandibular fragments and fix them to their stable counterparts. We avoid entering the oral cavity to minimize contamination. Although this method is rather imprecise, and for the most part has been supplanted by other techniques, it remains useful as a temporary means of stabilizing the anterior mandible.

Primary Bone Grafting

In the treatment of mandibular fractures characterized by loss of bone (in severely comminuted fractures with extensive devascularization or injuries resulting in direct loss of bone) consideration is given to (1) stabilization of the remnant mandibular segments according to their normal anatomic relationships, (2) reconstruction of the mandibular defect, and (3) provision of adequate soft tissue coverage.

All nonviable bone and soft tissue are debrided. If there are teeth on both sides of the defect, these can be used to help position the fragments in relationship to the maxillary dentition. Acrylic occlusal splints are extremely valuable for this purpose. Internal or external stabilization can be used to secure the fragments. We prefer a biphasic external appliance because it avoids a lot of cumbersome and rather irritating intraoral hardware. Furthermore, this appliance can be maintained during subsequent jaw reconstruction with bone grafts.

The question of placing a bone graft into an acute mandibular defect should be reserved for those rare instances in which (1) there has been minimal soft tissue trauma, (2) there is adequate soft tissue coverage, and (3) there is contamination.

Blast injuries to the jaw represent an absolute contraindication to primary bone grafting. The ideal situation exists in the comminuted mandibular fracture or those defects resulting from "clean blows" (e.g., machete, hatchet). For small defects, a corticocancellous bone graft from the iliac crest is excellent donor material. Some surgeons prefer a metallic mesh tray, which cups around the defect and is filled with cancellous bone chips. Both methods have their proponents as both work well. We prefer the former method because it contains minimal foreign body and does not require a secondary operation for tray removal. Absorbable synthetic trays, which do not require subsequent removal, are now available as well.

Large mandibular defects represent a major reconstructive problem and should probably be delegated to the management of post-traumatic sequelae. However, the recent techniques gained from our microsurgical experience allow the transfer of vascularized bone with the additional benefit of soft tissue for a composite reconstruction. The clinical application of this technique for acute traumatic defects remains limited to date.

Maxillary Fractures

Although the standard categorization of the maxillary fractures is represented by the Le Fort classification, it is infrequent that any patient presents with a "pure" form of the classic pathology. More commonly, a mixed type of injury is encountered with variable degrees of comminution of the involved structures. A characteristic not often associated with other facial fractures is the frequent occurrence of severe hemorrhage from the nose and nasopharynx. In most cases, bleeding usually stops with elevation of the head and the application of ice compresses. Occasionally, posterior and anterior nasal packs are necessary to control the hemorrhage. In the unusual circumstance, direct ligation or embolization of the internal maxillary artery or other branches of the external carotid system may be indicated.

Standard radiologic and CT assessment, while important, do not supersede the information gained from a detailed physical examination. The occlusion is particularly important as this represents a key in the operative management. Therapy is directed toward the restoration of functional dental occlusion. Some believe that equal emphasis should be given to esthetics, and we agree. Severely comminuted midfacial fractures can give rise to dishface deformities and elongation or shortening of the central facial height.

Direct wiring of the maxillary bone fragments and skeletal suspension have become the standard form of therapy, replacing older techniques such as chin straps, complicated head caps, and outrigger appliances. A stable mandible and a full complement of teeth simplify the management of these fractures. Broken or avulsed teeth, an edentulous jaw, and a fractured mandible are given first consideration. In these cases, the mandible is stabilized and custom acrylic occlusal splints, bite splints, spacers, or dentures are employed to guide the disharmonious segments into the proper position. The maxilla is "floated" into a functional occlusion with the mandible, and the two structures are thus immobilized by intermaxillary fixation. In this fashion, the maxilla is passively aligned to the mandible and then fixed to the stable facial skeleton by direct interosseous wiring or skeletal suspension. Care must be taken to ensure that the mandibular condyles are resting in their centric position at the completion of the reduction to avoid later temporomandibular joint problems (see Table 1).

Alveolar Fractures

Simple segmental fractures of the alveolus are manipulated into reduction and stabilized by direct ligature or arch bar fixation to the adjacent dentition.

An acrylic palatal-alveolar splint constructed from a plaster dental model is an ideal method for stabilizing comminuted tooth-bearing segments of the alveolus as well as palatal fractures. Occasionally, a distracted fragment may be recalcitrant to the manipulative reduction and alignment to the remaining dental arch. In these cases, we prefer a direct open reduction and interosseous wire fixation through the vestibular mucosa. Precise dental alignment is completed by the employment of a stiff single arch bar. Posterior segmental fractures of the alveolus may benefit from a combination of interosseous fixation and intermaxillary fixation of both arches. Fixation for a period of 4 to 6 weeks is usually employed. After that, the patient is kept on a mechanical soft diet for an additional 3 to 4 weeks to prevent loosening by occlusal forces during eating. The alternative method of applying upper and lower arch bars and elastic traction to guide the dental bearing fragment into position is often complicated by incomplete reduction, rotation of the fragment, or labial eversion. In addition, this method requires a class I type of occlusion to be successful.

Le Fort I Fractures

Transverse fractures of the maxilla can be managed by a variety of techniques, yet the prerequisite common denominator is primary establishment of correct occlusal relationships. This is accomplished by intermaxillary fixation. Arch bars are applied to the upper and lower dentition. The tooth-bearing maxillary fragment is disimpacted with Walsham forceps and brought into proper occlusion with the mandible. Elastics are applied, bringing the two components together. We like to orient the elastics forward from the maxilla to the mandible so as to overcome the tendency to an open-bite deformity. The maxillary fragment is reduced to its normal position with the facial skeleton. By placing a finger in the external meatus of the ear one can palpate the mandibular condyle to check its position in the fossa. It is important not to leave the condyle distracted after maxillary reduction, for reasons already explained.

In isolated Le Fort I fractures, reduction and intermaxillary fixation alone may provide sufficient stabilization. Some argue that it is necessary to fix the maxillary fragment to the stable facial skeleton in order to prevent a long-face deformity. However, comprehensive study of this concept has not borne out this statement, but it is probably safest to stabilize these fractures with suspension wiring. A variety of methods are available, and all employ the attachment of stainless steel wires to a stable part of the facial skeleton (infraorbital rim, lateral orbital rim, zygomatic arch), and then to the maxillary arch bar at a point of suspension. We prefer stabilization to the lateral orbital rim just above the zygomaticofrontal suture line. This approach is simple and places the suspension point more central and posterior to the others; it has the advantage of preventing the common posterior collapse of the maxillary dentition—a major cause of open-bite deformities in these fractures.

After the maxillary fracture has been reduced and stabilized to the mandible by intermaxillary arch bar fixation, the lateral supraorbital rims are exposed through bilateral brow incisions. A No. 26 wire is connected to a pull-out wire and passed through a small drill hole in the supraorbital rim. The two ends of the wire loop are passed through the temporal fossa attached to a long curved wire passer. The wires are delivered into the mouth at the level of the upper first molar on each side. After the maxillary reduction and the position of the mandibular condyles are checked, the wires are fastened to the maxillary arch bar and twisted until snug. The pull-out wire is brought out through the skin above the brow and attached loosely to a button.

Elastics securing the intermaxillary fixation are replaced with wires after 48 hours or when the teeth look and ''feel'' like they are in good occlusion. The teeth are left in intermaxillary fixation for approximately 4 weeks. During this time, a rigorous course of oral hygiene is implemented. Frequent mouthwashes and brushing are extremely important in preventing gum and dental disease. Dietary counseling is often necessary as intermaxillary fixation necessitates a liquid diet with attendant restriction of food intake and the disturbance of normal eating habits. The arch bars are left in place for 1 or 2 weeks after intermaxillary fixation is terminated. The diet is advanced to solid foods during this time. Careful frequent checks of the occlusion are made with special consideration given to the development of an open bite. Any shift of the dentition is treated by resumption of the intermaxillary fixation (with elastics, then wire) for an additional 2 weeks.

Le Fort II Fractures

These pyramidal fractures of the midface are best managed by direct interosseous wiring of the infraorbital rims and nasofrontal process followed by suspension wiring from the zygomatic process of the frontal bone. An intact mandible and correct occlusal alignment are prerequisites to fixation of the maxilla. Frequently, there are associated zygomatic and orbital fractures, which should be reduced and stabilized to the facial skeleton prior to management of the maxilla.

Injuries to the lacrimal sac and canaliculi should be suspected in all Le Fort II fractures. Function is usually maintained with proper fracture reduction. In severely comminuted fractures, exploration of the medial orbital wall and drainage of the lacrimal apparatus may be indicated (discussed previously).

Comminuted Maxillary Fractures

Severely comminuted fractures of the maxilla are reconstructed by piecemeal interosseous wiring through an intraoral approach. It is important to remove all bone fragments and foreign bodies (teeth) from the maxillary sinus to prevent possible infection. If the anterior maxillary wall is unstable, the sinus is packed with a rubber drain to provide additional support. The maxillary sinus pack is removed after 7 days, when the fracture segments have consolidated.

Panfacial Fractures

Combined fractures of the facial skeleton are the result of high-velocity impact usually sustained in automobile or motorcycle accidents. The tremendous force absorbed by the head in these injuries is frequently manifested by intracranial and cervical spine sequelae. The patients may not demonstrate any airway difficulties initially, but may soon succumb to the effects of massive hemorrhage and inevitable swelling. A cricothyroidotomy should be performed as a part of the initial trauma management.

The surgical philosophy employed in these injuries is reduction of the fractures into their anatomic positions, fixation to a stable support (usually the skull or a craniofacial outrigger appliance), and soft tissue repair.

In the acute situation, therapeutic priorities are given to the control of hemorrhage, ophthalmologic emergencies, and frontal bone or other fractures communicating with the cranial cavity. If massive swelling is present, definitive management of the remaining fractures is delayed for approximately 5 days, and supportive measures are employed (e.g., temporary stabilization of the fractures, wound closure, oral lavage).

Mandibular fractures are repaired first, followed by sequential reduction and stabilization of the zygomas, nasoethmoid region, orbital floors, and maxilla. Comminuted fractures are treated by direct interosseous wiring of the fracture segments with stabilization of the repaired "bloc" to a rigid support, such as an adjacent facial bone, the orbital rims, frontal bone, zygomatic arch, or an outrigger appliance. Considerable improvisation is required as these fractures rarely follow any stereotyped pattern. Intermaxillary fixation, with the reconstruction of a normal or "preinjury occlusion," correct projection of the facial parts, and facial symmetry, are key end points of therapy.

Blast Injuries to the Face

The devastating effects of a high-velocity projectile, as from a gun or a bomb, represent the most complex of facial injuries. Such injuries may produce extensive destruction of soft tissue, comminuted fragmentation of bone, loss of composite facial parts, and widespread impregnation of foreign bodies. These wounds are difficult to assess at the outset. Initial care is directed to the establishment of an airway and restoration of blood volume. Arteriography should be performed if there is suspicion of vascular injury. CT scan assessment is, at times, valuable, but may be clouded because of the deflections caused by metallic foreign bodies.

Operative management of these injuries is staged and consists of initial cleansing, minimal debridement, and hemostasis. Antibiotic and tetanus prophylaxis is instituted at the outset. Broad-spectrum therapy (penicillin, erythromycin, cephalosporin) is recommended.

As a rule, we do not close these wounds primarily because of the high propensity to infection and the indeterminability of tissue viability. Repeat wound exploration is performed in 24 to 48 hours, and further debridement of the devitalized bone and soft tissue is effected. Wound closure is planned as a secondary procedure, incorporating a multidisciplinary approach. First considerations are given to the re-establishment of bony relationships and appropriate drainage of the paranasal sinuses. Direct interosseous wiring, craniofacial appliances, acrylic splints, and intermaxillary fixation constitute the primary means of fixation for this purpose. Bone grafting is reserved for the reconstruction of the orbital walls, rims, and floor, and the major facial buttresses, provided adequate soft tissue coverage is available. Nasal, septal, palatal, and mandibular reconstructions are performed as delayed procedures after the initial wounds have healed.

After the facial skeleton has been repaired, the soft tissues are closed. Despite the impressive defects encountered, many of these wounds can be closed by approximation. Others may require the introduction of skin grafts, local or regional flaps, or simple skin-to-mucosa closure. Because of the nature of the injury, fibrosis of the soft tissues is a common sequela and can pose significant problems in later facial reconstruction. For this reason, it is advantageous for bony defects that are not reconstructed primarily to be supported with temporary obturator devices to check the tissue contraction. This is particularly applicable in the region of the anterior mandible, the maxilla, and the palate.

TRAUMA TO THE TORSO AND EXTREMITIES

TORSO TRAUMA: AN OVERVIEW

DONALD D. TRUNKEY, M.D.

Conceptually, the torso may be viewed as a cylinder that has an outer muscular coat to protect the viscera within. The upper torso and all of the posterior torso have additional bony protection. Ingeniously attached to the upper torso are the two shoulder girdles and upper extremities that deal primarily with work, food gathering, and other fine motor skills. The bottom part of the cylinder is the pelvis, which transmits the weight of the upper body and articulates with the two lower extremities that are primarily concerned with locomotion.

The upper 35 to 40 percent of the cylinder contains the thoracic viscera separated from the remaining abdominal viscera by the diaphragm. Traditionally, trauma to the torso has been divided into abdominal and thoracic components, but this is artificial because it is primarily based on division by specialty and does not recognize injury patterns, necessary treatment, or anatomy.

The torso may be divided into three sagittal zones: two lateral and one midline (Fig. 1). In general, trauma, blunt or penetrating, that involves the midline zone is more serious and more likely to be lethal than trauma in the lateral zones because the heart, great vessels, and spinal cord occupy this space. In many instances, the lateral zones do not require operative intervention, particularly when the upper torso is involved.

The torso may also be divided into three zones from the cephalad aspect to the rostral aspect (Fig. 2). Zone 1 comprises the torso from the nipples cephalad. Zone 2 is the area between the nipples and the umbilicus. Zone 3 comprises the remaining lower torso, including the pelvis. Zone 1 injuries, exclusive of the midline, do not usually require operative intervention. (Exceptions include injuries to the vessels where they extend over the bony thorax.) Midline zone 1 injuries have a high mortality rate whether caused by blunt or penetrating trauma.

Zone 2 injuries are particularly common following blunt trauma. These injuries are sustained from the steering column and are particularly prevalent in

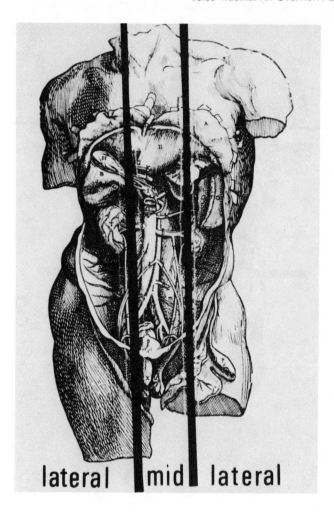

Figure 1 The torso divided into the three sagittal zones.

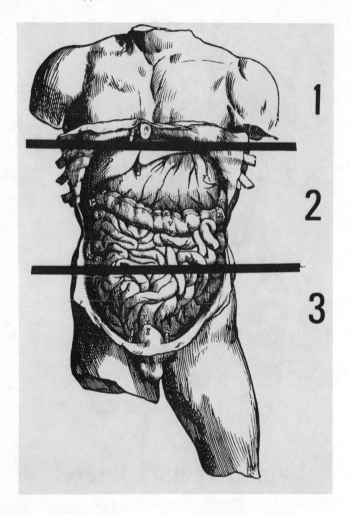

Figure 2 The torso divided into three zones from cephalad to rostral aspect.

the unrestrained driver. Examples of injuries in this zone include rupture of the myocardium, myocardial contusion, rupture of the liver, laceration of the spleen, and injuries to the pancreas and duodenum. Although penetrating injuries to the lateral portions of zone 1 may be managed nonoperatively because of the low pressure within the pulmonary parenchyma, zone 2 injuries almost invariably require exploration. Penetrating injuries to zone 3 also require exploration, but in blunt trauma, it may be prudent to take a more conservative approach. Because of the viscoelastic properties of the intestine, complete disruption is uncommon, and bleeding into the pelvis is best managed by alternative means.

In contrast to treatment of the extremities, which is directed primarily at restoring locomotion and other motor skills, primary goals of treatment in the bony torso are control of bleeding, correction of neurologic deficits, and restoration of pulmonary function.

It is a general axiom that if the organism has sustained enough kinetic energy from blunt trauma to damage one organ within the torso, others may also be injured. Similarly, a bullet or knife respects no artificial boundaries within the torso, such as the diaphragm, and may penetrate almost any organ on both sides of the diaphragm, depending on the velocity of the thrust and the trajectory.

The remainder of this section will address injury of individual organs and their treatment within the torso.

THE NECK

ERWIN R. THAL, M.D., F.A.C.S.

The management of neck injuries has undergone close scrutiny during the past decade. The time-honored dictum of mandatory exploration for all wounds that penetrate the platysma has been challenged by those who advocate a more conservative approach. Improvement in diagnostic techniques such as arteriography, endoscopy, and contrast radiology now allows better evaluation of potential areas of injury. Selective nonoperative observation has been recommended by many authors for patients with low risk of injury and no objective clinical signs. Current data would suggest there is a group of patients who seemingly do well in the initial post-injury period with nonoperative management. However, most trauma patients are not available for long-term follow-up, and hence the true incidence of long-term complications is not known.

Neck trauma is most commonly caused by penetrating injuries: stab wounds, gunshot wounds, and other sharp implements. The tract of a stab wound is more limited than that of a gunshot wound; however, innocuous-appearing cuts and lacerations have the potential to cause devastating injuries. Because the path of a gunshot wound is totally unpredictable, a more aggressive diagnostic work-up is necessary. This work-up includes a complete evaluation of all structures from the base of the skull to the clavicles.

Although blunt trauma involves the neck less frequently, it also has the potential to injure any anatomic structure. Blunt trauma is more likely to cause musculoskeletal instability such as a cervical fracture or dislocation, especially when associated with decelerating forces.

ANATOMY

The neck is divided into three anatomic areas. Zone 1 involves structures at the thoracic outlet: the subclavian vessels, major vessels in the chest, lungs, esophagus, and trachea. Zone 2 includes the area between the clavicle and the angle of the mandible. Injuries in this area are the easiest to evaluate and expose at operation. Zone 3 injuries are located between the angle of the mandible and the base of the skull. Exposure is much more difficult in this region.

When evaluating patients with neck injuries, consideration must be given to all anatomic structures. Whereas the vessels generally command the most attention following establishment of an adequate airway, one cannot overlook injuries to the pharynx, esophagus, nerves, thyroid, muscles, and thoracic duct.

INITIAL EVALUATION

The major concern in the management of any patient with a neck injury, whether blunt or penetrating, is establishment and maintenance of an adequate airway. This is often complicated by the possibility of an associated cervical fracture, with or without neurologic injury. It is essential that the airway be secured early, as soft tissue swelling and hematoma formation can turn a relatively easy procedure into a difficult challenge. If simple maneuvers such as chin lift, suctioning, and oral airway insertion fail, formal intubation via the endotracheal route with the neck in the neutral position should not be delayed. If this is not possible, a nasotracheal tube should be inserted, and failure of either of these procedures would warrant a cricothyroidotomy, which is preferable to tracheostomy in urgent situations. Tracheostomy is best performed in the operating room as an elective procedure. If an injury occurs in the trachea, it is acceptable to place the tube at the site of the injury. It is advisable to pre-oxygenate the patient with a bag-mask device before attempting intubation, a procedure that generally takes longer than anticipated.

If a cervical fracture is suspected, the neck must be immobilized in the neutral position until one can ascertain that there is no evidence of injury. The cervical collar can be removed to permit completion of the examination of the patient, during which in-lying traction is provided by an assistant. Following the physical examination, a lateral cervical spine film usually is sufficient, but subtle injuries may necessitate a CT scan for definitive recognition. It is essential that all seven cervical vertebrae, as well as the odontoid (dens), be visualized. If the patient's condition is unstable, the neck must be kept in the neutral position and the injury treated as a fracture until proved otherwise.

Penetrating wounds should not be probed, cannulated, or locally explored. Opening a tract may dislodge a clot and thus trigger uncontrollable bleeding. Occasionally, local exploration is performed in the operating room with all ancillary support available. Similarly, a nasogastric tube is not inserted until just before the induction of anesthesia. The gagging and retching also may precipitate excessive bleeding.

Arteriography is indicated for patients with penetrating trauma that is proximal to a major vessel regardless of the zone of injury. Generous proximal and distal visualization of the suspected area of injury is important. Cerebral arteriograms are obtained on all patients suspected of having carotid artery injuries. The acquisition of multiple views, the use of subtraction techniques, and image magnification are all helpful in identifying subtle injuries. Arteriograms of the ipsilateral carotid and vertebral vessels are obtained on all patients with stab wounds of the neck, and four-vessel studies (both carotids and both vertebrals) in nearly all patients with gunshot wounds, especially if the missile traverses the midline.

Depending on the likelihood of esophageal injury and the stability of the patient, contrast studies with barium may be obtained. On occasion, endoscopy is used to identify an esophageal injury. Recent experience with both contrast radiology and endoscopy tends to favor the radiologic study, although a small number of injuries were missed with both techniques.

It must be emphasized that patients with hemodynamic instability should not undergo extensive, time-consuming, preoperative studies. On rare occasions, if all diagnostic studies are normal, a patient may be managed nonoperatively, but most patients who have undergone arteriography are taken to the operating room for a formal exploration. The usual preoperative preparations are made, including the insertion of chest tubes, if indicated, in patients with zone 1 injuries. Perioperative antibiotics, usually penicillin or cephalosporins, are used if an injury to the airway or digestive tract is suspected. If neither of these injuries is present, the role of antibiotics is less clear.

GENERAL APPROACH

A generous vertical incision is made along the anterior border of the sternocleidomastoid muscle for injuries in zones 2 and 3. Proximal and distal control of the vessels is obtained by dissecting the vessels on either side of the injury and securing with a vascular loop or umbilical tape. If the patient is actively bleeding, direct pressure is applied and control obtained quickly. No attempt at further dissection or repair should be made until the anesthesiologist has fully resuscitated the patient with fluids and blood.

SPECIFIC INJURIES

The Airway

Injuries to the trachea are closed with a single-layer extraluminal nonabsorbable suture. If a tube has been placed through the injury and is still needed, it is not necessary to create another ostomy site unless it has been placed in the first tracheal ring. Larger defects may require either a fascial flap or a synthetic patch. A Jackson-Pratt drain attached to bulb suction or a soft Penrose drain is used for a short period of time or until drainage ceases.

Vascular Injuries

Common Carotid Artery

After gaining proximal and distal control, resuscitating the patient, and achieving hemostasis, the examiner assesses the extent of injury. Anticoagulation is not used unless there is a prolonged ischemia time and no associated injuries are present that would preclude its use. A shunt is rarely used, but can be inserted if it becomes necessary to occlude the vessel for an extended time.

Lateral repair of the vessel is preferred, but it is important to adequately debride all devitalized tissue. This may necessitate a limited resection and primary anastomosis. It is important to secure a smooth intimal surface without tension on the suture line. Some injuries require a patch graft utilizing a vein or ligated external carotid artery. If an interposition graft is used, autogenous tissue, from either a reversed saphenous vein or the cephalic vein, is preferable to prosthetic material. The repair is completed with 6–0 vascular suture after the Fogarty catheter has been carefully passed to remove all clots. Before the last suture is placed, the proximal and distal clamps are momentarily released to flush out any clot or debris that accumulates at the clamp site.

Internal Carotid Artery

The same principles apply to repair of this vessel, although the external carotid artery can be ligated and transposed to serve as an interposition graft in selected patients. If a subadventitial hematoma is present, a vertical arteriotomy is made over the area and the inside of the vessel inspected for injury.

Exposure of the distal internal carotid artery may be difficult to achieve. Access to an additional 2 cm of artery can be accomplished by dislocating the mandible and pulling it forward.

If the injury involves an inaccessible area, it may be necessary to ligate the distal segment and perform an extracranial-intracranial bypass. This bypass procedure is indicated if a cerebral collateral circulation seen on arteriography is inadequate or if the neurologic deficit has been present for less than 2 to 4 hours. In rare desperate instances, the insertion of a Fogarty catheter has been used to achieve hemostasis in an extremely high injury.

As long as there is no neurologic deficit present, primary repair should always be attempted if technically possible. If there is a severe neurologic deficit and no flow present at the time of operation, ligation without an attempt at revascularization is recommended. If the deficit is dense, but flow is present, vascular repair is performed.

External Carotid Artery

This vessel can be ligated if necessary. If the injury is near the take-off from the common carotid, it is repaired unless the patient's condition becomes unstable.

Subclavian Artery

Base-of-the-neck injuries require aggressive management. Uncontrollable hemorrhage often necessitates an emergency thoracotomy. The right subclavian artery, both subclavian veins, and the distal two thirds of the left subclavian artery can be exposed through a clavicular incision, which includes resection of the middle one-third of the clavicle. After the posterior periosteum and subclavius muscle are incised, the subclavian vein is easily identified anterior and inferior to the artery. The origin of the right subclavian, innominate artery, and proximal left common carotid artery may be exposed through a median sternotomy incision. The clavicular incision can be extended into a sternotomy incision for additional exposure. The proximal subclavian artery is best exposed by performing an anterior or lateral thoracotomy.

Standard techniques of repair are used. Occasionally it is necessary to construct a panel graft if suitable autogenous tissue is not available and prosthetic material is deemed inadvisable because of bacterial contamination. Attempts at venous repair are made unless the patient's condition warrants ligation.

Vertebral Artery

With the liberal use of arteriograhy, vertebral artery injuries have been diagnosed with increasing frequency. Again, in the stable patient an attempt is made to control this injury by performing proximal and distal ligation.

The proximal part is easy to expose at its take-off from the subclavian vessel. The distal end may be a bit more difficult, but can be ligated at the C1-C2 interspace where it is easily accessible once the bony canal is unroofed. The vessel can be similarly ligated between C2 and C6 by removing the costal face of the appropriate cervical transverse process. This area is exposed by retracting the sternocleidomastoid muscle and mobilizing the longus colli and longus capitis. Prior to ligation, it is important to know that a normal contralateral vessel is present and that no spinal cord branches take off from the ligated segment.

Venous Injuries

Injuries to the internal jugular vein are repaired if possible. Lateral venorrhaphy, patch venoplasty, and resection with anastomosis are all acceptable techniques. In severe injuries requiring excessive debridement that precludes primary repair, ligation is preferred. Venous interposition grafts are not recommended. Whereas both internal jugular veins can be ligated, this procedure is not advisable unless there is no other choice. Lesser veins can be ligated without concern.

Thoracic Duct

Thoracic duct injuries occur more commonly with penetrating trauma in proximity to the left subclavian vessels. When identified, the duct should be ligated. These injuries are rare, but should not be overlooked because complications such as persistent drainage and chylothorax can be difficult to manage.

Pharyngeal and Esophageal Injuries

Penetrating trauma in the zone 3 area may injure the pharynx. Careful evaluation preoperatively and inspection of the area at the operating table are important. These injuries are closed in two layers and the area adequately drained.

Esophageal injuries in the neck are uncommon. Diagnosis is facilitated by contrast radiologic studies. If strongly suspected, preoperative endoscopy, preferably with a rigid scope rather than a flexible scope, may demonstrate the injury. An intraoperative technique used to help identify an esophageal injury is to withdraw the nasogastric tube to the level of the suspected injury. Air is then injected down the tube after the wound has been filled with saline irrigation fluid, and bubbles appear in the irrigation solution at the site of injury.

Esophageal injuries are repaired with an inner absorbable layer and an outer nonabsorbable layer. The area must be adequately drained. For devastating injuries requiring extensive resection and debridement, as seen with some shotgun wounds, it may be necessary to perform a cutaneous esophagostomy for feeding purposes and a cutaneous pharyngostomy for salivary drainage. Secondary reconstruction can be accomplished after healing.

Nerve Injuries

A careful search is made for injuries to the major nerves including the vagus, phrenic, recurrent laryngeal, hypoglossal, spinal accessory, and brachial plexus. The injured nerve is debrided and repaired primarily, if possible, with interrupted fine silk placed in the perineurium. Occasionally free nerve grafts are used, but more commonly the nerve endings are tagged for later reconstruction if the situation does not lend itself to primary repair.

Thyroid

Thyroid injuries are unusual, and bleeding usually can be controlled with suture ligation. Massive injuries are debrided, and on rare occasions, a lobectomy may be necessary.

Muscle and Soft Tissue

All necrotic muscle and soft tissue needs to be debrided, but it is essential that the vessels have some type of soft tissue coverage prior to closure. Occasionally, it is necessary to transpose a muscle such as the levator scapulae to cover an exposed vessel. Sometimes this can be accomplished by use of a myocutaneous flap.

CHEST WALL

FRANK R. LEWIS Jr., M.D.

Blunt trauma to the chest wall is one of the most common problems seen in the emergency department and may produce injuries both in the chest wall and within the thorax. The injuries that result are principally a function of the magnitude of force and the time over which it is applied (energy dissipation), and the location and direction in which it is applied. A knowledge of these factors should always be sought, as they provide the experienced clinician with the likely diagnostic alternatives. Penetrating trauma, in contrast, produces a more limited range of problems, prinipally hemothorax and pneumothorax. These will be treated in a separate chapter.

CHEST WALL CONTUSION

The least severe injury occurring with blunt trauma is chest wall contusion in which there is local soft tissue swelling and interstitial hemorrhage. This causes local pain and some accentuation of pain with deep breathing and coughing, as well as splinting of intercostal muscles in the area, but it rarely causes serious ventilatory compromise.

Rib Fracture

The next most serious injury and overwhelmingly the most common, is rib fracture. Fractures may be single or multiple. The number of ribs broken, and to some extent their location, are an indication of the severity of trauma. The ribs most commonly broken, because of their relatively exposed position, are the fourth through the tenth. The first and second ribs are well protected by the shoulder girdle and their fracture indicates that the force and energy dissipation was massive. Similarly, the eleventh and twelfth ribs are short and less exposed and so are fractured less commonly.

Splinting is universally accompanied by rib fractures, and as a result, decreased respiratory excursions and hypoventilation are the major complications to be expected. Effective pain relief with opiates may allow deep breathing to some extent; they should be used judiciously, but their use will not restore normal vital capacity. Splinting will increase with the number of ribs broken. Hypoventilation, with inability to clear secretions, becomes a progressively greater problem. When severe, progressive atelectasis results, and pneumonia frequently follows.

Ultimately, if there are multiple rib fractures, or if multiple ribs are broken in two sites, instability of a segment of the chest wall develops, and paradoxical motion with ventilation, or "flail chest" will result. This condition results when the structural integrity of the chest wall is lost so that efforts at inspiration, with increased negative intrathoracic pressure, result only in the inward movement of the unstable portion of the chest wall. Flail chest is a particularly severe and potentially lethal injury because it reduces markedly the ability to generate negative intrathoracic pressure. It therefore affects both lungs equally, not just the side on which there are fractures. This compromise reduces vital capacity dramatically, often out of proportion to the degree of paradoxical motion which is seen on physical examination. Efforts by the patient to increase depth of ventilation and raise minute ventilation are relatively inefficient; they increase the paradox more than they increase alveolar ventilation, and, at the same time, increase oxygen consumption due to the increased work of breathing. When the patient reaches this precarious state, where effectively he has no ventilatory reserve, decompensation, respiratory distress, carbon dioxide retention, respiratory acidosis, and death can occur with relative suddenness. An awareness of this possibility should lead the surgeon to assess respiratory status with especial care in any patient with rib fractures, but particularly in those who are over the age of 60 years. One must have a high index of suspicion, and must examine both hemithoraces carefully when the patient is first seen. The best method of assessment is with the patient supine and the thorax fully exposed. As the patient breathes, the anterolateral thorax on both sides is carefully examined for absolute respiratory excursion as well as relative motion of the two sides. If the patient complains of any pain with ventilation, careful rib-by-rib palpation is carried out to determine where the fractures are and to define the extent of the problem. Clinical palpation is a better guide than a plain film of the ribs because the chest roentgenogram does not show the costal cartilage-to-rib separations, which are equivalent to bony rib fractures, and often constitute the second fracture in a rib, thereby producing instability.

Any patient who has more than two or three broken ribs should have his vital capacity measured. This provides the best guide to the degree of ventilatory compromise. Although the measurement is rarely done, it is extremely simple and requires inexpensive equipment. It is also the only test that allows one to predict the degree of ventilatory reserve and the likelihood of later decompensation. Normal vital capacity is 60 to 70 ml per kilogram body weight, or approximately 4,500 ml for a 70 kg adult. Minimally adequate vital capacity is 10 to 15 ml per kilogram, or 700 to 1,000 ml in the average adult. Anyone with less than this vital capacity should be intubated and ventilated or, at the very least, observed in an intensive care unit where optimal nursing care can be provided.

As mentioned previously, older patients are more prone to decompensation than young ones and should be observed particularly carefully. It should also be recognized that the impairment of ventilation becomes worse during the first 3 days after injury owing to increasing chest wall edema and decreased compliance. Patients with marginally adequate ventilation often will not decompensate until the second or third day. If this is a concern, the patient must be observed in an intensive care unit until the danger period has passed. Rib stabilization and improving vital capacity begins about day 10, initially slowly, and then more rapidly. Such functional improvement begins well before callus can be seen at the fracture sites on x-ray films and, no doubt, results from fibrosis at the rib ends. Patients who are intubated initially for flail chest normally require ventilation for about 2 weeks and in severe cases for 3 to 4 weeks.

In selected patients with massive flail chest injuries from fractures to eight or more ribs, I have undertaken internal fixation of the ribs as described by Thomas with flat metal plates (Jergesen plates) that are normally used for fracture reduction. This technique entails exposure of the ribs with a posterolateral thoracotomy, then reduction of the fractures; the flat metal plate is bent to conform to the rib curvature. The plate is then "strutted" to the rib using an encircling stainless steel wire of large size (No. 18). The adjacent ribs above and below are then "strapped" to the rib, which has been internally fixed, using doubled No. 1 chromic sutures so that a single plate stabilizes three ribs. If this fixation technique is used to stabilize six ribs on a given side, that is all that is necessary to improve ventilation markedly and to hasten weaning from the ventilator. Experience with this technique so far is small, but the results have been dramatic in a few patients.

Sternal Fracture

Sternal fractures result from the same types of trauma as rib fractures, but require much greater force to produce and are far less common. Isolated sternal fractures rarely cause ventilatory compromise, but are a cause for concern because of the likelihood of myocardial contusion when they are present. The pain with a sternal fracture is usually severe and produces marked splinting, just as with rib fractures. In addition, costal cartilage fractures or cartilage–rib separations are usually present in association and add to the ventilatory problems. When the sternal fracture is nondisplaced no specific therapy is indicated. When the fracture is offset or overriding, it should be reduced and the ends wired together to maintain reduction.

With sternal and rib fractures, internal thoracic bleeding must also be evaluated and treated as necessary. The fracture of a rib may transect the accompanying intercostal artery, and the sharp rib ends at the site of fracture may lacerate the lung, causing intrapleural bleeding. With sternal fractures the internal mammary arteries may be similarly torn.

Intrathoracic Injury

Injuries within the chest caused by blunt trauma, which should be suspected when chest wall damage is severe, are pulmonary contusion, cardiac contusion, and major vessel disruption. Most commonly this occurs at the aortic arch just distal to the left subclavian artery. Pulmonary contusion usually occurs in the lung just beneath the area of impact and corresponds to the area where the rib damage is greatest. Cardiac contusion, as noted previously, is seen when there is direct sternal trauma or sternal fracture, most typically from an unbelted automobile driver who is thrown into the steering wheel hub. Aortic arch disruptions result from sudden deceleration with massive energy dissipation. The typical history in such cases is a fall from a height of 30 or 40 feet or ejection from a car or motorcycle on striking a fixed object at high speed. Such injuries will be discussed in detail elsewhere.

PENETRATING TRAUMA

With penentrating trauma to the ribs damage is usually minor and, except for single fractures that occur at sites of bullet impact, they are uncommon. In contrast, problems that result are from pleural-cutaneous communications that cause an open pneumothorax, from penetration of a lung with resulting air leak and pneumothorax, and from intrapleural bleeding due to either pulmonary damage or transection of a systemic artery, usually intercostal or internal mammary. When the penetrating trauma also crosses the mediastinum a new range of problems must be considered, particularly cardiac and great vessel injuries, tracheal-bronchial injuries, and esophageal perforation. All of these will be discussed separately in this book.

HEMOPNEUMOTHORAX

FRANK R. LEWIS Jr., M.D.

Hemothorax is the term used to describe free blood within the pleural space, and pneumothorax, free air. After either penetrating or blunt trauma one may see either condition alone, or both simultaneously as hemopneumothorax. With penetrating trauma, air may enter the pleural space either through the defect in the chest wall if it is large, or from lung parenchyma that has been penetrated. With blunt trauma, pleural air is nearly always a result of a lung laceration produced by rib fracture. Rarely, with blunt trauma, the sudden increase in intrapulmonary pressure at the time of impact may result in rupture of blebs on the lung, which produces pneumothorax without any direct pulmonary damage.

Two subtypes of pneumothorax—open pneumothorax (sucking chest wound) and tension pneumothorax—deserve comment because of their special features.

Open Pneumothorax

Open pneumothorax occurs when large missile penetration of the chest wall occurs and free communication between the pleural space and the atmosphere is produced. This results in inability to generate negative intrathoracic pressure with breathing efforts, because air exchanges through the chest wall defect rather than the trachea. Since pressures on both sides of the thorax are equal owing to the ability of the mediastinum to shift, air exchange, even in the undamaged lung, is adversely affected and the condition can rapidly become lethal. Emergency treatment is to close the chest wall defect with whatever is available so that negative intrathoracic pressure and some degree of ventilation can be reestablished in the undamaged lung. Any type of occlusive dressing can be used, as long as it prevents air exchange. Definitive care is operative closure of the defect.

Tension Pneumothorax

Tension pneumothorax is the creation of a closed pneumothorax under some degree of positive pressure, such that the lung is totally collapsed and the mediastinum is shifted toward the opposite side. It is thought to result from a flap valve mechanism at the visceral pleural surface, such that air is allowed to move from the lung into the pleural space, but cannot return in the opposite direction. In actuality, it is most common in patients who are being ventilated with an endotracheal tube with positive airway pressure. The need for treatment is relatively urgent if respiratory compromise is severe, or if signs of decreased venous return to the heart occur owing to severe mediastinal shift and partial occlusion

239

of the vena cavae at the thoracic inlet and the diaphragm. Treatment is the same as for routine pneumothorax.

Hemothorax results from bleeding from the pulmonary parenchyma, the hilar pulmonary vessels, the heart and major systemic arteries in the mediastinum, or the intercostal and internal mammary arteries. Bleeding from the pulmonary parenchyma, which is most commonly encountered with penetrating and blunt trauma, is usually self-limited because of the low pressures in the pulmonary circuit. Bleeding that is persistent or large in volume most commonly comes from intercostal or internal mammary arteries, which are at systemic pressures. Penetrating trauma which crosses the mediastinum or passes close to the pulmonary hilum may cause cardiac or great vessel damage, or hilar vessel injury. Although infrequent, such injuries are relatively lethal due to rapid exsanguination.

The diagnosis of hemopneumothorax is difficult on clinical grounds; chest x-ray is usually required. It should be suspected in all penetrating trauma and moderate to severe blunt trauma. If breath sounds are decreased on one side, or if there is dullness to percussion in the lower hemithorax, one may suspect the diagnosis. Tracheal shift is often sought, but except with tension pneumothorax, it is infrequently seen. Any patient who has penetrating or blunt chest trauma and respiratory distress should be assumed to have the condition until proved otherwise.

Definitive diagnosis is by chest films and is usually obvious on an upright or supine film. In upright films the blood tends to lie at the bottom of the lung and can be mistaken for a high diaphragm. The distinction is usually made by seeing a meniscus wrapping around the lateral edge of the lung adjacent to the chest wall. In supine films the blood tends to layer out posteriorly; this gives a picture of increased density to the entire hemithorax. When uncertainty exists, right and left decubitus views will usually define whether or not free blood is present.

Pneumothorax is easily missed if it is small, as the lateral chest markings tend to be dark anyway, and one may be missed by an overpenetrated film. The radiographic line of the visceral pleura is quite subtle. If there is any question about the diagnosis, an expiratory chest film, slightly underpenetrated, will usually allow it to be defined clearly.

When patients present with thoracic trauma and are in marked respiratory distress, treatment should be undertaken immediately as outlined previously. In the great majority of situations this is not the case, and chest films can be obtained prior to institution of treatment.

Treatment for both hemo- and pneumothorax is tube thoracostomy; insertion of the tube is carried out under local anesthesia as soon as the diagnosis is made. A large bore (No. 36 or No. 40 F) siliconized straight tube with multiple side holes should be used in all cases. Right angle tubes have no place in emergency placement, as they are difficult to position properly and should only be placed when the chest is open. Foley catheters, Malecot tubes, and the like should be condemned as they are inadequate for draining the pleural space.

The tube should be placed in the lateral chest between the anterior and posterior axillary folds (pectoralis major and latissimus dorsi), at the level of the nipple or above. Placement lower than this runs the risk of inserting the tube through the diaphragm, possibly into the parenchyma of the liver or spleen, as the diaphragm rises to within an inch or so of the nipple line in expiration. It is much easier to use the nipple line as a marker, rather than count interspaces, as the position on the circumference of the chest will warrant use of different interspaces.

Anterior placement of tubes in the second interspace at the midclavicular line should always be avoided in the emergency setting, as one is working under multiple disadvantages. In this location one must go through the body of the pectoralis major, which may be more than an inch thick, and in women it creates a scar in the breast. The ribs separate poorly this close to the sternum and it is difficult to insert a large bore tube. Finally, the direction of the tube tends to hold the lung away from the chest wall, preventing full expansion. All of these problems are obviated with lateral placement, which is far easier for the physician and patient, and guarantees a "universal" tube which will evacuate air or fluid effectively. The final objection to an anterior tube is that it will not evacuate fluid.

After selection of the insertion site, the chest wall is prepped with an iodine containing antiseptic solution, and sterilely draped. We have found a 36 inch square drape with a 3 inch center hole ideal for this purpose. The skin, subcutaneous tissue, and the parietal pleura at the insertion site are infiltrated thoroughly with 1 percent xylocaine. A 2 to 3 cm incision parallel to the ribs is made and carried down through the subcutaneous tissue. The fascia of the chest wall is incised, but the incision is not carried into the pleural space. A large curved blunt-nosed clamp (Pean or large Mayo) is then inserted forcefully from the bottom of the incision into the pleural space, using the left hand grasped tightly around the clamp as a stop to prevent it penetrating more than a couple of centimeters through the parietal pleura. The jaws of the clamp are then spread to create an opening large enough to admit the fingertip, and a rush of air will usually be heard. The index finger is then inserted into the pleural space and swept circumferentially to insure that one is in the proper site, and that the pleural surfaces are not adhesed together. If they are, insertion of the tube may cause it to enter the lung parenchyma, creating further damage. The tube is then inserted, either directly or after grasping the tip with the curved clamp, to allow it to be directed. After entering the pleural space, the tube is directed posteriorly and superiorly until one feels it contact the mediastinum. The tube is moved back and forth until it is comfortably positioned and one is sure it is in the proper place and is not kinked.

A large No. 0- or No. 1-silk suture is then placed through both sides of the incision, either using a U-stitch, or a simple through and through stitch, and a single throw is placed. The tails of the suture are then wrapped several times around the tube and tied. At the time of tube removal, the knot holding the tube is cut, and the tails are unwrapped. When the tube is removed, the sutures may be pulled tight to close the incision and to prevent air entry into the pleural space.

The tube is connected to a chest suction unit at 20 cm suction and is then observed closely for amount and rate of bleeding as well as for the presence of a continuing air leak or not. In most cases there will be a rapid drainage of blood within the first few minutes and this will quickly decrease. If it continues, or if the air leak is massive, the patient may need to be prepared for surgery in order to repair the damage and control the bleeding via thoracotomy.

The usual indications for thoracotomy are the drainage of 1,000 to 1,500 ml of blood or more initially, a continuing rate of bleeding greater than 200 to 300 ml per hour, or a massive air leak such that the lung cannot be kept expanded. In 85 to 90 percent of cases this will not be necessary, and only the chest tube will be needed. Following insertion another chest film is obtained to verify position, evacuation of blood, and reexpansion of lung. Occasionally the hemothorax will be clotted, and a density will remain on radiography. Unless it is massive and interferes with lung expansion, thoracotomy for removal is not necessary since it will lyse spontaneously and be reabsorbed over several weeks, leaving no adverse sequelae.

After the chest tube has been secured, the patient may be admitted to the ward or intensive care, depending on his general status and other injuries. The presence of a chest tube alone is usually not enough to require admission to the intensive care unit, since most surgical wards have nursing staffs who are comfortable with management of tubes and suction units.

If the tube was inserted primarily for bleeding, it is left in place until the drainage becomes serous, and decreases to less than 75 ml per day. If it was inserted because of a pneumothorax, it is left in place until any air leak stops plus an additional 24 hours on suction. The suction is then discontinued and the patient is observed for a further 24 hours, followed by a chest film to verify full lung expansion. If there is no problem, the tube can be removed. Immediately following tube removal, an x-ray should always be obtained, and the patient should be observed in hospital for at least an additional 12 to 24 hours, followed by another chest film before discharge.

LARYNX, TRACHEA, BRONCHI, AND LUNGS

ROBERT F. WILSON, M.D., F.A.C.S.

LARYNGEAL INJURY

Clinical history is extremely important when diagnosing trauma of the larynx. The classic presentation is that of an individual who is involved in a motor vehicle accident in which he is pitched forward, striking his anterior neck on the steering wheel or dashboard. The increased use of off-road vehicles such as snowmobiles, dirt bikes, and all-terrain vehicles has resulted in an increase of laryngeal trauma from accidents involving guy-wires and fences.

Diagnosis on physical examination is often difficult. Characteristically patients with severe laryngeal injury present with local tenderness, subcutaneous emphysema over the neck, and voice changes. Except for local tenderness or crepitus, some patients may have minimal evidence of injury until an airway problem, heralded by inspiratory stridor, suddenly develops. The use of laryngoscopy for diagnosis must be considered carefully because the instrumentation itself may suddenly convert a partial obstruction into one which is complete.

In elderly patients the laryngeal cartilages may be calcified, and fractures of these structures may occasionally be apparent on plain x-ray films of the neck. Occasionally, routine cervical spine films may reveal that the hyoid bone is displaced cephalad. If one draws a horizontal line to the top of C3, the hyoid bone should be beneath this line. If the hyoid bone is above the line, this is presumptive evidence of laryngeal trauma. In the more subtle injuries, diagnosis may only be possible with a computerized tomography (CT) scan.

If an airway obstruction develops, emergency endotracheal intubation may be required, but this can cause increased laryngeal injury and, if not successful, result in complete airway obstruction. If endotracheal intubation is not possible, a cricothyroidotomy (coniotomy) may be life-saving. In the most severe injuries with total laryngotracheal separation, endotracheal intubation or cricothyroidotomy may not provide an adequate airway. Intubation over a bronchoscope may occasionally be helpful in such circumstances, but an emergency tracheostomy affords the most certain chance of salvage in such patients.

TRACHEAL INJURY

Blunt trauma to the cervical trachea except at its orgin is rare, but injuries following penetrating neck trauma are not unusual. Hemoptysis is virtually diagnostic of tracheal laceration. Mediastinal or subcutaneous emphysema usually indicates airway or pharyngoesophageal injury. In questionable cases, bronchoscopy can be diagnostic. Nevertheless, in some instances neck exploration for stabs or gunshot wounds will have been already planned since the injury has penetrated the platysma.

Exploration is usually performed through a sternocleidomastoid incision in order to rule out other cervical trauma or through a long collar incision about a centimeter above the sternum and clavicles if it is likely that only a tracheal injury is present. Most injuries can be repaired using interrupted 4–0 Prolene sutures. More extensive lacerations with actual loss of tracheal tissue may require mobilization of the trachea by means of releasing the hyoid muscles. With more severe injuries, local pleura or muscle should be used to reinforce the closure. The closure should also be protected for at least 7 to 10 days with endotracheal intubation or tracheostomy with the balloon placed below the repair.

Injury of the Distal Trachea or Bronchi

If there is massive subcutaneous or mediastinal emphysema and/or if there is a large pneumothorax that is not corrected by two large, well placed chest tubes which are bubbling vigorously, injuries to the distal trachea or major bronchi should be suspected. In such instances, bronchoscopy should be performed as soon as possible in order to rule out a tracheobronchial tear or proximal bronchial obstruction by a foreign body or secretions. Longitudinal tears of the trachea usually occur within 2 cm of the carina at the junction of the cartilagenous and membranous portions. Tears of the major bronchi are usually transverse and are particularly common at the origins of the upper lobe bronchi.

As a temporizing measure, a Carlens-type endotracheal tube may be inserted to control massive air leak. This double-lumen allows separate ventilation of each lung; however, aspiration of blood or secretions through these relatively narrow tubes can be difficult. In addition, one must have extensive training and experience in inserting double-lumen tubes to be able to do this quickly under emergency circumstances.

Surgical repair is indicated as soon as possible. Choice of right or left thoracotomy is determined primarily by the chest x-ray film and findings at bronchoscopy. The edges of the laceration must be carefully approximated using interrupted 4–0 Prolene or Vicryl sutures. The repair should be reinforced with a covering flap of pleura or intercostal muscle. Repeated postoperative bronchoscopy may be required to remove secretions that tend to accumulate distal to large bronchial tears.

If the bronchial tear is missed initially and the lung reexpands, the patient almost invariably develops bronchial stenosis with distal atelectasis and repeated infections that eventually require resection of the involved lung. This emphasizes the importance of a high index of suspicion and early bronchoscopy for diagnosis.

PULMONARY PARENCHYMAL INJURY

Pulmonary Contusion

The most frequent injury to the lung after blunt trauma is pulmonary contusion. Diagnosis of pulmonary contusion can usually be made from the history and findings of localized opacification on the initial chest roentgenogram; however, the extent of contusion is usually greatly underestimated on the x-ray film.

Hypoxia is often the first clinical evidence of severe lung contusion, but this may be minimal when the patient is first seen. The arterial PO_2 tends to deteriorate progressively over the next 24 to 48 hours as edema increases in the area of the parenchymal lung injury. If the contusion is large enough, or is bilateral, a significant fall in compliance with increased difficulty in breathing and tachypnea may also be seen. If there are segmental fractures of three or more ribs or a fractured sternum, a significant flail chest is often seen.

Treatment is primarily directed at maintaining adequate ventilation and preventing atelectasis; this is effected by promoting deep breaths and coughs. If chest pain prevents adequate coughing, intercostal nerve blocks with 0.5 percent marcaine to the involved ribs, as well as to the two ribs above and below the injury and to any residual tender spots, often provide dramatic pain relief for 6 to 8 hours or longer. If the patient still has trouble bringing up his secretions, nasotracheal suction or even bronchoscopy may be required. The use of diuretics, salt-poor albumin, and steroids are advocated by some, but are extremely controversial and could be harmful. Fluid overloading must be avoided.

Endotracheal intubation and ventilatory support should be considered if the arterial Po_2 remains below 60 to 80 mm Hg on 40 percent oxygen, or if the PCo_2 exceeds 50 mm Hg in the face of normal arterial bicarbonate levels. Ventilatory support is also recommended with large pulmonary contusions and/or flail chest if the patient has concomitant shock, massive transfusions, two or more other associated injuries, coma, fracture of eight or more ribs, or severe preexisting pulmonary disease.

Pulmonary Hematoma

The clinical appearance of a pulmonary hematoma resulting from a missile or stab wound is often not different from a contusion. However, the hematoma is likely to appear more dense and more discrete on x-ray film. There is some debate on the best management of large hematomas resulting from high velocity missile wounds. Some surgeons believe that immediate thoracotomy should be performed to remove the involved segment or lobe; however, the majority of authors still favor a conservative approach and remove the involved lung only if there is severe or continuing hemorrhage, air leak, or infection.

Severe Pulmonary Laceration

Pulmonary lacerations are common after extensive rib fractures. Although a lung injury is seldom visible on the chest roentgenogram, it is usually manifested clinically by a major hemothorax or a sustained air leak. A thoracotomy is indicated for the pneumothorax if it is large and persistent, particularly, if a major air leak is also present. A thoracotomy is indicated for hemorrhage, if (1) the entire hemothorax is opacified, if (2) the patient has shock which is persistent or which develops as the hemothorax is being evacuated, if (3) there is rapid removal of more than 1,500 to 2,000 ml of blood, if (4) blood loss exceeds 200 to 300 ml per hour for more than 4 to 6 hours, or if (5) the patient has significant hemoptysis.

If there is moderate to severe hemoptysis, or if it is likely that the pulmonary hilum is injured, the patient should not be turned for a standard posterolateral thoracotomy, but should have the surgery done in a supine position. This prevents intrabronchial blood from the injury flooding the dependent lung. The lateral position also reduces venous return and may increase the severity of shock in hypovolemic patients.

In most instances the lung lacerations can be oversewn with deep horizontal vicryl mattress sutures or stapled with the TA-55 or TA-90 stapler. In a few patients, lobectomy may be required to control a severe air leak or bleeding, particularly, if the laceration extends into the hilum.

INTRABRONCHIAL BLEEDING

Intrabronchial bleeding, which manifests as hemoptysis, is poorly tolerated and can lead rapidly to death by flooding dependent alveoli. The arterial Po_2 may fall rapidly and severely before there is any other clinical evidence of airway or alveolar dysfunction. In some instances, hemoptysis due to a lung tear may be associated with systemic air embolism, which is discussed in the chapter by that title.

Patients with moderate to severe hemoptysis should be positioned so as to facilitate dependent drainage of the blood out of the trachea. The uninvolved lung must be kept as free of blood as possible. Nasotracheal suction and/or bronchoscopy should be used as often as necessary to keep the bronchial tree clear and the lung expanded. If bleeding is severe, insertion of a Carlen double-lumen endotracheal tube by a skilled individual should be performed as soon as possible. This tube can be used to confine the bleeding to one lung and thus protect the uninvolved lung. In some instances, bleeding may be controlled by occluding the involved bronchus with a Fogarty arterial balloon catheter or by packing it with gauze.

If severe intrabronchial bleeding continues, or if there is evidence of air embolism, a thoracotomy should be performed promptly. To reduce drainage of blood into the dependent lung, the thoracotomy should be performed with the patient supine and the bronchus to the involved lobe or the hilum clamped as soon as possible. The involved lung must then be completely repaired or resected.

AIR EMBOLISM

DONALD D. TRUNKEY, M.D.

Systemic air embolism has not been commonly diagnosed and treated. Traditionally, air embolism was thought to be the presence of air on the right side of the systemic circulation that leads to ineffective right heart stroke volume and pulmonary hypertension. Systemic air embolism is most often associated with a bronchopulmonary venous fistula caused by blunt or penetrating trauma, primarily laceration of the lung from a fractured rib.

In our experience, systemic air embolism occurs in 14 percent of all major thoracic injuries. The incidence of air embolism following penetrating versus blunt upper torso trauma is 3:1. Patient survival is more likely following penetrating trauma (slightly greater than 50%) than after blunt trauma, which has a survival rate of 20 percent.

DIAGNOSIS

The primary reason the syndrome is underappreciated and therefore undertreated is the subtlety of the presenting signs and symptoms. They fall into four categories, and the patient may present with any combination of these findings.

1. Lateralized or focal neurologic findings in the absence of obvious head injury. This results from air in the cerebral circulation and can be confirmed by air seen in the retinal vessels during fundoscopic examination.
2. The second presentation is hemoptysis. Although hemoptysis is associated with many pulmonary injuries, when it is present, one must have a high index of suspicion for a bronchopulmonary venous fistula. With adequate blood volume and negative airway pressure, hemoptysis is not infrequent. With positive-pressure ventilation, however, the pressure differential favors entry of air into pulmonary veins with resultant air embolism.
3. Sudden cardiovascular collapse shortly after endotracheal intubation. This represents air in the coronary circulation and is aggravated by the positive-pressure ventilation that is usually applied immediately after intubation.
4. The fourth presentation is froth that is obtained during aspiration of arterial blood for blood gas determinations. This is associated with 100 percent mortality.

Approximately two-thirds of patients have signs or symptoms of air embolism on, or shortly after, presentation to the emergency room. The remaining one-third usually manifest their symptoms within the first 24 hours of admission, although symptoms may occur as late as 5 days post injury.

SURGICAL MANAGEMENT

Treatment of patients who have definite signs and symptoms on admission, is relatively straightforward; they require emergency thoracotomy. Ideally, the thoracotomy should be performed in the operating room, but if the patient is dead or dying on presentation, thoracotomy in the emergency department is indicated. In many instances, it is obvious which thorax is involved; I prefer to do the thoracotomy on the ipsilateral side. For example, if there is a penetrating wound of the left thorax or a flail chest involving the left hemithorax, a left anterior thoracotomy should be done. A left anterior thoracotomy is my preference for other resuscitative efforts. In some instances, the offending bronchopulmonary venous fistula is in the contralateral lung from the obvious injury, or it is difficult to determine which side is involved. If such is the case, a left anterior thoracotomy can be extended across the sternum into the right thorax so that bilateral anterolateral thoracotomies, which give excellent exposure, are used. The primary objective is to open the involved hemithorax as soon as possible so as to clamp the hilum of the lung and thus reduce the inoculum of air to the left atrium. After the hilum has been clamped, further resuscitation (which may include cardiac massage) should be carried out. Before cardiac massage is given, it should be noted whether or not there is air within the coronary circulation. This observation is not only to help confirm the diagnosis, but also to aid in treatment. If air is the suspected cause of circulatory collapse, it is prudent to administer epinephrine, either endotracheally or intravenously, to increase systemic pressure and empty the microcirculation of the microbubbles. If internal cardiac massage is being carried out, holding the ascending aorta with the thumb and index finger for two or three strokes helps to evacuate the coronary artery air. It is also important to vent the ventricle and/or the aortic arch with a needle to remove as much of the accumulated air as possible.

Once resuscitation has been achieved and the hilum of the lung is clamped, definitive surgery, in the majority of cases, consists of oversewing the pulmonary laceration. If the penetrating injury to the lung parenchyma is deep, thorough exploration down to and including the hilum are mandatory. The gastrointestinal anastomosis (GIA) stapler has been excellent for opening wound tracts quickly while preventing air leaks and bleeding. In instances of extensive trauma, lobectomy or even pneumonectomy may be necessary. The rest of the operative procedure is routine, as with any thoracotomy.

Postoperative complications, which result from the initial air insult and cause dysfunction of other organs, may require the usual supportive measures.

THE HEART

DAVID V. FELICIANO, M.D.
KENNETH L. MATTOX, M.D.

INCIDENCE OF INJURY

The number of cardiac injuries has increased in recent years, and an annual incidence of 40 to 50 injuries is not uncommon in urban trauma centers. The major factors contributing to this include the increased number of penetrating truncal wounds, increased number of early survivors from motor vehicle deceleration accidents, and improvements in prehospital care and transport.

Penetrating cardiac injuries are usually caused by knives or missiles outside of the hospital or, on rare occasions, by misplaced indwelling central venous catheters in the hospitalized patient. Blunt cardiac injuries are invariably related to cardiac compression between the spine and steering wheel in a deceleration-type accident and should be looked for in all patients with significant associated thoracic injuries such as a first-rib fracture, sternal fracture, or flail chest.

PRESENTATION

Prehospital mortality for penetrating cardiac injuries is approximately 75 percent, and of most of these victims die as a result of tamponade or exsanguination within 4 or 5 minutes of wounding. Because of the small number of patients with blunt cardiac rupture, it is difficult to give an accurate figure for prehospital mortality in this group. In Parmley's oft-quoted review (Circulation 1958, 18:371), only 6.5 percent of patients with this lesion were reported to have lived more than 30 minutes.

Patients with perforation resulting from cardiac injury of either type present with either cardiac tamponade (70% to 80% of patients) or hemorrhage (20% to 30% of patients). Patients presenting with tamponade often have a dusky or deathly appearance and exhibit extreme anxiety about their condition. On physical examination, the presence of hypotension, distended neck veins, and somewhat muffled heart sounds is characteristic. It should be noted that a young trauma patient with either a tension pneumothorax or tension hemothorax may present with similar physical findings. The absence of breath sounds on one side of the chest should help to distinguish these conditions from cardiac tamponade; in addition, most patients with tension hemothorax have collapsed neck veins. As patients with tamponade are being evaluated, the central venous pressure steadily increases. This is in marked contrast to the usual trauma patient whose central venous pressure usually falls once the original stimulation of venous line and urinary catheter insertion is completed. A significant fall in blood pressure may

249

be delayed until immediately before the patient suffers cardiac arrest. Whereas a paradoxical pulse (exaggeration of the normal inspiratory fall in blood pressure) has been said to be of value in the diagnosis of cardiac tamponade, several large series of penetrating cardiac wounds have noted that only 10 to 35 percent of patients actually demonstrate this sign.

Most patients with cardiac perforation and hemorrhage as a presentation have suffered precordial penetrating wounds. These patients generally arrive in profound shock with a massive unilateral hemothorax secondary to communication between the cardiac wound and pleural cavity. A large "caked" hemothorax outlining the lateral margin of the collapsed lung is often present on the initial chest film.

MANAGEMENT OF PENETRATING WOUNDS

There are several options in management of the patient who presents with tamponade or hemorrhage. Included among these are emergency center subxiphoid or parasternal pericardiocentesis, emergency center thoracotomy, or subxiphoid pericardial window to confirm the diagnosis of a tamponade in the operating room.

Pericardiocentesis performed with an 18-gauge spinal needle may be of temporary therapeutic value even if only 20 to 30 ml of blood is removed from the pericardial sac. The major disadvantages of this technique are the high incidence of puncture of previously uninjured cardiac chambers and a 50 percent false-negative rate in actually making a diagnosis of cardiac tamponade. In our center, pericardiocentesis is reserved for the few patients who are awake, alert, and first demonstrating a significant fall in blood pressure. If pericardiocentesis is to be performed as a temporizing maneuver in order to allow for transport of the patient to the operating room, the insertion of a plastic catheter through the hollow needle in the pericardial sac will allow for repeated aspirations prior to thoracotomy.

Patients who are profoundly hypotensive (BP under 70) or who have suffered cardiac arrest secondary to tamponade or hemorrhage on arrival are best treated by emergency center thoracotomy in hospitals where the operating room is geographically distant. Once the patient is intubated, a left anterolateral thoracotomy is performed in the fifth intercostal space just beneath the male nipple. In females, the breast is pulled upward toward the shoulder, and the incision is made where the nipple used to be. When the precordial wound has been in the right parasternal area, some consideration may have to be given to performing a bilateral anterolateral thoracotomy at the same level. These incisions may then be connected by transverse division of the sternum using a Gigli saw. This bilateral anterolateral thoracotomy allows for wide exposure of both sides of the heart and the proximal great vessels. In the hypotensive or arrested patient, minimal bleeding occurs from the sides of the thoracotomy incision, and a standard chest wall retractor is rapidly inserted with the handle lying toward the surgeon. This allows for easier exposure if a sternal transection has to be performed. The second maneuver in the emergency center thoracotomy for the hypotensive or arrested patient is clamping of the descending thoracic aorta to maintain coronary and cerebral arterial flow. The surgeon lifts the left lung out of the hemithorax by cupping his left hand (with the palm facing the ceiling) around the lung. Once the left lung has been elevated, an assistant on the right side of the patient can hold the lung out of the surgeon's way. At this point the surgeon should spread a DeBakey aortic clamp above and beneath the mid-descending thoracic aorta, which lies on the vertebral bodies. It should be noted that the diameter of the vessel in the hypovolemic arrested patient is only about 2 cm and in no way resembles the large structure frequently depicted by medical artists. When the aorta has been exposed, the surgeon can hook his left index finger around it and pull it out from the posterior mediastinum. In this way, clamping is then performed under direct vision and eliminates both aortic and esophageal injuries. The clamp is applied, the time is noted, and the left lung is allowed to drop back into the thorax. If no obvious lung injury is present and the pericardial sac is filled with dark blue blood or shows a perforation oozing blood, a pericardiotomy must now be performed. Distention of the pericardial sac stretches the mediastinal pleura and makes it extremely difficult to grab with a forceps. It may be necessary, therefore, to "hook" the pericardium with one blade of a straight Mayo scissors and then grab it with the forceps. The pericardial sac should be opened with a scissors in a longitudinal directional above the left (or right) phrenic nerve from the diaphragm below to the great vessels above. A scalpel should not be used to open the pericardial sac as inadvertent injury to the left anterior descending coronary artery may result. If the pericardial sac is still tight around the heart following the longitudinal pericardiotomy, a transverse cut anteriorly up to the sternum helps to free the heart in many cases. The surgeon should now manually evacuate all the clot in the pericardial sac and swing the heart over into the left hemithorax if only a left anterolateral thoracotomy has been performed. Once the heart is in view, the surgeon should inspect the right ventricle and right atrium, the chambers that are most commonly injured by penetrating wounds. The surgeon should not try to lift the heart as entry of air into a left-sided cardiac perforation may result in sudden fatal coronary air embolism. Most atrial wounds can be temporarily sealed by the application of a Satinsky vascular clamp and then sewn with a running 5-0 polypropylene suture. Wounds of the ventricles are generally tamponaded by the surgeon's or assistant's finger, and horizontal mattress sutures of 3-0 polypropylene or polyester are then placed under the finger and tied by the assistant. When a wound lies next to a major coronary artery, the mattress suture is placed beneath the artery in preference to ligation.

Several techniques are available for handling large cardiac wounds. The insertion of a 5-ml or 30-ml balloon catheter into a large or inaccessible (posterior) defect may allow for control of hemorrhage until a pursestring suture can be applied around the hole. Sutures placed on either side of a large defect and pulled together may allow for control of hemorrhage until cardiopulmonary bypass can be instituted. Finally, occlusion of the superior vena cava and inferior vena cava by the assistant's fingers or vascular clamps slows the heart and finally stops it, allowing for a quick repair of a large defect without precipitating exsanguination. If this latter technique is used, all air is evacuated from the ventricle by allowing hemorrhage through the hole prior to tying the final suture. The technique of creating ventricular fibrillation by the use of internal paddles is no longer recommended.

Once cardiorrhaphy has been completed, internal cardiac massage using the palms of two hands may be necessary. Warm saline poured over the heart may prevent ventricular fibrillation, which is often associated with the hypothermia of shock and resuscitation. If ventricular fibrillation occurs, defibrillation with internal paddles at 20 watt-seconds should be performed. When the patient has a satisfactory rhythm, the descending thoracic aorta is gradually declamped as infusions of fluid, blood, and bicarbonate are administered. The use of vigorous inotropes such as intravenous adrenalin should be avoided at this point as they inevitably cause rupture of a ventricular repair. In some patients, complete declamping may take 15 to 30 minutes. The stable patient is then moved to the operating room, where the transected internal mammary vessels are ligated and all clot is washed out of the pericardial and pleural cavities. The edematous heart infrequently allows for pericardial closure following a vigorous resuscitation and is left open in many patients.

A subxiphoid pericardial window performed through a short, upper midline, abdominal incision in the operating room is used to confirm the diagnosis of a cardiac injury in some trauma centers. We only use this technique as part of an exploratory celiotomy when proximity of an upper abdominal or costal margin missile or knife wound mandates pericardial exploration. If suspicion of a cardiac injury is high as the patient reaches the operating room, a left anterolateral thoracotomy should be performed.

Some patients, especially those with tamponade, may be in stable enough condition to be moved to the operating room without dramatic emergency center intervention such as the performance of a pericardiocentesis or thoracotomy. In the "stable" patient with a small precordial stab wound, a standard median sternotomy incision may be used as clamping of the descending thoracic aorta is not likely to be necessary. All other patients—including those with gunshot wounds, those who are in unstable condition and may require an aortic cross-clamp, and those with midline celiotomy incisions in whom fecal contamination may be present should have the previously described left anterolateral thoracotomy performed.

On rare occasions, cardiopulmonary bypass may be required to complete cardiac repairs. Examples would be ventricular holes too difficult to repair in the beating heart, rupture of the emergency center repair, or ventricular failure second to transection or compression of a main coronary artery. In the latter instance, emergency aorto-coronary-artery grafting may be lifesaving.

In patients with penetrating cardiac wounds, certain factors adversely affect survival. Included among these are gunshot wounds (as compared to stab wounds), a prolonged period of prehospital cardiopulmonary arrest, injuries involving two chambers, and associated abdominal injuries. Any of the aforementioned causes the expected survival rate of 60 to 65 percent (if vital signs are present on admission) to decrease.

Because of the significant incidence of internal cardiac injuries such as VSDs, valve injury, or internal fistulas which have been discovered on late follow-up of patients who survive penetrating cardiac wounds, our present recommendation is to perform 2-D echocardiography on all patients with persistent murmurs after cardiorrhaphy. If any abnormality is present on echo, cardiac catheterization is then performed to help plan the operative approach using cardiopulmonary bypass.

MANAGEMENT OF BLUNT INJURIES

The spectrum of blunt cardiac injuries includes myocardial contusion, myocardial infarction, myocardial rupture, and internal cardiac defects.

Myocardial contusions occur in drivers with compression from the steering wheel in deceleration-type accidents, as previously noted, or in individuals who have received some other type of direct blow to the sternum. Significant findings on physical examination may include the imprint of the hub of the steering wheel on the patient's sternum, ventricular arrhythmias, or congestive heart failure. The diagnosis is suspected from these findings and can generally be confirmed on electrocardiogram or by the measurement of CPK isoenzymes (CPK-MB analysis). Electrocardiographic findings that are common with contusion include nonspecific ST and T wave changes, sinus tachycardia, premature beats, and heart block. Myocardial injury is confirmed if the CPK-MB is 5 percent or more of the total CPK activity; this was found to be elevated in approximately two-thirds of patients with myocardial contusion in one recent study (Snow N et al. Surgery 1982; 92:744). Radionuclide scanning has also been used to confirm the presence of myocardial contusions in recent years, but results have been somewhat disappointing to date; in contrast, 2-D echocardiography and radionuclide angiography have been used successfully to document the diagnosis of contusion. The treatment of myocardial contusion is the medical treatment of its complications. This may include drug control of arrhythmias or congestive heart failure, insertion of pacemakers to control heart block, or use of the intra-aortic balloon pump for severe cardiac failure.

Transmural infarction from blunt cardiac injury is a rare entity and is best diagnosed by classic ECG findings, radionuclide scanning, or 2-D echocardiography. Treatment involves observation in a monitored unit and management of the same complications associated with contusion.

Myocardial rupture generally occurs at the atrial insertion of the venae cavae (right atrium) and pulmonary veins (left atrium) or in the left atrial appendage. These injuries generally occur in deceleration-type accidents, whereas rupture of the right ventricle at the origin of the pulmonary artery occurs more commonly with direct precordial blows. In almost every case, rupture of the left ventricle is seen only in the autopsy room. Patients with myocardial rupture present with tamponade and have excellent survival rates if they do not suffer cardiopulmonary arrest in the prehospital period and if the diagnosis is rapidly recognized during evaluation in the emergency center. Techniques for repair are exactly the same as those used for penetrating wounds from missiles and knives.

A variety of internal disruptions from blunt cardiac trauma including VSDs, valvular tears, and papillary muscle tears have been reported in the literature. As with penetrating wounds, 2-D echocardiography should be used to evaluate any patient with severe blunt cardiac injury who has a persistent murmur while under observation. Cardiac catheterization can be used to verify the presence of an internal lesion, as previously noted.

THE ESOPHAGUS

KENNETH L. MATTOX, M.D.
DAVID V. FELICIANO, M.D.

Injury to the cervical, thoracic, or abdominal esophagus is rarely the sole indication for surgical exploration of that area. Other associated organ injuries are usually the indication for cervical exploration, thoracotomy, or laparotomy. On rare occasions, perforation of the esophagus is the result of an ingested foreign body. Iatrogenic perforation from endoscopy with forceful dilation of an achalasia produces mediastinal pain associated with fever and possible sepsis and requires surgical intervention. Endoscopy and barium contrast esophagography are antecedent to the diagnosis of esophageal injury and do not play a definitive role in the decision making process with regard to exploration or choice of treatment. Although a high index of suspicion for esophageal injury may have existed, this injury is most often found inadvertently at the time of repair of other organ injuries.

CERVICAL ESOPHAGUS

Although the cervical esophagus is occasionally injured iatrogenically during endoscopy, intubation, or insertion of the esophageal obturator airway, most injuries to the cervical esophagus are secondary to penetrating wounds. At neck exploration for a missile or knife tract, the surgeon encounters a tear in the esophagus with retraction of the muscular ends. The nasogastric tube in the esophagus is encountered by the exploring finger, confirming the hole in the esophagus. Such injuries should be closed in two layers with (1) an inner layer of absorbable suture for hemostasis and (2) an outer layer of permanent suture of the surgeon's choice. A drain should be placed near the repair and brought out away from the carotid artery. If a concomitant arterial and/or tracheal injury is present, the involved structures are repaired, and a muscle flap of sternocleidomastoid or pectoralis muscle is interposed between the esophagus and trachea and/or carotid. Drainage of the esophageal repair should be through the side of the neck opposite to the repair of the associated injury. Should an esophageal fistula occur, it will close spontaneously in 5 to 15 days.

THORACIC INLET

Esophageal injuries at the thoracic inlet are often present with associated tracheal and major vascular injury. When the patient has concomitant injuries to the trachea and/or vascular structures, the esophageal injury is best managed by a lateral cervical esophagostomy which creates a controlled fistula. The tracheal and/or vascular injury is repaired with a muscle flap interposed between that repair and the lateral cervical esophagostomy. Placement of gastrostomy and feeding jejunostomy tubes completes the immediate treatment. Following recovery, a simple esophageal closure is accomplished under local anesthesia if the fistula has not already closed spontaneously.

THORACIC ESOPHAGUS

The esophageal injury is frequently discovered in the supine patient through an anterior incision (median sternotomy or anterolateral thoracotomy). The associated injuries should be repaired and the anterior incision closed. The patient is then turned to the appropriate lateral decubitus position and a posterolateral incision made to expose the esophageal injury. A rib is excised during the incision in order to create an intercostal muscle flap sufficiently large to cover the two-layer esophageal repair. The viable muscle flap is positioned to encircle the esophageal repair, and the pleura is closed over the repair if possible. Drainage tubes are placed near the esophageal repair, and the chest is closed. In the case of a patient with extensive injuries to the thoracic esophagus, a lateral cervical esophagostomy, tube gastrostomy, and feeding jejunostomy should be performed in addition to the lateral esophageal repair.

Grillo has emphasized a pleural or muscle flap coverage of the repair, and Urschel has recommended exclusion of the esophagus at the esophageal gastric junction (Fig. 1) with a ligature of umbilical tape. Popovoski has modified Urschel's technique by recommending an absorbable suture, which later renders the esophagus amenable to dilation via the cervical stoma. For either technique, the vagus nerves should be protected outside the tie. In selected destructive injuries to the esophagus from massive caustic injury or high velocity missiles, management that includes a side-cervical esophagostomy, esophagectomy, oversewing of the esophagogastric junction, tube gastrostomy, and feeding jejunostomy may prevent the serious complication of multiple mediastinal infection, with its inevitable morbidity and mortality. Reconstruction with gastric or colon bypass is indicated at a later date.

INTRA-ABDOMINAL ESOPHAGUS

The intra-abdominal esophagus is very short, but it is occasionally injured when there is a penetrating wound(s) near the esophageal hiatus. With such injuries, shock, hemorrhage, and associated wounds are common. Lateral esophagorrhapy is accomplished, and a gastric serosal patch with partial wrap-around

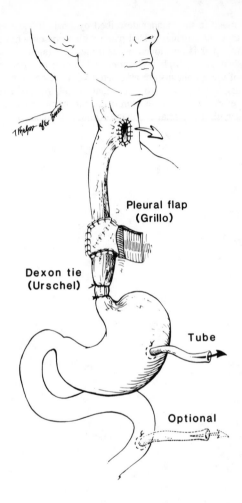

Figure 1 Drawing depicting management of complex thoracic esophageal injury by lateral cervical esophagostomy, pleural flap coverage of esophagorrhapy, temporary occlusion of distal esophagus, tube gastrostomy for drainage, and tube jejunostomy for feeding.

is indicated, much in the manner described by Thal. If the esophagus cannot be closed without narrowing, a Thal patch with a Nissen wrap-around is indicated, and the repair is positioned beneath the diaphragm. This repair should be accomplished over a Maloney esophageal bougie (greater than 35 F).

Injuries of the esophagus are associated with a high mortality rate (about 50%) from missed injuries or from secondary breakdown of a repair. It is imperative, therefore, that a proper plan of management be thought through before a patient with a potential esophageal injury is taken to surgery.

THE GREAT VESSELS

DONALD D. TRUNKEY, M.D.

Injuries to the great vessels (arteries) of the thorax are rarely reported since most exsanguinate at the time of injury. Injury to the great veins in the upper thorax is probably more common than we recognize. A widened mediastinum is often indicative of injury to a great vein that has tamponaded. At San Francisco General Hospital, 85 percent of the arteriograms performed for widened mediastinum are negative for aortic or great vessel injury. How many of these represent venous injuries is unknown. During a recent 12-year period we treated five innominate vein injuries, nine subclavian vein injuries, and three axillary vein injuries. Eighty-three percent of these were due to penetrating trauma and 17 percent were due to blunt trauma.

DIAGNOSIS

Penetrating injuries to the great vessels and the thorax should be obvious. A stab wound or gunshot wound to the neck or chest should alert the clinician to the possibility of arterial or venous injury. Even more remote wounds to the abdomen can transgress the diaphragm and cause injury to the great vessels. Complete disruption of a great vessel secondary to blunt trauma is usually associated with massive hemorrhage and exsanguination. On the other hand, if the injury causes disruption and retraction primarily of the media and intima, and if the adventitia is still intact, survival is possible. On initial x-ray examination, these patients are seen to have widened mediastinum, obscuration of the aortic shadow, left pleural cap, lower neck hematoma, or swelling and hematoma formation in the infra- and supraclavicular spaces. Distortion of the airway with subsequent airway obstruction can occur.

SURGICAL INCISIONS

Various intrathoracic and base-of-the neck incisions have been described for gaining access to the great vessels. Since the overwhelming majority of these patients are in shock, or may have associated injuries, I strongly favor keeping the patient in a supine position and selecting a midline incision. If a left anterior thoracotomy has not been performed already in the emergency room, I prefer a midline sternotomy incision with the option of extending the incision more cephalad along the border of the sternocleidomastoid muscle on either side. A second option is to carry the incision along the top of the clavicle, with or without resection of the medial half of the clavicle, to gain access to the proximal sub-

259

clavian artery and vein. Axillary injuries are best managed by an infraclavicular incision or a combine supra- and infraclavicular incision (S-shaped) that resects the medial half of the clavicle to gain proximal control.

Left subclavian injuries present a problem because the proximal vessel is posterior in the chest and may be difficult to reach through a median sternotomy. One option is to perform the "trap door" incision in which the left anterior chest is opened in the third or fourth intercostal space, the upper sternum is split, a supraclavicular incision is made, and the clavicle is resected. This procedure allows the chest wall to be opened like a "trap door." An alternative is a left anterior thoracotomy incision to obtain proximal control, followed by a separate supraclavicular incision with or without clavicular resection. Some authors have described emergency access to the left subclavian artery at its origin by performing anterior thoracotomy in the third intercostal space while the patient is in the emergency room. In my experience it is almost impossible to diagnose such an injury without arteriograms, even with a high index of suspicion. In the case of cardiac arrest or a moribund patient, a standard left anterolateral thoracotomy is preferable. The options then include cutting the costocartilage cephalad to gain access to the left subclavian artery, if that vessel is injured, or to extend it as a sternotomy and convert it to a trap door incision. A third option is to extend the incision into the right chest (butterfly incision), and thus gain excellent access to all vessels in the chest.

SURGICAL MANAGEMENT

Penetrating Wound

Penetrating wounds to the intrathoracic great vessels almost invariably lend themselves to lateral repair since larger arterial wounds are incompatible with survival. In the case of venous injury, it is preferable to repair the innominate vein, but ligation can be tolerated by the patient. The latter is performed when there are extensive associated injuries demanding the surgeon's attention and when venous repair would take too long. Injuries to the subclavian and axillary vessels may be extensive and require either end-to-end anastomosis or even graft replacement. In my experience the subclavian artery is one of the most difficult arteries to repair because it lacks elastic fibers in the media. End-to-end anastomosis under any tension is doomed to failure, and it is better to attempt graft replacement, preferably with autogenous tissue, or with either polytetraflouroethylene (PTFE) or Dacron. If there is associated injury to hollow viscera such as esophagus or trachea, it is far preferable to use autogenous tissue or to ligate the vessel. If the vessel is ligated and the patient subsequently has signs of ischemia or claudication in the arm, extraanatomic bypass from the opposite extremity or neck may be done at a later date.

Blunt Injury

Blunt injury to the innominate, left common carotid, or subclavian artery may pose more difficult operative management. In most of these instances, the adventitia is the only intact portion of the vessel wall as the media and intima usually have retracted. Therefore, grafts are often necessary. If more than one of the great vessels is injured, heparin-bonded shunts or cardiac bypass should be considered. Cardiac bypass may be contraindicated because of associated injury, particularly closed head injury and increased risk of hemorrhage in the fully heparinized patient. Repair of the left subclavian artery is not mandatory, and the patient will tolerate ligation. I have also ligated the common carotid since there is usually excellent collateral circulation in the young, healthy individual.

Injury to the Thoracic Aorta

Patients with injury to the thoracic aorta should have arteriography prior to operative treatment. Most patients present with a widened mediastinum, but other indications for arteriography have been outlined previously. Aortography of the entire thorax is necessary because, in rare instances, the patient may have disruption of the thoracic aorta in more than one place. The most common site of disruption is just distal to the ligamentum arteriosum (approximately 85% to 90%); other sites of disruption are at the aortic valve and the aortic hiatus (approximately 5% each). Patients with injury to the aortic valve area require cardiopulmonary bypass and repair of the valve, or replacement if the valve is severely damaged. Controversy exists whether extracorporeal bypass or shunts are useful in the surgical repair of the descending thoracic aorta. Although both techniques may allow more time for the procedure to be done, there is no evidence that either prevents paraplegia. The complication of paraplegia is more dependent on the arterial anatomy to the spinal cord, and bypass does not avoid this complication. In my experience, a patient with a disrupted aorta commonly has associated injuries, and it is prudent to avoid heparinization when possible. When clamp repair technique is used, the occluding clamps should be placed as close to the injury site as possible to avoid unnecessary occlusion of intercostal arteries that may provide flow to the spinal cord.

Arterial monitoring proximal to the injury site is necessary to avoid hypertension and overdistention of the left ventricle. Anticipated hypertension is managed by bleeding the patient of 1 to 2 units of blood just prior to placing the proximal clamp. Additionally, hypertension is managed with an afterload-reducing agent such as nitroprusside. Prior to removing the clamps after a graft has been placed, the autologous blood is retransfused. In general, I prefer to place a short segment of Dacron graft to repair a thoracic aorta deficit as the aorta usually can not be primarily repaired.

THE DIAPHRAGM

RICHARD E. WARD, M.D.

The diaphragm is a muscular organ that separates the thoracic cavity from the abdominal cavity. It is attached to the tenth, eleventh, and twelfth ribs posteriorly and laterally and to the costal cartilages anteriorly. It is innervated by the phrenic nerves, which run through the mediastinum along the posterior pericardium and branch in a radial fashion to extend out over the leaves of the diaphragm. The anterior central portion of the diaphragm is the inferior wall of the pericardium, and thus the diaphragm is in direct contact with the inferior surface of the heart. Through muscular extensions of the diaphragm in the posterior central portion called the crura run the aorta and the esophagus. To the right of these structures courses the inferior vena cava above the liver. The arterial supply of the diaphragm originates from branches of the intercostal arteries, and the venous return is via the phrenic veins, which empty into the inferior vena cava.

The diaphragm is important in respiration and, along with the intercostal musculature, is considered the primary muscle involved in respiration. The diaphragm's semispheric shape, with its concave surface facing the abdominal cavity and its convex surface facing the thoracic cavity, allows it to increase the volume of the thoracic cavity with contraction and decrease the volume with relaxation. Thus, the diaphragm moves inferiorly on inspiration, and its convexity becomes more pronounced on expiration. This results in excursion of the dome of the diaphragm over a wide area within the thoracic cavity. The dome of the diaphragm may be at the level of the twelfth rib on deep inspiration and rise to the level of the seventh rib on forced expiration. Because of this wide excursion and the fact that the abdominal viscera move in conjunction with the diaphragm, penetrating injuries to the chest or fractures of the seventh rib or below may injure the abdominal viscera. Thus, although the diaphragm is a discrete anatomic barrier between the abdominal and thoracic cavities, it does not prevent injury of the abdominal viscera in patients with lower thoracic trauma.

Injuries to the diaphragm occur in two ways: (1) by penetration, and (2) by blunt disruption. Penetrating injuries to the diaphragm must be considered as an indicator of potential damage to viscera in both body cavities, but do not represent significant disability to the patient in his immediate post-injury course. If unrepaired, they represent a threat of disability in the long-term post-injury course. They may be a site for herniation of abdominal viscera; incarceration, obstruction, or strangulation may follow. For this reason, it is important to identify and repair penetrating injuries to the diaphragm. Blunt disruption to the diaphragm occurs after blunt injury in which severe forces are dissipated in the abdominal cavity, forcing the abdominal viscera into the chest and rupturing one leaf of the diaphragm. This is most often seen after motor vehicle accidents, but it can also be seen in patients who have fallen from great heights. These occur more often on the left side because the liver is not situated there to absorb forces and buttress the diaphragm. They may be a source of respiratory embarrassment if the abdominal viscera herniate into the left chest. This can occur in the immediate post-injury period or any time subsequent to that if the injury is not appreciated. Injuries to the right diaphragm generally do not create acute respiratory difficulties, but may be recognized later as eventration of the diaphragm or a high-riding right diaphragm on chest roentgenogram as the liver fills the rupture in the diaphragm and migrates into the chest.

Evaluation and resuscitation of the injured patient must follow principles established in other sections of this book. Specifically, patients with penetrating thoracic injuries below the level of the seventh rib or penetrating abdominal injuries with abnormalities on their chest film must be considered to have diaphragmatic injury as well. Those with penetrating thoracic injury require evaluation of their abdominal cavity for abdominal injury. Those with penetrating upper abdominal injury generally require exploration with close attention paid to inspection of the diaphragms. Evaluation of the patient who has experienced blunt abdominal trauma must include chest roentgenogram—and close attention must be paid to both diaphragms. Any blurring of the diaphragmatic margin may be indicative of diaphragmatic injury. Likewise, one must be careful not to mistake a distended stomach herniated into the left chest through a diaphragmatic tear for a pneumothorax. The lung is displaced superiorly into the apex of the chest with herniation of abdominal contents, whereas it collapses medially toward the hilum with pneumothorax. Respiratory distress caused by a distended stomach in the left chest is easily remedied by placement of a nasogastric tube. Most patients with blunt disruption of their diaphragm have other associated abdominal injuries and thus other indications for abdominal exploration. Therefore, the diagnosis of diaphragmatic disruption is often made in the operating room rather than during the preoperative work-up. Occasionally, this is not true, and the diagnosis is made late in the patient's hospital course or after discharge from the hospital, at which time the patient suddenly becomes short of breath after abdominal straining and herniation of abdominal viscera into the chest is confirmed radiologically. Occasionally, diaphragmatic disruption is identified on routine post-injury chest films of a patient who has no symptoms.

Therapy of diaphragmatic injuries requires operative repair. In the acute post-injury phase, this is best accomplished through the abdomen because the most frequent associated injuries affect organs in the abdominal cavity and are best approached through a laparotomy incision. These associated injuries are generally more life-threatening than the diaphragmatic injury. Those blunt disruptions that are identified late in the post-injury course may be repaired through the chest if time and the patient's course indicate no associated intra-abdominal injury. During exploration of the abdomen for any injury, whether it be blunt or penetrating, careful attention should be paid to the diaphragms. Palpation of the diaphragms must be undertaken to ensure that there are no injuries to these structures. Penetrating injuries should be closed, generally with one or two interrupted sutures. These should be stout with high-tensile strength absorbable sutures of the polyglycolic acid variety or nonabsorbable sutures. Catgut sutures are not recommended. Occasionally, troublesome bleeding occurs from the edges of the diaphragm. This can generally be controlled by means of figure-of-8 sutures or a locking running closure. Because of the potential for a pneumothorax once the abdominal cavity is opened, a small soft rubber catheter can be placed through the hold in the diaphragm and evacuated while the patient is being held in inspiration by the anesthetist. If these two maneuvers are accomplished while the final sutures are being tied and the catheter is removed as the suture is being tied in place, the incidence of significant pneumothorax will be small. In patients who have disruption of a hollow viscus and significant spilling of its contents, as well as a diaphragmatic injury, special care must be paid to irrigation of the thoracic cavity to remove all visceral contents and prevent empyema.

Repair of blunt diaphragmatic injuries is somewhat more difficult. These can occur in a radial fashion extending from central tendon to the lateral wall or can be manifest as tearing of the lateral wall away from the attachment to the ribs. Careful inspection of the injury must be undertaken to define the limits of the rents. Often these are difficult to expose posteriorly as they lie behind the superior pole of the spleen or the dome of the liver. With traction inferiorly on the spleen and the stomach on the left or the dome of the liver on the right, the most posterior portion of the rent should be identified. A long 0-suture placed at the most posterior portion of the tear and, after tying, used as a traction suture to expose the rest of the incision is useful. One can then successively place figure-of-8 sutures the entire length of the tear, cutting the previously placed suture and using the most recently placed suture as a traction suture. As in the case of a penetrating injury, one should place a tube through the tear into the thoracic cavity, decompress the thoracic cavity after all but the last suture is tied in place, and, while placing suction on the decompression tube and having the anesthetist place the patient in full inspiration, one should remove the tube and tie the last suture so that the diaphragm is air-tight. Occasionally, if the diaphragm is torn off its attachment to the ribs, sutures may have to be placed around the ribs as there is essentially no tissue available to hold sutures adjacent to the ribs. Figure-of-8 sutures placed through the muscular leaf of the diaphragm and then placed around the ribs facilitate a sturdy repair.

Postoperative care is the same as for any patient who has sustained major life-threatening injury. Chest films obtained postoperatively are essential to determine the presence of residual pneumo- or hemothorax. Thoracostomy tubes may be necessary in some patients, and use of chest tube drainage and prophylactic antibiotic therapy should be considered in patients with significant spillage of enteric contents into the chest. Patients who have large blunt disruptions of their diaphragm with subsequent repair often have paresis of that hemidiaphragm. If they have had other significant injury with large amounts of fluid resuscitation and require ventilatory support, they may be ventilator-dependent for a longer period of time than patients who have normal diaphragms. This fact should be kept in mind when considering whether to extubate patients or while weaning patients from ventilatory support.

Careful evaluation of patients with lower thoracic and upper adominal penetrating injury, as well as those with major abdominal blunt injury, allows the physician to identify the great majority of diaphragmatic injuries. Whether this occurs prior to operation or in the operating room is immaterial as long as careful inspection of the diaphragms and repair are undertaken. There is little morbidity or mortality associated with the repair of the diaphragm, whereas the morbidity associated with the unrepaired diaphragm is significant.

THE SPLEEN

C. JAMES CARRICO, M.D.

The spleen is the organ most frequently injured following blunt trauma and ranks second behind the liver as the source of life-threatening hemorrhage following injury. Until two decades ago, lack of appreciation of the immunologic importance of this organ and the belief that the spleen frequently failed to heal properly following repair resulted in routine splenectomy for virtually all splenic injuries. Concern about postsplenectomy sepsis (overwhelming postsplenectomy infection—OPSI) prompted reappraisal of this approach. This has resulted in a wide range of approaches to the patient with a potential injury to the spleen. Some propose that routine splenectomy remains the only rational treatment. At the other end of the spectrum are those who advocate extensive blood transfusion prior to operation and suggest that "uncontrollable" blood loss is the only indication for an operative approach to the injured spleen. This chapter will briefly review the information that has caused reappraisal of the approach to the patient with an injured spleen. The options available to the surgeon responsible for such a patient will be categorized and the risks and benefits of each of these approaches addressed. At the conclusion of the chapter, an attempt will be made to formulate a rational approach based on these risks and benefits.

POSTSPLENECTOMY SEPSIS

The recent trend toward conservative management of splenic injury is due in large part to concern over postsplenectomy sepsis. The incidence of such overwhelming infection following splenectomy for certain hematologic diseases is high. For instance, thalassemia carries a 25 to 30 percent sepsis rate following splenectomy. However, the mortality from overwhelming sepsis in young healthy people following splenectomy for trauma is significantly lower. It is probably between 0.5 and 1.0 percent. It is probably higher in children than in adults. These statements are based on analysis of several large series primarily involving children. In these series the incidence of sepsis following removal of a previously normal spleen ranges from 1 to 3 percent. The mortality for children who develop such sepsis ranges from 30 to 50 percent. Thus, the risk is significant, but the true incidence needs to be kept in perspective when making choices regarding management of the patient with an injured spleen.

OPTIONS AVAILABLE

For the patient with a high probability of spleen injury, the surgeon can choose from three basic options: (1) to operate on all such patients and perform splenectomy, (2) to carry out abdominal exploration on the patients with the highest probability of injury, deal with any other abdominal injuries that may be present, and attempt to preserve all or part of the spleen whenever practical, (3) to observe such patients in the intensive care unit, vigorously support the circulation with fluid and blood infusion, and operate only if "forced." The choice of approach should be based on a rational weighing of the risks and benefits of each (to be discussed).

Routine Splenectomy

Routine splenectomy is the treatment for which the most historical information is available. The mortality for splenic injuries in patients with multiple injuries ranges from 10 to 18 percent. The majority of these deaths result from associated injuries and make comparison between groups extremely difficult. For purposes of these comparisons, it is appropriate to focus on patients with isolated injuries to the spleen, among whom the immediate postoperative mortality following splenectomy is much less than 1 percent. Although many series are reported with essentially no immediate postoperative mortality, let us assume that the immediate operative mortality following splenectomy for isolated injury approximates 0.5 percent. We can then construct a "worst case" calculation of the overall risk. To the immediate operative mortality of 0.5 percent, we will add the risk of dying from overwhelming infection. If we take the highest reported incidence of overwhelming postsplenectomy infection following removal of a previously normal spleen (3 percent) and assume the highest reported mortality rate of 50 percent, we begin to approach this number. The number needs to be modified by the effectiveness of pneumococcal vaccine in preventing death from overwhelming infection following splenectomy. The efficacy of the vaccine is about 33 percent because it covers only about 85 percent of pneumococcal strains, and many of the cases of overwhelming infection following splenectomy are not due to pneumococci. Accounting for all these factors yields an overall long-term mortality of 1.5 percent for routine removal of the spleen for isolated splenic injury (Fig. 1). This long-term mortality is the major disadvantage of routine splenectomy. It may be possible to improve on this outcome using the other approaches to be discussed. *However, approaches that are proposed as an alternative to routine splenectomy must equal or better this long-term outcome.* The advantages and disadvantages of this approach are obvious. It minimizes the probability of missed intra-abdominal injuries. On the other hand, it results in a large number of "nonproductive" laparotomies and carries the combined short- and long-term risks already outlined.

Nonoperative Management

The variables of this approach (nonoperative management) are more difficult to quantify. To determine the risk-benefit ratio, data are needed on the immedi-

Early operative mortality

0.005

+

(Incidence OPSI × mortality × [1 − vaccine efficacy])
(0.03 × 0.67) = 0.010

=

1.5 per 100

Other modalities must equal this

Figure 1 Long-term risk for isolated spleen injury treated by splenectomy.

ate outcome of the nonoperative approach, the probability of missing (or delaying treatment of) an associated injury, the percentage of people in whom splenic function is eventually preserved, the impact of prolonged marginal perfusion on other organs, the risk of added blood transfusions, and the cost of prolonged hospitalization. Data from large trauma centers have demonstrated that 20 percent of adults with a splenic injury (following blunt trauma) have an associated visceral injury requiring operative repair. Therefore, in adults the risk of missing a serious associated injury appears to argue heavily against a nonoperative approach. In children, the data are not so clear. Reports from large trauma centers suggest that the incidence in children is less than in adults, but still high. In contrast, reports from children's hospitals with a vast experience with blunt trauma and single system injuries suggest a lower incidence.

The success of this approach in preserving the spleen depends on the severity of the injury, and most of the data that is available addresses the success of this technique in children. In series with a predominance of multiple injuries, splenic function is preserved in roughly 75 percent of patients who are successfully managed. In more recent series (dealing almost exclusively with isolated injury to the spleen), splenic function is preserved greater than 90 percent of the time. The incidence of late bleeding from the spleen is exceedingly low and, when present, has occurred almost uniformly within the first week. The incidence of hepatitis and other consequences of transfusion is not available since most of these series are relatively small. However, the risk of transfusion complications (for instance, viral hepatitis risk: 1 to 2 percent per unit transfused with 20 percent progressing to chronic hepatitis) may become a factor in patients receiving one or more blood volumes.

Overall, this approach has been successful in children with low-energy blunt trauma when managed by individuals with considerable expertise. Under these circumstances, the outcome appears to satisfy the criteria stated previously.

However, a more general application of this approach to adults or to children with higher-energy injuries, penetrating injuries, and hemodynamic instability seems likely to produce a combined short-term and long-term outcome significantly worse than that from routine splenectomy.

Selective Operative Management with Spleen Repair

Data on which to base an analysis of the risk and benefit of this approach are relatively sparse since this approach is the newest of the three outlined. Questions that need to be answered in order to analyze this approach include the following. What percent of spleens can be preserved by this approach? What is the incidence of rebleeding after repair? What is the efficacy of splenic function after repair? What is the average transfusion requirement? What is the number of nonproductive laparotomies? What is the average length and cost of hospital stay? What are the optimal criteria for surgical exploration?

Partial answers to many of these questions are available. With experience and *adequate mobilization of the spleen*, the majority of spleen injuries in children are ameanbel to surgical repair. Exceptions are injuries with "pulverization" of the spleen and with major hilar vascular disruptions. A smaller proportion of splenic injuries in adults are easily repaired. (However, the long-term impact of splenectomy in adults appears to be less than in children, and the number of associated organ injuries appears to be higher.) The average transfusion requirement for children treated by this method appears, from some early reports, to be significantly less than for children treated initially nonoperatively and subsequently requiring spleen repair or splenectomy. The success rate following early operation is predictably higher than that following delayed operative intervention. (This last observation is obviously imbalanced since some of the patients in the conservatively treated group with simpler injuries never undergo operation.) Most important, the rebleeding rate following spleen repair is well below 10 percent and appears to be decreasing as more experience is gained. As in patients who are treated nonoperatively, virtually all episodes of re-bleeding appear to occur within the first week. Current evidence suggests that adequate protection against overwhelming postsplenectomy sepsis can be obtained if one-third of the spleen and its arterial supply are maintained intact. Several techniques for preservation of splenic function in patients who undergo splenectomy are being explored. Among these are the implantation of thin slices of spleen in omental pockets. Although such implants do appear to be able to remove damaged red blood cells, adequate proof of their ability to remove encapsulated bacteria is not yet forthcoming, and this approach must be considered experimental.

It is predicted that the foregoing selective approach will result in a significantly lower long-term incidence of overwhelming postsplenectomy infection than that of routine splenectomy. It seems probable that it will have a lower incidence of missed injuries and lower total blood requirement than nonoperative management. These and other considerations suggest that, particularly in adults and in children with multi-system injury, this approach should have an overall better short-term and long-term outcome than either of the other two approaches.

RECOMMENDED APPROACH TO PATIENTS WITH POSSIBLE SPLENIC INJURY

Realizing that as more data accrues, it will become easier to choose from among the courses just outlined, I currently recommend the following approach to patients with potential spleen injury, based on their overall clinical presentation. For the purpose of discussion, they are separated into several arbitrary groups.

Penetrating Trauma

In general, these patients (adults and children) with penetrating trauma should undergo exploratory laparotomy. For gunshot wounds, in particular, this principle is adhered to in the majority of trauma centers throughout the country. In the opinion of most, the high incidence of injuries requiring surgical attention supports this approach. For stab wounds to the abdomen, some exceptions exist. The primary exceptions are superficial wounds to the back in hemodynamically stable, otherwise asymptomatic patients and anterior stab wounds in patients who show no evidence of hemodynamic instability, peritoneal signs, or intra-abdominal blood loss.

Blunt Trauma

Patients who have experienced blunt trauma confined to the abdomen, who are hemodynamically stable, and in whom an abdominal examination reveals no peritonitis and minimal findings have traditionally been treated by observation. This approach has been very successful, and there seems little reason to change. If, for whatever reason, such patients should undergo a CT scan which reveals an "asymptomatic" injury to the spleen, this should not alter the predetermined course of observation. Development of significant abdominal findings or evidence of ongoing blood loss would be an appropriate indication for operative intervention and attempted splenic repair in these patients.

At the other end of the spectrum of blunt abdominal trauma are those patients (adult or children) with high-energy abdominal injuries who have evidence of peritonitis, pneumoperitoneum, or other intra-abdominal problems requiring operative repair. In this group of patients, rapid celiotomy with attempt at spleen repair is generally agreed to be the appropriate approach. The same approach is appropriate for individuals with continued cardiovascular instability in the face of vigorous intravenous resuscitation and in patients with ongoing transfusion requirements. There is some debate about what constitutes sufficient transfusion requirement to justify a laparotomy. It is my opinion that if the ongoing blood loss has an intra-abdominal cause (that is, if the patient's blood requirement cannot be explained based on extra-abdominal injuries), laparotomy, hemostasis, and appropriate attempts at spleen salvage will result in optimal long-term function with minimal short-term negative consequences.

The third group of patients present a more difficult decision. These are the patients who have usually (but not always) had a high-energy injury and either an equivocal physical examination or a physical examination of the abdomen that is rendered unreliable by the patient's mental status or accompanying injuries. In this group of patients, it is believed appropriate to consider adults and children separately. In the *adult*, the risk of associated intra-abdominal injuries is high, the long-term immunologic effects of splenectomy may be less than in children, and the practicality of spleen repair decreases with time. For these reasons, if a significant intra-abdominal injury can be identified, exploratory laparotomy is recommended. In this group of patients, I use peritoneal lavage as my first screening test. If the peritoneal lavage reveals over 100,000 red blood cells per cubic millimeter or other evidence of peritoneal injury, I proceed with laparotomy. If peritoneal lavage reveals essentially no red blood cells, I generally follow a course of careful observation. If the peritoneal lavage is equivocal, the patient is a candidate for CT scan or other tests that are more satisfactory than peritoneal lavage at diagnosing retroperitoneal and other occult injuries.

The major controversy evolves around *children* with the presentation just described, particularly those with high-energy injuries and equivocal or indeterminate abdominal examination. Most agree that further diagnostic procedures are indicated. Part of the debate centers around which procedures are best. It is proposed here that the approach be based on the patient's hemodynamic status. If the patient has had significant hypotension or is requiring ongoing intravenous therapy for cardiovascular support, I would recommend a determination of whether the patient has intra-abdominal bleeding. If intra-abdominal bleeding is present, I would recommend exploratory laparotomy. For this group of patients, peritoneal lavage would appear to be the initial diagnostic test of choice. The course of action based on the result of lavage is then similar to that exercised in the adult. If, on the other hand, the patient's cardiovascular status is stable, imaging techniques designed to identify specific organ injuries would appear to be a better initial diagnostic choice. If the CT scan (or other imaging technique) demonstrates an injury that requires surgical exploration, the course is obvious. If the patient has other system injuries that require operative intervention and a spleen injury is identified, the argument for celiotomy and spleen repair seems strong, since such patients carry a high mortality and can ill afford ongoing bleeding or delayed or missed injuries. If the extensive work-up reveals only an isolated injury to the spleen and the patient remains stable without signs of significant blood loss, careful observation may be justified.

OPERATIVE APPROACH TO SPLEEN REPAIR

Several excellent reviews of the operative approach to spleen repair are available and details are beyond the scope of this chapter. However, a few points deserve emphasis.

1. Repair of the spleen is usually possible except when the spleen is "pulverized" or in the face of major vascular hilar disruption.
2. Even if spleen repair is possible, it should not compromise the patient's probability of short-term recovery. This suggests that in patients with prolonged severe hypotension and in patients with multiple intra-abdominal or extra-abdominal injuries, attempts at spleen repair should not be extensive. If one patient in a hundred fails to survive the short term because of time and effort devoted to attempted spleen repair, the potential advantage is lost.
3. The most crucial step in repair of the spleen is adequate mobilization. A brief visit to the dissecting room to review the anatomy of splenic attachments can greatly enhance the surgeon's ability to rapidly and adequately mobilize the spleen. In the vast majority of patients (particularly in children), the spleen can be mobilized and brought virtually into the midline with ease.

THE LIVER

JOHN A. WEIGELT, M.D., F.A.C.S.

The liver is the second most commonly injured organ following blunt abdominal trauma and is the most commonly injured organ in patients with penetrating trauma of the abdomen. Diagnosis of liver injuries is not difficult since blood loss resulting in hypovolemic shock is the most common finding. Penetrating injuries to the abdomen requiring exploratory laparotomy usually present little diagnostic challenge. Blunt injuries of the liver are usually diagnosed by abdominal paracentesis or peritoneal lavage. At present, noninvasive diagnostic tests play virtually no role in the management of liver trauma.

MANAGEMENT OF LIVER TRAUMA

At least 70 percent of all liver injuries can be managed with little difficulty. Anatomic descriptions of common liver injuries include simple capsular tears, simple lacerations, stellate or multiple lacerations, avulsion, or crush injuries, and hepatic venous injuries.

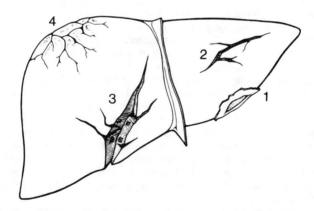

Figure 1 1) Capsular tear, 2) Simple laceration, 3) Stellate, multiple laceration, 4) Stellate laceraton with crush injury.

The management of liver trauma depends upon the severity of the injury, especially in relation to the presence of active bleeding and devitalized liver tissue.

Nonbleeding Laceration

The most common liver injury is a nonbleeding laceration. Such injuries are managed by simple drainage, regardless of the severity of anatomic disruption. A large stellate laceration of the liver dome is treated by drainage in the same manner as a simple laceration of the liver edge. It is not advisable to surgically explore a complex laceration that is not actively bleeding; closed suction drainage is preferable to ensure effective removal of blood and bile. Injuries of the inferior right hepatic lobe are drained with a single drain in Morison's pouch. A laceration in the dome of the liver without inferior penetration requires a second drain adjacent to the injury in addition to the subhepatic drain. For injuries of the left hepatic lobe, the closed suction drainage tube is placed in the left subhepatic space. All drains are brought out through separate stab wounds away from the laparotomy incision. The drains should remain in place until blood and bile drainage ceases or becomes minimal, usually within 1 to 5 days.

Bleeding Lacerations

A bleeding laceration of the liver parenchyma is the next degree of injury. The first priority is to control blood loss. A highly successful technique for achieving hemostasis is manual compression of the liver or "hepatic tamponade" with laparotomy packs. An injury can be packed for hemorrhage control while the rest of the abdomen is explored for associated injuries. Once extrahepatic injuries are identified and repaired, or at least controlled, attention can again be directed to the liver injury.

Temporary packing often controls hepatic hemorrhage and converts the bleeding laceration into a nonbleeding laceration, which may be managed by drainage alone. If bleeding continues despite packing, other hemostatic techniques must be used. One technique is to occlude the porta hepatis (Pringle maneuver). This requires placing a vascular clamp or soft tape around the hepatic artery, portal vein, and common bile duct. Temporary occlusion of blood flow in this manner may permanently stop the parenchymal bleeding or at least aid in control of hemorrhage. The amount of time this occlusion may be safely continued is controversial. Hepatic ischemia is reduced by releasing the occlusion for 1 to 2 minutes every 15 to 20 minutes.

If bleeding continues after this maneuver, the next step should be a controlled exploration or "tractotomy" of the liver laceration. The laceration is enlarged sufficiently to permit adequate exposure of injured vessels within the liver.

The liver capsule is incised with the electrocautery at the site of injury, and the liver substance is dissected by finger fracture technique, which permits tactile identification of blood vessels and bile ducts. These are ligated with 3–0 silk. Larger vessels and bile ducts are doubly ligated with simple ligatures and transfixion sutures of 3–0 or 2–0 silk. Small metallic clips may help to control bleeding in smaller vessels and bile ducts, but are not dependable for larger structures. The liver injury is systematically explored in this fashion until hemostasis is achieved. The Pringle maneuver is continued throughout this dissection.

Once the "tractotomy" is completed, the liver edges may be approximated with absorbable liver sutures. An omental pedicle is placed within the "tractotomy" to cover the raw surfaces of the liver and aid in local hemostasis. This dissection technique is peferable to blindly placed large liver sutures. The large liver sutures may control the bleeding by pressure, but may also lead to the formation of an intraparenchymal hematoma that can cause an intrahepatic abscess or hematobilia.

Avulsion-Crush Injury

Avulsion-crush injuries usually are a result of blunt trauma. Debridement of devitalized hepatic tissue is the most important aspect of treatment. Dissection techniques, previously described, are used to control hemorrhage. Manual control of the bleeding liver parenchyma is usually possible; this facilitates suture ligature of vessels and bile ducts. A Penrose drain wrapped tightly around the liver parenchyma may be helpful for temporarily controlling hemorrhage while identifying and suturing bleeding vessels. A large liver clamp (e.g., Lin hepatic compression clamp) usually is not helpful in these cases because the line of resection often does not allow enough room for the clamp to be placed properly. Debridement of devitalized liver tissue should be complete to avoid postoperative hepatic necrosis and suppuration. An omental pedicle may be used after debridement to cover the raw liver surfaces and promote hemostasis.

Adequate drainage for the larger liver injuries is imperative. True dependent posterior drainage is preferable and is best achieved by twelfth rib resection that is done from within the abdomen. The dissection is easily performed through the bed of the twelfth rib and extended through the muscular layers. Penrose drains are sewed together with a Keith needle. The needle is then pushed through the dorsal skin to identify the site for the external skin incision. The skin incision is not made until after the abdominal cavity is closed, and the patient is rolled on the opposite side to expose the twelfth rib area on the side of the injury. The Penrose drains placed earlier are now brought out through the skin incision and secured. This technique ensures the most dependent drainage and the least chance for retained fluid and/or blood.

An alternative choice for drainage is the use of large sump drains that have filtered air vents. These drains should be placed as dependently as possible through

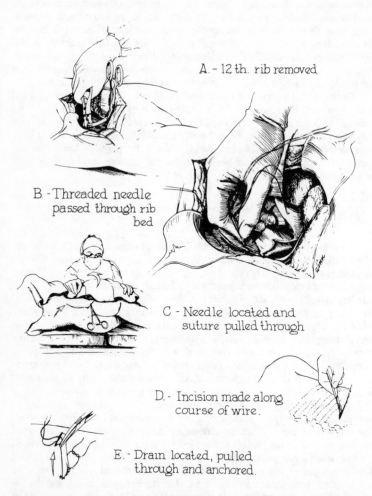

A. - 12 th. rib removed

B - Threaded needle
passed through rib
bed

C - Needle located and
suture pulled through

D. - Incision made along
course of wire.

E. - Drain located, pulled
through and anchored.

Figure 2 Reproduced with permission from Coln D. A technique for drainage through the bed of the twelfth rib. Surg Gynecol Obstet 1975; 141:608–609.

separate stab incisions. This method is not as reliable as dependent twelfth rib drainage with several Penrose drains in the postoperative management of large resectional debridements of the liver.

Liver-Packing Technique

When bleeding cannot be readily controlled or a coagulopathy develops, it is often necessary to pack the liver injury to control hemorrhage by tamponade and stabilize the patient's condition. Simple laparotomy packs can be used for this purpose. Packs should be placed under the liver first and then over the dome of the liver. The packing must be sufficiently tight to tamponade the bleeding without occluding the vena cava and impairing venous return. A total of 10 to 20 packs are often needed. Once the packing is complete and bleeding is controlled, the abdomen is closed. The patient is taken to the intensive care unit and transfused with appropriate blood components to correct volume deficits and coagulopathies. The packs are usually removed 48 to 72 hours after coagulation function has returned to normal. The patient is returned to the operating room, the packs are removed, and the operation is completed. It is often unnecessary to do much at the second operation except remove the packing and establish drainage.

Hepatic Artery Ligation

Hepatic artery ligation is an adjunctive technique for controlling liver hemorrhage. Ligation is easily performed by dissecting out the appropriate artery in the hepatoduodenal ligament. The common right or left hepatic artery can be ligated, depending on the site of injury. It is important to remove the gallbladder, especially when the right hepatic artery is ligated, to avoid morbidity from subsequent gallbladder necrosis. Hepatic artery ligation may not be helpful as the most common source of troublesome bleeding is the venous system.

Hepatic Vein Injury

Injuries to the hepatic veins with or without vena cava involvement are difficult to manage successfully. Early operation, identification of injury, and control by suturing results in the best outcome. Bleeding can only be controlled if adequate exposure of the injured area is obtained. Occasionally, an intracaval shunt may be helpful in isolating the injured area from its major blood supply; however, a shunt is infrequently required. Recently, hepatic tamponade with laparotomy packs has been used to control hemorrhage instead of immediately

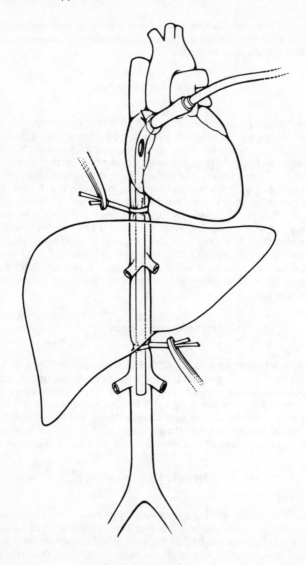

Figure 3 Atrial caval shunt placement.

placing a shunt. If bleeding is not controlled by liver packing, a shunt may be used. Ideally, a shunt should be used before coagulopathy or hypothermia develops, and it should always be placed in a deliberate, step-by-step fashion as outlined below.

1. Liver bleeding is controlled by packing and manual pressure.
2. A Pringle maneuver is performed.
3. The midline incision is extended into a median sternotomy, which allows isolation of the supradiaphragmatic vena cava and the right atrium.
4. The infrahepatic vena cava is encircled with a vascular tape just above the renal veins, taking care to avoid injury to any lumbar veins.
5. A 36 F plastic chest tube is used to fashion an intracaval shunt. An extra hole is made in the chest tube before shunt placement. This hole corresponds to the level of the left atrium after shunt placement.
6. The right atrial appendage is grasped with a Babcock clamp and a 2–0 silk pursestring suture is placed. Three equidistant guy sutures are placed around the atrial pursestring suture. The tip of the atrial appendage is cut off and the shunt is inserted. The guy sutures are used to stabilize the atrium during shunt placement. Care is taken to backbleed the shunt to remove all air before the pursestring is tied around the shunt. A clamp is initially placed over the end of the shunt exiting the heart, but this end of the catheter can also be used to infuse blood or fluid.
7. The introduction of the shunt into the vena cava should be guided by the operator's hand to ensure that the shunt does not pierce the vessel wall and create more damage. Once the shunt is in the vena cava, the vascular tapes above and below the liver are secured around the shunt to achieve vascular isolation of the hepatic venous injury and any associated retrohepatic vena caval injury.

An intracaval shunt can also be placed without opening the chest. A special shunt with a balloon at one end may be used to avoid encircling the suprahepatic vena cava. Inserting the shunt from below is not easy, and good backflow occlusion is not always obtained by the balloon catheter. For these reasons, the cardiac insertion method is preferred in the approximately 1 percent of liver injuries for which the shunt is needed.

After vascular isolation is established, the liver should be completely mobilized from its ligamentous attachments in order to repair the parenchymal and vascular injuries most effectively and accurately.

POSTOPERATIVE CARE

Postoperative care of patients with liver injuries involves blood transfusions, correction of coagulopathies, and respiratory and nutritional support. If a large amount of liver parenchyma has been resected, patients must be observed for hypoglycemia, thrombocytopenia, and hypoalbuminemia in the immediate postoperative period. Early complications are related to the massive amount of blood transfusions often required, and late complications are usually caused by infection.

PANCREAS AND DUODENUM

CHARLES F. FREY, M.D.

Injury to these organs, which constitutes no more than 3 to 12 percent of abdominal injuries, if overlooked or not treated appropriately at operation, is associated with a high morbidity and mortality. In the absence of disruption of the major pancreatic duct, the complications of pancreatitis, pancreatic fistula, pseudocyst, and pancreatic ascites seldom occur. Duodenum, common duct, and major pancreatic ducts may be injured separately or in combination. The incidence of combined injury of major pancreatic duct and duodenum is about 20 percent. When all three structures are injured, prompt recognition and appropriate therapy are essential to the patient's survival.

Factors affecting survival following pancreatic or duodenal injury include the number of associated injuries and, in particular, involvement of major vascular structures, the liver, and the colon. The wounding agent also affects mortality. Shotgun wounds and blunt trauma are generally more serious than a stab wound. The mortality rate for pancreatic or duodenal injury is reported to be 16 to 20 percent. Half of all deaths from pancreaticoduodenal injury occur within 24 to 36 hours after injury and are invariably associated with hemorrhage from injured major vessels, liver, or spleen. Injury to the duodenum and pancreas have little to do with the fatal outcome in these early deaths. Late deaths are usually secondary to sepsis and are often seen in patients in whom there is associated colonic or other gastrointestinal tract injury that causes bacterial contamination of the duodenal and pancreatic wound. Most importantly, these deaths are, for the most part, preventable and often result from overlooked or inappropriately treated pancreatic or duodenal injuries. Our highest priority in managing the patient with pancreatic or duodenal injury is to control hemorrhage from associated injury prior to attending the pancreatic or duodenal injury. Our next objective is the restoration of enteric and ductal integrity of the pancreas, duodenum, and common bile duct of the injured patient.

DIAGNOSIS

Penetrating injury of the abdominal cavity is usually obvious, and if the wound enters the peritoneal cavity, operative exploration is necessary. If penetrating injury is associated with signs of peritonitis or shock, operative celiotomy is mandatory. Identification and evaluation of pancreatic or duodenal injury is made intraoperatively.

Recognition of injury to the pancreas or duodenum following blunt trauma is a challenge to the clinician, both preoperatively and intraoperatively. When the patient has signs of peritoneal irritation, laparotomy is indicated. The presence

281

or absence of pancreatic or duodenal injuries is then assessed at operation. In patients with blunt abdominal trauma, the presenting signs and symptoms sometimes do not accurately reflect the seriousness of injury. Most often this occurs when the pancreatic or duodenal injuries occur in the absence of associated injuries to other intra-abdominal structures. The paucity of clinical signs and symptoms in some patients may be due to the fact that the duodenal rupture is retroperitoneal or the duodenal wall is necrotic from crush injury, but no leakage of intraluminal contents has occurred. In the case of rupture of the major pancreatic duct, insufficient time may have elapsed for the development of pancreatitis or the extravasation of significant amounts of pancreatic juice.

Assessment of the Pancreatic and Duodenal Injury

Injury to the pancreas is significant when the major pancreatic duct has been fractured (Fig. 1). Disruption of the major pancreatic duct leads to leakage of enzymes, local inflammation, and ductal obstruction. The complications of pancreatic injury all result from injury to the major pancreatic duct and include acute and chronic pancreatitis, pancreatic fistula, pancreatic ascites, pseudocyst, and abscesses. In the absence of injury to the major pancreatic duct, these complica-

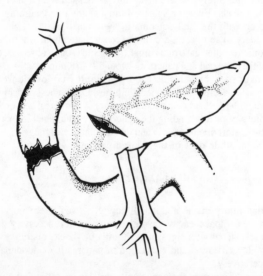

Figure 1 Major injuries to the duodenum and proximal pancreatic duct are depicted. The laceration of the distal pancreas, as depicted, is not significant as the major pancreatic duct is intact.

tions are rarely seen. Therefore, it is of paramount importance in the preoperative and intraoperative assessment of the patient with suspected pancreatic injury to determine whether the major pancreatic duct is intact. Conversely, what constitutes major injury to the duodenum is well understood and consists of obstruction by hematoma, necrosis of the wall with delayed leakage of contents, or disruption of the duodenal wall.

In penetrating abdominal injury, it is inappropriate to take time preoperatively to attempt to identify specific injuries involving the pancreas or duodenum as these organs can be examined at operation. Likewise, patients who have experienced blunt trauma who present with hypotension or an acute abdomen also come to operation and have no need for preoperative identification of specific injuries. Isolated injuries to the pancreas or duodenum usually are not associated with evidence of shock. Patients initially may have only mild tenderness over the upper abdomen, and further preoperative assessment is needed to establish the presence or absence of duodenal or pancreatic injury.

Laboratory Findings

Frequently, the serum pancreatic enzyme amylase and its isoenzymes and lipase are elevated in pancreatic injury. Serum elevation of amylase, including the isoamylase P, or increased urinary excretion of amylase is not the sine qua non of pancreatic injury. Any upper gastrointestinal enteric perforation, including a duodenal disruption, may release pancreatic enzymes normally destined for the gastrointestinal tract into the free peritoneal cavity, where they are absorbed by the abdominal lymphatics and returned to the blood through the thoracic duct. The result is elevation of serum enzymes in the absence of injury to the pancreas itself. Amylase is also released from the parotid gland if there is a facial injury. The isoamylases of the pancreas and parotid gland are not the same and may be used to differentiate the source of elevated serum levels. The isoamylase of the pancreas and intestine are one and the same. Therefore, the pancreatic isoamylase is of no value in distinguishing between obstruction of the major pancreatic duct or an upper gastrointestinal enteric perforation; either can produce elevation of the pancreatic isoamylase in serum and in peritoneal lavage returns.

Peritoneal Lavage

The retroperitoneal position of the pancreas and a large portion of the circumference of the duodenum may result in the retroperitoneal containment of air, fluid, and pancreatic juice following disruption of the duodenum or major pancreatic duct, at least temporarily. The retroperitoneal location of the duodenal contents and pancreatic juice prevents their uptake in the lavage fluid when lavage is performed soon after injury. Likewise, an initially intact but necrotic duodenal wall from a crush injury prevents egress of lumina contents and is not identified on lavage returns.

Usefulness of Serum and Urinary Amylase Determination

Serial determinations of the serum or urine amylase showing a progressive elevation over time may be helpful in identifying patients with isolated pancreatic or duodenal injury who often have equivocal abdominal findings and, because of the absence of associated injuries causing hemorrhage or peritonitis, no compelling indication for immediate operation. If the serum or urinary amylase progressively increases on the basis of determinations made ever 3 to 4 hours or if the levels remain elevated, duodenal or pancreatic injury should be suspected, and further diagnostic studies of the pancreas or operation is indicated. A cautionary note: serum amylase may not become elevated for 24 to 36 hours after injury of the pancreas even with total fracture or obstruction of the pancreatic duct. Surgery is not indicated on the basis of a single amylase elevation or if the initially elevated serum amylase declines on serial determinations.

Role of Water-Soluble Contrast Studies, Endoscopy, or Endoscopic Retroscopic Cholangiopancreatography (ERCP)

Water-soluble contrast material or endoscopy may be used to define the presence or absence of duodenal hematoma or duodenal rupture. ERCP is an underutilized but accurate means of preoperatively assessing the presence or absence of injury to the major pancreatic duct. Ultrasound and CT scan are less helpful in identifying a major pancreatic injury. Although ultrasound and CT scan are capable of identifying hematomas and swelling of the pancreas soon after injury, they provide no information about the integrity of the major pancreatic duct, which is the single most important factor determinant of a major pancreatic injury.

PREOPERATIVE PREPARATION

Preoperative preparation is similar to that of any other suspected intra-abdominal injury and has been discussed elsewhere in this text. I would emphasize, however, that blood should be sent for typing and crossmatch, and venous access should be secured through two cut-downs. A urinary catheter and nasogastric tube are placed, and a CBC, urinalysis, chest film, and one-shot IVP are obtained.

OPERATIVE EVALUATION

Priorities

The abdomen is entered through a midline abdominal incision which gives access to the pancreas, duodenum, liver, spleen, and other major vascular structures. The small bowel is eviscerated to allow inspection of the abdomen and retroperitoneum.

First priority is given to control of bleeding, usually from injuries to the liver, spleen, and major vascular structures. Hemorrhage from these sources has the potential to reach exsanguinating proportions, and its management takes precedence over pancreatic and duodenal injury. Injury to these latter structures is rarely associated with exsanguinating hemorrhage. Half the deaths from pancreatic and duodenal injury occur in the first 24 to 36 hours postinjury and are the direct result of hemorrhage from injury to associated structures.

Inspection

In the absence of, or following control of, hemorrhage, the pancreas is inspected through the gastrohepatic mesentery and the base of the mesocolon. Whenever retroperitoneal hemorrhage, hematoma, crepitus, induration, or bile staining is visualized in the pancreas, periduodenally, or at the base of the mesocolon, an injury to the major pancreatic duct or duodenum should be suspected. Likewise, if the pancreas itself is severed or transected more than half its diameter, it should be assumed that there is injury to the major pancreatic duct.

Although the body and tail of the pancreas can be visualized through the gastrohepatic ligament and base of the mesocolon, the head of the pancreas and the retroperitoneal duodenum are best examined after a Kocher maneuver is performed. When extended from the foramen of Winslow to the mesenteric vessels, the head of the pancreas and the first, second, and third portions of the duodenum can be visualized anteriorly and posteriorly by medially rotating the duodenum. The Kocher maneuver also permits bimanual palpation of the head of the pancreas. An area of pulpification indicates the probability of duct transection.

When hematomas are visualized through the gastrohepatic ligament or the base of the mesocolon, at the ligament of Treitz, the lesser sac should be opened through the gastrocolic ligament. To further evaluate hematomas, areas of pulpefaction, or loss of substance in the body and tail of the pancreas, the inferior border of the pancreas to the left of the superior mesenteric vessels may be mobilized and rotated superiorly, permitting bimanual palpation and inspection of the posterior surface of the gland.

In many patients, loss of integrity of the major pancreatic duct is obvious. In patients who are hemodynamically stable and in whom it is uncertain whether ductal injury has occurred, the major pancreatic duct may be visualized by intubating the ampulla of Vater through a duodenotomy or the associated duodenal laceration, if present, and contrast material injected. A pancreatic ductogram provides definitive information as to whether the major pancreatic duct is intact. The leakage of pancreatic fluid from small tributory ducts usually resolves in 4 to 6 weeks if managed by drainage alone.

TREATMENT

Objectives and Rationale

1. The control of hemorrhage, usually from associated injuries, takes top priority in management.
2. Resection of the distal pancreas should not exceed 80 percent of the gland in order to avoid, particularly in young patients, iatrogenic pancreatic exocrine or endocrine insufficiency. It is often difficult to judge accurately the percentage of pancreas to be resected because of variability in the size of the uncinate process. Therefore, resection of the distal pancreas should not be carried beyond the superior mesenteric vessels.
3. Eighty percent of duodenal injuries can be handled by debridement and simple closure. When there is significant loss of tissue or crush injuries for more than 75 percent of the circumference or devascularization of the duodenum, individualization of the operation based on the anatomy of the injury is essential.
4. When the common bile duct, duodenum, and major pancreatic ducts are transected, pancreaticoduodenectomy effectively restores intestinal and ductal integrity with a lesser mortality than less definitive procedures and provides long-lasting good results with less than a 20 percent chance of exocrine or endocrine insufficiency.

In summary, after control of hemorrhage, restoration of enteric and ductal integrity with preservation of function should be the major objective in the management of patients with pancreatic and duodenal injuries.

Factors Affecting Mortality

Most deaths occur within the first 48 hours of injury, the result of hemorrhagic shock from associated injuries. Sepsis, the second most common cause of death, is more often seen in patients who were in hemorrhagic shock preoperatively and/or had associated bowel injuries. Complex injuries involving the major pancreatic duct, common bile duct, and duodenum and overlooked injuries to any of these structures or delay in operative treatment also contribute to a fatal outcome. Mortality may exceed 40 to 50 percent in patients in whom preoperative therapy has been delayed for 24 hours or longer.

Isolated Duodenal Injuries

Local debridement and duodenal closure in two layers provide definitive therapy in 80 to 85 percent of patients with penetrating duodenal injury, most of whom have wounds that are not extensive. Tube duodenostomy or gastrostomy is of doubtful benefit in these patients. Segmental resection and end-to-end anastomosis with a two-layer closure is indicated in patients who have lost more than 75 percent of the circumference of the duodenal wall. Patients with blunt injury to pancreas and duodenum have a higher percentage of these circumferential injuries than are seen in patients with penetrating trauma to the duodenum.

Should segmental resection of the duodenum be indicated and the site of injury be close to the common bile duct and the ampulla, the common bile duct should be intubated with a Bakes dilator to prevent injury to the common bile duct or ampulla. Patients who have a major loss of duodenal tissue may require diversion of the gastric secretion from the duodenum to avoid a destructive fistula if the duodenal closure is tenuous. This can be accomplished by performing a gastrojejunostomy and stapling the pylorus shut. A duodenostomy tube may be used as well.

Injury to the Pancreas in Blunt Trauma

The most common site of injury to the pancreas is that portion of the neck that overlies the superior mesenteric vessels. Resection of the distal pancreas at the neck removes 60 to 65 percent of the pancreatic mass. The likelihood of exocrine or endocrine insufficiency when 35 to 40 percent of the pancreatic mass is retained is small. When the major pancreatic duct is disrupted to the left of the superior mesenteric vessels, I recommend resection of the distal pancreas, which includes tail or body and tail, of the pancreas. If the patient is in stable condition, I believe it is worthwhile to try to preserve the spleen when distal pancreatic resection is performed and thus avoid the late complications of infection associated with splenectomy. This can be accomplished if the splenic vein is preserved during removal of the tail, or body and tail, of the pancreas. When the major pancreatic duct is fractured to the right of the superior mesenteric vessels, distal resection carries the risk of producing endocrine or exocrine

insufficiency. Therefore, I prefer to (1) oversew the proximal severed end of
the pancreas with interlocking mattress sutures, (2) individually ligate the pancreatic duct, and (3) anastomose the distal segment of the pancreas with an end-
to-side pancreatic jejunostomy, utilizing a precise duct-to-jejunal-mucosa anastomosis (Fig. 2). I believe that this anastomosis is essential to the success of this
procedure. I strongly disagree with the placement of Roux-en-Y jejunal limb
over a fresh pancreatic laceration, in lieu of a duct-to-jejunal-mucosa anastomosis, nor do I use a Roux-en-Y limb to drain both the proximally and the distally

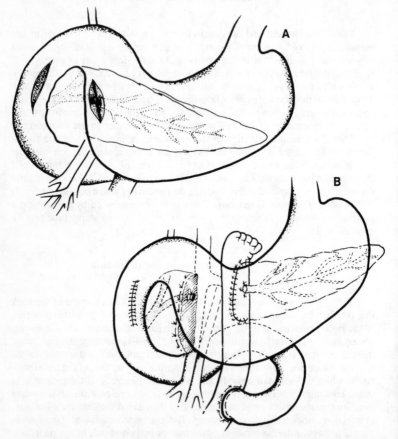

Figure 2 *A,* Combined injury of the duodenum and the proximal major pancreatic duct.
B, Recommended repair of combined injury of the duodenum and proximal major pancreatic duct.

fractured segments of the pancreas. Such a double anastomosis increases the likelihood of leakage, abscess formation, and fistulization.

Combined Major Duodenal and Pancreatic Injury

The ampulla of Vater can be intubated with a Fogerty irrigating catheter through the already opened duodenum and a pancreaticogram obtained on the operating table. If the injury to the major pancreatic duct is to the right of the mesenteric vessels, as previously described, the Roux-en-Y jejunal limb is used to drain the distal pancreas end-to-side. The proximal end of the severed pancreas is oversewn. The pancreatic duct should be individually ligated. If the associated duodenal injury involves more than 75 percent of the duodenal circumference or if a large duodenal defect has been created by the injury, segmental resection and end-to-end repair of the duodenal wound may be necessary. If the segment of injured duodenum creates such a large defect that a secure end-to-end anastomosis or closure cannot be obtained, a diverticularization can be performed. Some authors have advocated duodenal diverticularization for the management of patients with major pancreatic ductal injury. This is nonsense. Duodenal diverticularization addresses duodenal injury, but not injury of the major pancreatic duct.

Combined Biliary Tract and Duodenal Injuries

These injuries are infrequent, comprising less than 5 percent of all duodenal injuries. An end-to-end duodenoduodenostomy and choledochojejunostomy using a Roux-Y limb may be feasible.

Pancreaticoduodenectomy may be necessary if there is extensive loss of duodenum. Failure to establish enteric and ductal integrity is usually fatal. Under these circumstances, lesser procedures are no substitute for pancreaticoduodenectomy. The procedure is made easier by preserving as long a length of common duct as the fracture site permits. The patient's nutrition is enhanced if the antrum of the stomach is preserved, as described by Longmire. Care should be taken in excising the uncinate process. A replaced hepatic or a replaced right hepatic or accessory right hepatic in 25 percent of patients may originate from the superior mesenteric artery and traverse the uncinate process, where it may be encountered during resection of the uncinate process. Reconstruction after pancreaticoduodenectomy includes an end-to-side anastomosis between the body or tail of the pancreas and a Roux-en-Y jejunal limb. I strongly believe that a duct-to-jejunal-mucosa anastomosis provides few leaks and preserves function of the distal segment of pancreas. The common duct is anastomosed to the jejunum end-to-side distal to the pancreatic anastomosis. A duodenojejunostomy, end-to-side on the jejunal limb distal to the two previous anastomoses, completes the operation.

Major Biliary Tract and Pancreatic Injuries

Injuries to the major pancreatic duct in the head of the pancreas are best treated by oversewing the proximal severed end of the pancreas and anastomosing the distal pancreas to the jejunum in a Roux-Y fashion. Transection of the

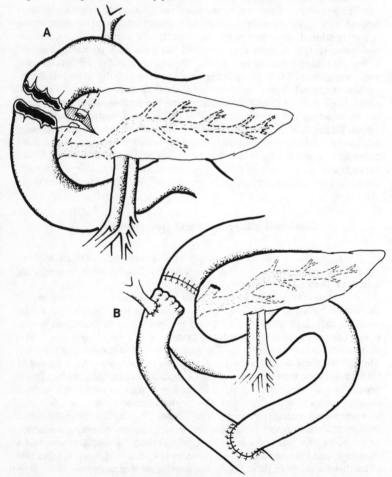

Figure 3 *A*, Combined injury of the duodenum and common bile duct. *B*, Reconstruction with Roux en Y choledochojejunectomy for combined injury of the duodenum and common bile duct.

bile duct can be dealt with by either choledochojejunostomy on a Roux-Y jejunal limb or choledochoduodenostomy.

Combined Bile Duct, Pancreatic, and Duodenal Injury

When the major pancreatic duct in the head of the pancreas has been transected as well as the common bile duct and duodenum, the most effective method of restoring ductal and enteral integrity and continuity is pancreaticoduodenectomy (Figs. 3 and 4). Attempts to treat this lethal combination of injuries by drainage alone or some compromise procedure only adds to the mortality associated with these major injuries. The positive long-term results of pancreaticoduodenectomy should further encourage qualified surgeons to employ pancreaticoduodenectomy in the combined duodenal bile duct and pancreatic injury. Only one in five patients requires exocrine or endocrine therapy.

POSTOPERATIVE CARE

Patients subjected to surgery for duodenal and pancreatic injuries should be decompressed by nasogastric suction until bowel function returns. Parenteral nutrition is an essential part of the postoperative management of these patients

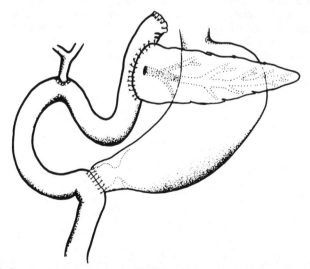

Figure 4 Reconstruction after pancreaticoduodenectomy for combined injury of the duodenum, common bile duct and major pancreatic duct.

with severe injuries who have a high incidence of complications during what may be a protracted postoperative course.

COMPLICATIONS

Injury to the major pancreatic duct may result in obstruction of the duct or leakage of pancreatic fluid. When injury to the major pancreatic duct is unrecognized, acute pancreatitis, chronic pancreatitis, pancreatic abscess, pancreatic fistulas, and pancreatic pseudocysts may result. Pancreatic fistula is the most common early complication associated with pancreatic trauma. Pancreatic abscess is the most serious. If the duct becomes obstructed, acute or chronic pancreatitis may develop. When there is leakage of the pancreatic secretion from the distal pancreas, this may form a collection; this collection becomes walled-off from surrounding structures to form a pseudocyst or, if not contained, a pancreatic fistula. Pseudocysts are the most common late complication of pancreatic injury following blunt abdominal trauma. Complications of duodenal injury include intra-abdominal abscess, duodenal obstruction, and fistulas. There is controversy whether the adjunctive procedures, jejunostomy and gastrostomy, should be employed during the operative management of most duodenal injuries. Although the reported incidence of duodenal fistula seems to be the lowest for those cases in which jejunostomy and gastrostomy are employed, this positive effect seems balanced by an increased incidence of intra-abdominal abscess, approaching 20 percent. When duodenal decompression is used selectively, the incidence of intra-abdominal abscess is lower, but there is a trade-off in that the incidence of duodenal fistula seems to be increased.

DUODENUM, SMALL INTESTINE, AND COLON

RICHARD A. CRASS, M.D.

CLASSIFICATION AND IMMEDIATE CARE

Injuries to hollow viscera are more commonly the result of penetrating rather than blunt trauma. There is a 95 percent incidence of visceral injuries in abdominal gunshot wounds. Thus, there are no special diagnostic problems with gunshot victims since exploratory laparotomy is indicated in every case. Abdominal films in such patients are most valuable if they are supplemented by injection of 100 cc of Hypaque to provide a one-shot IVP and to demonstrate bilateral renal function prior to exploration. If renal injury is found, repair or nephrectomy can be planned.

Abdominal Stab Wounds

Abdominal stab wounds with peritonitis or unexplained volume loss also present no special diagnostic problems, since all such patients should have exploratory laparotomy. However, special studies are helpful in the case of an abdominal stab wound if the patient is in stable condition and free of peritoneal signs. Abdominal films in these patients may demonstrate free air, the most sensitive film being an upright film taken after the patient has been upright for 15 minutes. If such studies are not possible, the next best view is a left lateral decubitus film. If these films are negative, the physician has the option either to admit the patient to the hospital and monitor vital signs, CBCs, and further physical findings or to undertake further diagnostic tests in the emergency department. Small bowel contents and blood are commonly not irritating to the peritoneal surfaces. However, delaying exploratory surgery in the patient with abdominal gunshot wounds or stab wounds for observation may be hazardous. One runs the risk of acute peritonitis or hemodynamic instability, which would necessitate surgery on a patient whose condition has been further weakened. Considering the low incidence of visceral injuries in stab wounds to the back, it is appropriate to take a conservative approach with these patients. For anterior stab wounds of the abdomen in stable patients without peritonitis, most trauma centers utilize local wound exploration with or without supplemental peritoneal lavage. We rely exclusively on the local wound exploration with the philosophy that, "If the weapon went into the peritoneal cavity, so do we." To reduce the frequency of unnecessary laparotomy, many centers utilize diagnostic peritoneal lavage in patients found, on local wound exploration, to have peritoneal violation. Unfortunately, some colon and diaphragmatic injuries do not bleed enough to result in a positive lavage if the classic cutoff of 100,000 RBC per cubic millimeter is used. Therefore, some centers advocate a lower cutoff of 50,000, 20,000, or even 10,000 RBC per cubic millimeter and this results in a greater number of false-positive lavage results. Therefore, we do not advocate peritoneal lavage in the evaluation of penetrating abdominal trauma.

Blunt Injuries to the Bowel

Blunt injuries to the bowel are often difficult to evaluate. Although colon injuries usually present with obvious peritoneal signs, small bowel and duodenal perforations often present with an unremarkable physical examination. Especially difficult are retroperitoneal duodenal injuries and duodenal hematomas. It is not an unusual occurrence for a trauma victim with a small bowel perforation to have such a benign examination that he is sent home from the emergency room, only to return hours later with established bacterial peritonitis. With blunt abdominal trauma, the keys to diagnosis are a high index of suspicion, serial physical examinations, and monitoring of vital signs, CBCs, and amylase determinations. If the patient requires orthopaedic or neurologic surgery, making physical examination unreliable or impossible, then peritoneal lavage or abdominal CT should be performed. Such studies are frequently indicated if the patient has a pelvic fracture, an equivocal physical examination, or a decreasing hematocrit without an obvious source of blood loss. If the patient is hemodynamically unstable, laparotomy rather than lavage should be performed. Computed tomography is more advantageous than peritoneal lavage in that it identifies and quantitates injuries and associated hemorrhage and provides imaging of the retroperitoneum. CT is an exquisitely sensitive indicator for free air; if contrast is routinely given by nasogastric tube, the study identifies contained retroperitoneal duodenal injuries. CT allows the nonoperative management of some liver injuries that, if studied by lavage alone, would lead to surgical exploration. If CT is not available or if the physician chooses diagnostic peritoneal lavage instead, and a duodenal injury is suspected (on the basis of elevated serum amylase or epigastric pain without peritonitis), a Hypaque upper gastrointestinal study (UGI) should be performed. A Hypaque UGI is also indicated if food intolerance following injury suggests the possibility of a duodenal hematoma.

In addition to routine resuscitation, insertion of a nasogastric tube, laboratory tests, and typing and crossmatching of blood, all patients suspected of having a bowel injury should receive preoperative antibiotics. Included are victims of abdominal gunshot wounds and stab wounds who will undergo laparotomy. With the low incidence of bowel injury associated with blunt trauma, we do not use antibiotics unless a bowel injury has been proved preoperatively. Although a combination of an aminoglycoside and clindamycin or metronidazole theoretically provides the best coverage for enteric organisms, cefoxitin alone has nearly the same coverage with less potential for nephrotoxicity and is our current choice.

CONDUCT OF EXPLORATION

The Abdomen

A midline exploratory laparotomy is recommended for all abdominal trauma. When operating for penetrating or blunt trauma, simple "running" of the bowel is usually sufficient for identification of bowel injuries. This should be done at least twice, and if an injury is found, the search should intensify for additional injuries since an "odd" number of holes is unusual. If a central abdominal hematoma is encountered, the duodenum should be mobilized by an extended Kocher maneuver to search for injuries. Hematoma adjacent to the ascending or descending colon should prompt full mobilization of that side of the colon to search for injuries. In penetrating trauma, hematoma around the rectum should be entered with a limited mobilization of the rectum supplemented by intraoperative proctoscopy if indicated. Blunt rectal trauma is rare. It is best not to explore pelvic hematomas caused by blunt trauma since this may result in release of the tamponade of pelvic tissues and in hemorrhage that is difficult or impossible to control. If rectal bleeding is found in such patients, intraoperative proctoscopy is indicated.

The Duodenum

Treatment of duodenal injuries must be individualized according to the extent of injury and the presence or absence of associated injury to the pancreas. For simple, small, nondevitalizing injuries, simple two-layer closure is sufficient. If the surgeon is concerned about the integrity of the repair, temporary decompression of the duodenum with a 10 F Foley catheter duodenostomy may be prudent. Such a duodenostomy should be placed within a pursestring suture through a surgically created stab wound and never through the repair. For more extensive injuries to the duodenum, especially if associated with pancreatic and/or biliary injuries, it is preferable to "diverticularize" the duodenum. This is accomplished by stapling the proximal duodenum with the TA-55 stapler (3.5-mm staples) and performing an antecolic gastrojejunostomy. The only time we resort to pancreaticoduodenectomy is for extensive, devitalizing, combined pancreatic and duodenal injuries of which repair is impossible.

Small Intestine

Most small bowel injuries can be handled by a simple two-layer closure. One-layer closures should be avoided since they can result in troublesome postoperative mucosal hemorrhage. For extensive injuries, certain injuries on the mesenteric side, and multiple injuries in a short segment, small bowel resection and reanastomosis is indicated. Because of the rich blood supply and paucity of luminal bacteria in the small bowel, these anastomoses usually heal without incident. Jejunostomy or ileostomy is never indicated for small bowel injuries. Small bowel mesentery injuries are common in blunt and penetrating trauma and usually are simple to manage by suture ligation of bleeding points. It is important not to compromise the blood supply to the small bowel. If the blood supply to the small bowel has been compromised by the injury or repair, it is often necessary to resect the affected bowel. We have found fluoroscein angiography to be extremely useful in determining whether or not to resect small bowel, and in delimiting the extent of resection. For proximal mesenteric injuries, with injury to the superior mesenteric artery and/or vein with extensive bowel compromise, an attempt at vascular repair is indicated. If there is any questionably viable bowel left behind or if a vascular repair has been performed, a second-look operation is generally prudent at 24 hours. Abdominal closure in small bowel injuries can be routine; the skin is left open only if there has been a delay in exploration leading to established peritonitis.

Colon

Because of fecal content and poorer blood supply than in the small bowel, colon injuries are more difficult to manage than small bowel injuries. Over the past century, the mortality of colon injuries in armed conflicts has decreased from 90 percent during the Civil War to 13 percent during the Vietnam conflict. This improvement is the result of many factors including routine laparotomy, faster evacuation of combat casualties, and a policy of mandatory colostomy from the period of the Second World War onward. More recently the necessity of mandatory colostomy for civilian colon injuries has been questioned. Most combat wounds are caused by high-velocity gunshot wounds and schrapnel with attendant fecal soilage of the peritoneal cavity and devitalizing injuries of the colon. Approximately 85 percent of civilian colon injuries are caused by low- or medium-velocity gunshot wounds and stab wounds, with blunt trauma accounting for the rest. It has been shown unequivocally that small colonic wounds from low- or medium-velocity gunshots and stab wounds with absent or minimal fecal contamination, no shock, and no major associated injuries can be managed safely by primary repair without colostomy. More controversial is whether, given the same conditions, ileocolostomy for significant right colon injuries requiring resection is prudent. There is no compelling evidence in trauma, as opposed to general surgical teaching, that an ileocolostomy is a safer anastomosis than a left-sided colocolostomy. My policy in recent years has been to choose an end ileostomy and mucous fistula instead of primary anastomosis for most right colonic injuries requiring resection. For other colon injuries not suitable for repair, I favor division of the colon through the injury or resection of the injured segment with end-colostomy and mucous fistula. An exception to this policy is reparable lesions of the distal sigmoid that do not meet the criteria for primary repair and which, if divided, would leave the patient with a Hartmann pouch, making later restoration of continuity difficult. In such cases, I repair the injury and protect the repair with a proximal end colostomy and mucous fistula. Although some groups favor exteriorized repair, my experience with this procedure has shown poor results with infrequent healing of the exposed suture line.

For colon repairs, there is no evidence that a two-layer closure is necessary; I favor a one-layer closure with interrupted simple or Gambee 4-0 silk sutures. Rectal injuries are a special type of colonic injury and require different therapy. Because of their potential for catastrophic pelvic cellulitis, all rectal injuries necessitate proximal fecal diversion with a divided colostomy. Injuries should be repaired, if possible, either from above or, if low, by transanal repair if the injury can be exposed with anal retractors. All extraperitoneal rectal injuries should be drained. The presacral drains are placed through an incision posterior to the anus and carried just anterior to the coccyx to enter the presacral space. Unless there is an inaccessible rectal wound that might leak irrigant and feces into the perirectal spaces, I favor distal segment irrigation to remove feces from the rectum. I close the fascia in colon injuries with monofilament, interrupted, nonabsorbable sutures. The skin is packed open, with a delayed primary closure planned for postoperative day 5 if the wound is not soupy.

POSTOPERATIVE CARE

No special postoperative measures are necessary with most small bowel and duodenal injuries. A tube duodenostomy, if placed, should be withdrawn in stages, 9, 10, and 11 days postoperatively. For all bowel injuries, perioperative antibiotics should not be administered longer than 24 to 48 hours postoperatively. If a colostomy has been created, we plan restoration of continuity 4 to 6 weeks following injury. If a repair has been made in the distal segment, contrast studies should be performed to demonstrate the absence of leaks prior to restoration of continuity.

THE UTERUS

GERALD O. STRAUCH, M.D.

The management of uterine injury depends on whether the injury is blunt or penetrating and whether the patient is or is not pregnant.

THE NONGRAVID UTERUS

Injuries to the nonpregnant uterus are uncommon, and blunt injury is rare. If blunt injury occurs, the setting is one of massive pelvic disruption, and the uterine injury is almost incidental to injuries of associated pelvic structures, namely, the pelvic girdle and its associated vasculature, the urinary tract, and the colorectum. The uterus is resected, if required, or repaired with absorbable sutures if control of uterine bleeding is all that is needed.

Penetrating injuries of the uterus can occur as a result of transvaginal instrumentation or impalement, but such injuries are almost always isolated injuries that are managed according to well-established gynecologic principles and procedures. They are rare in the victim of multiple system injury.

For the traumatologist, almost all penetrating injuries of the nongravid uterus are bullet wounds that require suture to control bleeding. Substantial bites of the uterine wall with interrupted absorbable sutures ordinarily suffice for this purpose. Hysterectomy is an option, but is rarely required for most bullet wounds sustained from low-velocity weapons, as is the usual situation in civilian injury.

THE PREGNANT UTERUS

Management of abdominal injury during early pregnancy differs little from that in the absence of pregnancy. Abundant data attest to the rarity of injury as a cause of spontaneous abortion during early pregnancy. The physiologic and anatomic changes associated with early pregnancy are not sufficiently great to alter the management from that for the nongravid uterus.

On the other hand, pregnancy beyond the first trimester affects injury management substantially. The more advanced the pregnancy, the greater is its potential for altering the pattern of injury and response to injury. The most important factors in late pregnancy that bear on treatment following injury are (1) uterine size, (2) alterations in the vascular system, and (3) status of the fetus. The enlarged uterus in late pregnancy is more vulnerable to injury because of its size, causes compression of the small bowel into a more confined intra-abdominal compartment, and may aggravate the effects of hypovolemia following injury.

Blunt and penetrating wounds of the uterus are not uncommon when abdominal injury occurs in late pregnancy. Most blunt injuries are incurred in auto-mobile accidents. Uterine rupture is rare, but placental separation is not uncom-mon. Gunshot and knife wounds of the abdomen in late pregnancy frequently cause uterine wounds; in non-gravid women other abdominal organs are injured less frequently.

Because the small bowel is forced into a contracted space in late pregnancy, penetrating wounds that involve the small bowel may be more impressive in terms of the amount of damage incurred to small bowel and mesentery. The uterus of late pregnancy can severely reduce venous return to the heart, by compression of the inferior vena cava, when the injured woman in late pregnancy is supine. Maternal blood volume in late pregnancy is increased about 30 percent over normal values. Because the increase in plasma volume exceeds the increase in red blood cell mass, hematocrit levels in late pregnancy are commonly in the "mildly anemic" (average 35%) range compared to normal values. Cardiac output in late pregnancy is increased 30 to 40 percent over normal values. Uterine blood flow is enormously increased to supply the metabolic needs of the fetus. In the presence of maternal hemorrhage, uterine blood flow may be diminished to as little as half the normal flow because of selective uterine arterial constriction, which favors maternal survival but simultaneously jeopardizes the fetus.

Injury to a woman in late pregnancy requires consideration of the fetus in the treatment plan since a second life is threatened by the circumstances.

Strategic to the management of the severely injured woman in late pregnancy is the concept that *the most effective efforts to save the life of the mother constitute also the best means of saving her unborn child*. Another important rule is that the *general priorities of management are the same in this setting as they are for all victims of multiple systems injury*.

Resuscitation in Late Pregnancy

Because of the reduced venous return that may accompany the supine position, positioning the patient is important. The left lateral decubitus position is preferred to prevent vena caval compression by the uterus. If the patient must be maintained supine, elevation of the right hip and manual displacement of the uterus to the left may alleviate compression of the inferior vena cava.

Because of the pathophysiologic responses to injury in late pregnancy, the fetus may be rendered severely hypoxic when maternal hypoxia is only minimal. Accordingly, special efforts must be made to provide generous maternal oxygenation.

Similarly, severe maternal hemorrhage may not be reflected by evidence of hypovolemia in basic maternal hemodynamic parameters because of the combination of the normally high maternal blood volume and the uterine artery vasoconstriction; however, the fetus may be concurrently subjected to severe hypoxia caused by diminished uterine blood flow. If maternal shock supervenes, fetal mortality occurs in 80 percent of cases. Therefore, the need for aggressive maternal blood volume replacement and for appropriate hemodynamic monitoring cannot be overstressed. Specifically, early institution of central venous pressure monitoring is of critical importance, and monitoring of pulmonary artery pressures should be seriously considered.

If a pneumatic compression garment (MAST, PASG) is used for resuscitation, inflation of the abdominal compartment should be omitted.

Early obstetric consultation is essential so that appropriate fetal monitoring, which may dictate important management decisions, can be instituted.

Blunt Injury in Late Pregnancy

Management of blunt abdominal injury in late pregnancy requires recognition of some special facets pertinent to specific injuries in this setting. The enormous pelvic blood supply predisposes the patient to severe hemorrhage in pelvic fracture. Interestingly, uterine rupture is uncommon. Placental abruption may pose a serious threat to both mother and fetus from hemorrhage or the coagulopathy of disseminated intravascular coagulation. Premature labor is commonplace in survivors of severe automobile collisions, and intrauterine death of the fetus may occur. The close cooperation of a surgeon and obstetrician is critical to optimal decisions.

If diagnostic peritoneal lavage is felt to be appropriate, it is performed cephalad to the umbilicus, using an open technique to avoid injury to the uterus.

Abdominal operation is dictated by assessment of the abdomen essentially independent of the pregnancy except for considerations regarding cesarean section, which will be discussed subsequently. Axiomatic is the concept that an aggressive approach to operation in these circumstances is the safest strategy. After the fetus has been removed, a ruptured uterus can be repaired with interrupted absorbable sutures, assuming the rupture is not extensive. Superficial uterine tears can be controlled with sutures also. Under special circumstances, bilateral hypogastric artery ligation may salvage a bleeding uterus that might otherwise require hysterectomy, particularly if salvage of childbearing capacity is a high priority; however, this maneuver is by no means totally reliable and must be undertaken with a high degree of circumspection. Hysterectomy is indicated *only* when uterine repair is not possible.

Penetrating Wounds in Late Pregnancy

The principles applying to management of penetrating wounds of the abdomen are unaltered by late pregnancy. Gunshot wounds of the abdomen rarely cause maternal mortality because the uterus is chiefly the organ injured, and injuries to other organs, which may be much more life-threatening, only occur in about 20 percent of cases. Fetal damage and mortality are high, depending on the specifics of the injury. Stab wounds of the uterus are less common than gunshot wounds.

Indications for operative intervention applicable to any patient with a penetrating abdominal wound remain valid in late pregnancy. At operation, the principles pertaining to blunt injuries described earlier also apply to penetrating wounds. Although fetal injury and mortality are common, emptying of the uterus at operation is contraindicated if fetal injury or death is the sole indication. Celiotomy does not complicate subsequent vaginal delivery, even if labor occurs in the early postoperative period.

Indications for Cesarean Section

Cesarean section for injured women late in pregnancy is indicated (1) if the fetus is in jeopardy from hypoxia and (2) if the risk of fetal death from hypoxia exceeds the risk of death from prematurity after delivery. Fetal survival after delivery is over 50 percent if gestational age is over 28 weeks. Fetal death, in itself, is *not* an indication for cesarean section. Decisions regarding cesarean section in the patient whose abdomen has not been explored or in the patient whose injuries have necessitated prior celiotomy are ordinarily dictated by fetal monitoring. During the course of abdominal injury performed because of maternal injury and not primarily because of fetal distress, cesarean section may be required because of uterine rupture; mechanical blockage of the approach to the pelvis by the enlarged uterus in the presence of injuries to pelvic structures mandating repair, diversion, or resection, or sudden or impending maternal death.

On rare occasions, cesarean section may be considered following maternal death. In such an event, delivery as soon as possible after maternal death is critical, and it is essential that no more than 15 minutes ensue between maternal death and delivery. Fetal salvage following postmortem cesarean section is inversely related to the interval between maternal death and delivery. Survival of the infant, if the interval is more than 15 minutes, is highly unlikely. Other important factors that may influence a decision regarding postmortem cesarean section are the cause of the mother's death, the course of resuscitation and pathophysiologic events prior to maternal death, and the assessment of the condition of the fetus prior to maternal death.

GENITOURINARY TRACT

JACK W. McANINCH, M.D.

KIDNEY INJURY

The first indication of kidney injury on assessment in the emergency room is the presence of microscopic or gross hematuria. Dipstick methods of determining the presence of hematuria have proved to be satisfactory and should prompt immediate excretory urography and staging of the injury.

Blunt traumatic injuries caused by automobile accidents, falls, or blows to the abdomen may cause significant damage to the kidney and represent at least 80 percent of all renal injuries seen in most urban hospitals. In rural hospitals, 90 to 95 percent of kidney injuries are caused by blunt trauma. Bed rest and observation is successful in managing 95 percent of these *blunt* traumatic injuries. The patient should be maintained on strict bed rest until the gross hematuria has cleared, and then ambulation should be allowed to a limited extent. Hospitalization is usually unnecessary after the gross hematuria clears. The patient must be carefully monitored for falling hematocrit and evidence of retroperitoneal bleeding. Should gross hematuria return after ambulation is allowed, reassessment of the injury is indicated.

Penetrating injuries account for approximately 20 percent of renal injuries in urban settings such as San Francisco. These generally occur from gunshot wounds and stab wounds. All penetrating renal injuries require operative exploration, unless the staging process indicates that the renal injury is minor. Indications for operative exploration in renal injury are (1) excessive and persistent retroperitoneal bleeding, (2) pulsatile retroperitoneal hematoma, (3) urinary extravasation, (4) significant nonviable tissue, and (5) vascular injury. Clinical judgment must be exercised in applying these indications for operation. In a patient who is otherwise in stable condition following blunt injury, slight urinary extravasation would not necessitate renal exploration when additional indications for operation are not present. The large retroperitoneal hematoma incidentally discovered at exploratory laparotomy calls for an intraoperative excretory urogram, which will give information regarding the injured kidney as well as the presence of a normal contralateral kidney. Should the injured kidney not appear normal on this excretory urogram, renal exploration would be indicated. Careful preoperative staging of the injury by means of excretory urography and computed tomography helps to identify patients who can be managed nonoperatively.

The operative approach for exposure of an injured kidney requires a transabdominal incision, which allows the surgeon to expose the renal vessels and control them with vessel loops. Massive bleeding should be controlled by vascular clamps applied to the individual vessels. The kidney is then exposed by reflecting the colon off the hematoma, and the hematoma can be entered without fear of exsanguinating hemorrhage. Repair of the injured kidney is successful in 90 percent of cases. Total nephrectomy is seldom necessary.

The nonviable tissue should be removed and hemostasis obtained by means of fine figure-of-8 chromic sutures on individual bleeding points. The collecting system should be closed and made watertight and the defect covered with renal capsule or omental pedicle graft. Drains are left in the area only when a watertight closure of the collecting system cannot be accomplished.

Postoperatively these patients should be allowed to ambulate as soon as the gross hematuria has cleared. The mean hospital stay for patients who undergo surgery for renal injury is less than 7 days. Patients who have gross hematuria and are managed nonoperatively should be hospitalized and remain at bed rest until the gross hematuria is cleared and then allowed ambulation and discharge with restricted activity. Patients with microscopic hematuria should be well staged and discharged home with restricted activity levels. Excretory urography should be done 2 to 3 months following injury to evaluate the status of healing and functioning renal parenchyma.

URETERAL INJURY

A ureter may be injured by a penetrating object (bullet or knife), surgical mishap, or blunt trauma. Blunt trauma is rare, and the other two types of injury are approximately equal in incidence.

In penetrating injuries of the ureter, microscopic hematuria is present in 80 percent of cases and leads one to suspect injury. The surgically injured ureter usually causes obstruction and severe pain in the postoperative period. Excretory urography and retrograde ureterograms establish the diagnosis.

Penetrating injuries to the ureter require surgical reconstruction, in most cases by ureteroureterostomy consisting of resection of the injured area and a primary repair. In such cases, internal stents using double-J catheters are recommended. In cases of surgical injury to the ureter that have been discovered within 2 weeks of operation, re-exploration and surgical management of the injury is recommended. Lower ureteral injuries may require ureteroneocystostomy. Mid and upper ureteral injuries can be managed by transureteroureterostomy or ureteroureterostomy. Internal stents to maintain alignment and patency of the ureter are recommended in all repairs except the transureteroureterostomy procedure.

Drains should be left in the retroperitoneum following reconstruction. Internal stents are generally left in place for 4 to 6 weeks, and following excretory urography, they can be removed endoscopically through the bladder. Excretory urography should be performed approximately 3 months after reconstruction to ascertain ureteral patency.

BLADDER INJURY

Approximately 10 percent of pelvic fractures are associated with bladder rupture. Gross hematuria is present in most, and the diagnosis is established by a filling cystogram utilizing at least 300 cc of contrast material in the bladder. Injuries to the bladder are classified according to site of rupture, and these sites, in decreasing order of frequency are extraperitoneal (50%), intraperitoneal (30%), and combined (20%).

Patients who have bladder rupture should undergo surgical exploration and repair of the bladder. A transabdominal midline incision in the lower abdomen can be utilized, and exposure of the bladder should be done in the midline. One should carefully avoid entry into any lateral pelvic hematomas that exist. The bladder should be opened in the midline and inspected from within. Extraperitoneal lacerations are then closed from inside the bladder with a single layer of interrupted 2–0 chromic suture. Intraperitoneal bladder rupture should be closed in two layers of running sutures. A suprapubic cystostomy should be left in place for 8 to 10 days. Virtually all these bladders return to full function and, during the early healing phases, should be monitored carefully for potential urinary infection. X-ray studies are seldom indicated unless the patient has complaints that suggest problems.

URETHRAL INJURY

Approximately 5 percent of pelvic fractures are associated with urethral injury usually at the prostatomembranous junction. In addition, straddle injuries occur to the deep bulbar urethra and pendulous (anterior) urethra. The best indication of urethral injury is the finding of blood at the urethral meatus on initial examination. Passage of a urethral catheter is contraindicated when urethral injury is suspected. Urethrography should be the initial study performed and will establish the diagnosis.

Virtually all urethral injuries are the result of blunt trauma and occur in men. When penetrating injuries are seen, operative exploration and reconstruction of the specific injury is generally indicated. Female urethral injuries are uncommon.

The initial management of blunt traumatic disruption should be suprapubic cystostomy. This should be done by open exploration of the bladder through a lower midline abdominal incision. Exposure of the bladder should be confined to the midline so that lateral pelvic hematomas can be avoided. Only a small cystostomy incision is needed to permit inspection of the inside of the bladder for potential rupture. Manipulations in the deep pelvis should be avoided and no drains should be left in place because either measure can introduce infection in the perivesical hematoma. Associated long bone fractures of the lower extremity, if present, are treated by stabilization and fixation.

Patients with complete prostatomembranous urethral disruption invariably develop a stricture at the site of the disruption, but this can be repaired electively 2 to 3 months following injury. This repair can be accomplished by a combined transpubic perineal approach, by endoscopic urethrotomy, or by perineal urethroplasty. With this delayed approach to therapy, only 20 percent of these patients become impotent, but this is thought to be secondary to nerve and vascular damage at the time of the initial injury. Incontinence seldom occurs, but is a recognized complication of the injury. Secondary stricture formation following urethroplasty may occur in 15 to 20 percent of cases and often can be managed by endoscopic urethrotomy.

Patients with anterior urethral injury (bulbar and pendulous) who are managed by initial suprapubic cystostomy should have a voiding cystourethrogram approximately 2 to 3 weeks following injury; if no extravasation is noted, the patient should be allowed to continue voiding per urethra. Most of these patients develop relative strictures in the area of injury, but most do not require operative intervention or reconstruction. Should operative correction be indicated, endoscopic urethrotomy is usually successful.

GENITAL INJURY

Penile rupture, although uncommon, demands immediate diagnosis and correction. The patient gives a history of a loud cracking sound while engaging in sexual activity, and in all cases an erection is present. A transverse tear in the tunica albuginea that surrounds the erectile bodies occurs due to the force applied to the area. Immediate detumescence occurs, and a hematoma develops on the penile shaft. Surgical correction of this lesion should be performed and simply involves controlling the bleeding and reapproximation of the tunica albuginea with interrrupted polyglycolic acid sutures. Patients so treated experience normal return of erections and sexual function.

Blunt trauma to the scrotum results in large hematoceles and testicular rupture. Testicular rupture is best diagnosed by ultrasonography of the involved side, which will demonstrate areas of relative lucency of the echogenic patterns within the testicle parenchyma. Surgical correction of the ruptured testicle should be done by a transcrotal approach with evacuation of the hematoma and repair of the injury. The nonviable parenchyma that extrudes freely into the scrotal space should be removed, and the tunica albuginea of the testicle should be approximated with a running polyglycolic suture. These testicles heal after reconstruction and are useful for hormone production and cosmetic appearance. It is unlikely that spermatogenesis would return to testicles after such an injury.

Major skin loss to the penis and scrotum occurs from avulsion injuries, burns, gunshot wounds, and stab wounds. Urethrography should be done to determine whether concomitant urethral injury is present. Management should be aimed at reconstruction, using all available attached skin that can be salvaged. When local skin is not available, split-thickness skin grafts can be used to cover the testicles and penis. When the wound appears to be severely contaminated, testicles can be placed in subcutaneous pouches on the medial aspect of the thigh. Later scrotal reconstruction can then be performed. Third-degree burns of the penile shaft and scrotum should undergo total skin excision with immediate replacement by split-thickness skin grafts. With these methods, acceptable cosmetic and functional results can be expected.

THE PELVIS

DONALD D. TRUNKEY, M.D.

Pelvic injuries can be the most difficult torso injuries to treat. The potential for long-term disability is enormous owing to the frequent involvement of pelvic nerves that control extremity, bladder, anorectal, and sexual functions. In addition, the pelvis serves an important function in the transmission of weight from the torso to the lower extremities. Thus, injury to the pelvis often leads to permanent orthopaedic disability.

The most difficult immediate treatment problem encountered in severe pelvic injuries is hemorrhage which can be devastating and uncontrollable. Postmortem studies show that hemorrhage occurs principally as a result of laceration to veins in the posterior pelvis and small arterioles associated with fractures to cancellous bone. The bleeding occurs into the soft areolar tissue of the retroperitoneum, a huge potential space extending from the respiratory diaphragm to the mid thigh. This potential space and low tissue pressure accounts for the massive hemorrhage frequently associated with Type I and II fractures which involve the posterior elements (Table 1). Type III fractures are not usually associated with extensive hemorrhage unless a bony fragment lacerates a major vessel.

It is extremely important to rule out injuries associated with pelvic fractures since these may determine treatment priorities. Approximately one-third of pelvic fractures will have associated genitourinary injuries such as torn urethra or ruptured bladder. Because both of these injuries usually mandate suprapubic drainage it is prudent to waive consideration for peritoneal lavage or a computed tomography (CT) scan of the abdomen; exploratory laparotomy at the time of suprapubic cystostomy rules out associated intra-abdominal injury. Although associated rectal injury is not as common as associated genitourinary injury, its presence also mandates exploratory laparotomy and fecal diversion.

In my experience the majority of pelvic injuries (approximately 75%) become hemodynamically stable after the initial resuscitation. Some of these may require internal fixation if they have significant pubic diastasis, or major disruption of posterior elements or of the acetabulum. The remaining 25 percent of injuries can represent significant hemorrhagic problems but it is important to rule out bleeding from other intraperitoneal injuries before assuming the bleeding is from the pelvic fracture. Current methods for ruling out intraperitoneal hemorrhage include diagnostic peritoneal lavage, CT, and exploratory laparotomy. I favor CT unless there is already an indication to do a laparotomy such as suprapubic cystostomy or fecal diversion. Diagnostic peritoneal lavage often yields a false positive reading when the pelvic hematoma is large because of the diapedesis of red blood cells into the peritoneal cavity.

I would further characterize the 25 percent of injuries in patients with sig-

TABLE 1 Classification of Pelvic Fractures

Type	Characteristics
I	Comminuted (crush) injury
	3 or more major components involved (rami, ilium, acetabulum, sacrum)
	Often unstable
	Usually are combinations of Type II A, B, C, D
II	Unstable injury (requires immobilization or traction to reduce hemorrhage and/or maintain position of weight bearing portion of pelvis)
	A Diametric fracture with cranial displacement of hemipelvis (Froman and Stein, 1967; Malgaigne, 1847)
	B Diametric fracture, undisplaced
	C Open book (sprung) pelvis
	D Acetabular fracture
III	Stable injury (immobilization usually unnecessary except for symptomatic relief)
	A Isolated fracture
	B Fracture of the pubic rami

nificant hemorrhage into two categories: those who are hemodynamically unstable and those who require six units of blood within 8 hours of initial resuscitation. The first group show signs of hypotension, external bleeding, tachycardia, decreased urine output, and a falling or unstable hematocrit. If the bleeding is external, presumably due to a compound fracture, I favor packing with gauze pads or strips. If the external bleeding is an exsanguinating hemorrhage, exploratory laparotomy and control of the distal aorta are indicated, as is packing with gauze pads. Major vessel injury within the pelvis must then be ruled out; appropriate repair or ligation must be performed, if such an injury is found. Operative arteriography may help in locating the bleeding. If no major arterial bleeding source is found and the pelvic hematoma is contained it is prudent to not explore it.

If the patient is hemodynamically stable and has no associated intraperitoneal injury that is bleeding, but has lost more than six units of blood from the pelvic fracture, I would advocate performing arteriography. Expeditious placement of an external fixator to the pelvis to minimize venous bleeding can be done prior to arteriography. If the arteriogram is positive several options exist. If a major arterial bleeder is demonstrated such as the common iliac, external iliac, or hypogastric artery then operative repair is indicated. More commonly, the injury is to a branch of the superior gluteal or pudendal artery, in which case I favor embolization to the offending vessel with Gelfoam or similar substance. Only rarely is operative ligation necessary for these posterior vessels.

If the arteriogram is negative, which it will be in the majority of cases, treatment is directed toward minimizing venous hemorrhage. This is best achieved by application of pelvic external fixators such as the A–O or Hoffman apparatus. In some instances a posterior plate (internal) across the sacroiliac joint may also be necessary. An alternative approach is to stabilize the fracture externally with the pneumatic antishock garment inflated to approximately 40 mm Hg. This approach is associated with more complications including skin necrosis and compartment syndromes. In either instance internal fixation can be performed in a few days if indicated.

Compound fractures of the pelvis are particularly vexing, and all must be treated by diversion of the fecal stream, even if the rectum is not injured. This measure is necessary to minimize contamination of the open wound and prevent pelvic sepsis. Patients with compound pelvic fractures treated with fecal diversion have a 25 percent mortality rate, whereas, if fecal diversion is not accomplished, the mortality rate is increased to 50 percent. It is also imperative to debride devitalized tissue and provide adequate drainage. The latter is best accomplished with multiple drains.

TRAUMA TO THE EXTREMITIES

THE EXTREMITIES

ROBERT E. MARKISON, M.D., F.A.C.S.

This chapter will focus on trauma to the soft issues of the upper and lower extremities. Special emphasis will be placed on injuries to the hand. Optimal results are obtained when a single team manages problems related to soft tissue cover, peripheral nerve injuries, vascular compromise, and musculocutaneous disruption.

THE HISTORY

Routine history provides an essential base for evaluation of the injured extremity. Information must include (1) age, (2) height and weight, (3) hand dominance, (4) occupation, (5) avocations, (6) employment history, (7) previous extremity injuries, (8) allergies, (9) medical problems, (10) current medications, and (11) precise time of last food or drink. As regards the recent history, the following questions should be raised: What happened? When did it happen? How did it happen? What was the amount of blood loss? How did the patient initially treat the injury? What was the date of the last tetanus immunization?

PHYSICAL EXAMINATION

How complete a physical examination is performed is determined by the patient's overall status. Injured extremities have a relatively low priority in the patient with multiple wounds whose condition is unstable. In such cases it is sometimes necessary to transport the patient to the operating room immediately, with only minimal imaging. More often there is time for a thorough physical examination. This evaluation should not include prolonged specialty-type examinations, but the examining team should limit its immediate concern to questions of viability and gross deformities of the extremities. Further direct investigations are carried out after the patient's general condition is stable. For

310

purposes of this discussion, it is assumed that the patient's condition is stable and he is able to communicate with the examiner.

Inspection. Full exposure of all four extremities is necessary and so all clothing and jewelry should be removed. The following should be noted during the initial examination: (1) wounds, (2) attitude, shape, and size of the injured extremity, (3) color, (4) spontaneous movements, and (5) patient's subjective response to the injured part. Rapid bleeding from extremity wounds is recognized during the primary survey and controlled by pressure, although the need for proximal tourniquet control of bleeding is rare.

The attitude or posture of the proximally injured extremity reflects fracture or dislocation, depending on the presence of angular and/or rotational distortions. Further assessment of attitude of the hand and foot may indicate disruption of musculocutaneous units. For example, the supinated hand in repose has a gentle increase in curve to the fingers and minimal interphalangeal flexion of the midpositioned thumb. The hand looks as if it were holding an egg. If this expected attitude is disturbed by the combined presence of a distal palmar surface forearm laceration and an extended finger, the diagnosis of divided flexor tendons is confirmed. This finding obviates exploration of the wound in the emergency room, since complete operative exploration is required.

Perception of shape and relative size of an injured extremity is valuable in assessing interstitial bleeding. A fractured femur can result in as much as 1,500 cc of interstitial blood in the thigh. Color assessment of distal parts determines whether there is time for imaging studies before definitive repairs are made. A cyanotic finger, for example, with division of both flexor tendons requires immediate repair to include digital arteriorrhaphies, digital neurorrhaphies, and flexor tenorrhaphies. However, a patient who has divided flexors with a pink fingertip may be treated with simple skin closure and elective repair of flexors within 7 days with a good result. Lack of spontaneous movement suggests proximal nerve lesions or musculotendinous disruptions. The examination is not complete without assessing the patient's pain response to injury. Anxious patients with painful wounds often benefit from nerve blocks to reduce postoperative discomfort.

Functional Testing. Functional testing should proceed from the proximal to the distal extremities as the patient is asked to move parts through a range of motion at each joint. When pain limits active motion and thereby examination of parts that are distal to forearm, hand, leg, or foot lacerations, use of the flexor and extensor tenodesis effects is desirable. Tenodesis refers to the position assumed by one or more distal parts when the tendons are stretched by passive movement of a joint. Upper extremity extensor tenodesis effects are demonstrable by stabilizing the elbow and flexing the wrist. With 70 to 90 degrees of passive wrist flexion, the thumb pulls into full extension with the index finger. The remaining fingers are 10 to 20 degrees from full extension at the metacarpophalangeal joints, but are fully extended at the proximal interphalangeal and distal phalangeal joints. Therefore, a laceration at the wrist or hand dorsum that causes an increased drop in any of the fingers signals the presence of an extensor tendon division. Upper extremity flexor tenodesis effect is seen when the elbow is stabilized and the wrist is cocked back into 60 or 70 degrees of extension. Tenodesis then brings the fingers in convergence toward the scaphoid, the interphalangeal joint of the thumb flexes 45 degrees, the pads of the long ring and middle fingers touch the palm, and the index fails the thenar eminence by 2 to 3 cm. With a palmar wrist laceration, failure of the thumb interphalangeal joint to flex suggests division of the flexor pollicis longus tendon.

If the tenodesis effect findings are not conclusive, functional testing proceeds with evaluation of individual motor units, from the proximal to the distal extremity. As motor deficits may result from injury to the tendons, the nerves, or both, a review of major upper and lower extremity motor nerves is appropriate here.

There are four upper extremity motor nerves; the first is the musculocutaneous nerve, C5 to C6, which supplies the coracobrachialis, the long and short heads of the biceps, and the brachialis. A palsy of this nerve leads to loss of forearm flexion and reduction of the power of supination of the forearm. The deep raidal (posterior interosseous) nerve, C6 through C7, innervates the thumb, wrist, and finger extensors. The classic "dropped" or flexed wrist posture of radial palsy, which indicates injury to this nerve, is easily recognized. The ulnar nerve, C8 through T1, innervates several extrinsic hand motors, consisting of the flexor digitorum profundus to the ring and little fingers and flexor carpi ulnares, as well as 15 of the 20 intrinsic muscles of the hand. Ulnar palsy therefore results in a clumsy hand and weak grip, inability to cross the fingers, and flexion of the thumb interphalangeal joint (Froment's sign) to assist a weak pinch. The median nerve, C6 through C7, innervates all the superficial finger flexors, the index and long finger profundus flexors, the flexor carporadialis, and the muscles of the thenar wad. Median palsy, depending on its level, at the very least causes thenar motor deficit with the inability to pronate and oppose the thumb or, at higher levels, failure of thumb and finger flexion.

Three principal motor nerves serve the muscles of the leg. The femoral nerve innervates the anterior thigh muscles, and palsy is reflected by weakness in thigh flexion and leg extension. Medial thigh muscles are innervated by the obturator nerve, and a palsy results in adduction deficit. The tibial nerve innervates the posterior thigh muscles and reflects its palsy by loss of thigh extension and leg flexion. The tibial nerve continues as the posterior tibial and innervates the plantar flexors and toe flexors. Foot dorsoflexors and toe extensors are the motor territory of the deep peroneal nerve. Intrinsic foot muscles are innervated primarily by the medial and lateral plantar branches of the posterior tibial nerve.

Palpation. Palpation, the next step in examining the extremities, involves consideration of (1) temperature, (2) presence or absence of sweat, (3) pulses, (4) sensation, (5) turgor, and (6) pain on passive motion. Temperature and sweat both reflect perfusion as well as sympathetic nervous system activity. Sweat is also an important indicator of peripheral nerve division. Within seconds of nerve transection, sweating is eliminated through the nerve's sensory territory. Since patients are often diaphoretic from anxiety, the contrast of a dry, denervated field as seen by sidelighting can be dramatic. A simple test, called "pen drag," can be useful. This consists of drawing the body of a nontextured, plastic ballpoint pen across the sensate area and the area in question and comparing the amount of friction. Sensate areas grip the pen, whereas dry, denervated areas allow the pen to slip along, as if drawn across silk. Two-point discrimination is also valuable and can be done with a paper clip. Either of these tests is preferable to causing needless anxiety by sticking pins into the extremities of patients. Sensory denervation in the hands and feet of small children can be assessed by soaking the part in warm water: insensate areas do not wrinkle.

Pulse examination proceeds from proximal to distal and is measured on a scale of 0 to 4+, with 4+ being normal. A history of vascular disease or claudication may explain pulse deficits, which may be verified with a Doppler examination. The Allen test in the hand and its equivalent in the foot are useful in comparing the blood flow between the radial and ulnar arteries, and the anterior and posterior tibial arteries, respectively. The test can be performed in a conscious or unconscious adult by exsanguination of the part, occlusion of both arteries, and comparison of filling times when they are opened in turn. The rate of normal hand filling is equal from both the ulnar and radial vessels at 2.4 seconds on the average. Similarly, the anterior and posterior tibial arteries fill the foot at an almost equal rate in less than 3 seconds. Tissue turgor should also be assessed, since it may warn of a developing compartment syndrome (to be discussed). Pain on passive motion may further support this impression.

Tourniquet Examination. Direct probing of wounds is seldom required if an adequate physical examination has been completed. The goal of the physical examination is to atraumatically diagnose nonvisible structural division that requires operative repair. If questions remain, tourniquet examination is appropriate. This examination is best carried out by a physician who is part of the operating team. After the sensory examination has been performed and recorded, the wound is anesthetized with a field or digital block. The physician must avoid placement of digital blocks beyond the distal palm or plantar surface when blood supply to the finger or toe pads is compromised. Anesthetic volume placed in the base of such a digit may shut off the already decreased flow for a period sufficient to cause necrosis. Cast padding is applied to the proximal extremity and a blood pressure cuff is wrapped over this, The part is elevated for 1 minute, and the cuff is then inflated to 250 mm Hg. Even the most compliant patient cannot be expected to tolerate more than 10 or 15 minutes of touniquet examination. Therefore, skin preparation drapes, instruments, lighting, and expertise must all be adequate. Minimal wound extension is made along proper lines to gain adequate visualization of structures. A minimum of $2 \times$ loupe magnification is required. Depending on findings, definitive care may involve simple placement of skin sutures or simple approximation of skin edges to allow for later repair of divided structures. Dressings and splints are applied after closure, and the blood pressure cuff is released.

IMAGING TECHNIQUES

Imaging of the wounded extremity begins with plain roentgenograms for exclusion of fractures. It is helpful to request bilateral radiologic studies of childrens' extremities to avoid confusion between injury and normal patterns of development. Prior to sending the patient for roentgenography, it is appropriate to routinely flag gunshot wounds and other deep penetrating injuries with radiopaque markers. Several points should be considered in obtaining x-ray studies:

1. Multiple views may be required, since shards of glass in particular may be difficult to locate in the hand or foot.
2. In every significant injury related to glass wounding, x-ray studies should be obtained, since glass is clearly seen on film in 90 percent of cases.
3. Routine roentgenograms of animal and human bite wounds occasionally reveal the presence of tooth fragments in the soft tissues or joints.
4. Plain films are helpful in the evaluation of high-pressure injection injuries from paint, which is radiopaque, or grease, which is radiolucent. These injuries usually occur in the hand with the substances entering the palmar surface of the finger and travelling the flexor sheaths of the fingers to break through into one or more of the deep spaces of the hand. Immediate exploration is required and incision planning is aided by the pattern of infiltration revealed by the roentgenography.

Angiography often plays a vital part in the assessment of blunt and penetrating trauma to the extremities. The presence of distal pulses is reassuring, but does not rule out the possibility of proximal vascular disruption. It has been estimated that 20 percent of arterial divisions are associated with normal distal pulses. A high index of suspicion and aggressive angiography help to diagnose vascular problems before vascular insufficiency occurs. Indications for angiography include (1) posterior knee dislocation, which is associated with a 60 percent incidence of popliteal artery injury, (2) gunshot and penetrating wounds in proximity to major vessels, (3) extremities injured at multiple levels with distal ischemia, in which multiple vascular exposures would be impractical and injurious, (4) certain fractures, particularly supracondylar fractures of the humerus, major femoral fractures, and some tibial and fibular fractures, (5) complex injuries of the hand in which microvascular repairs may be necessary, (6) acute ischemia from arterial drug injection injuries, which may benefit from interventional radiologic techniques, such as the use of thrombolytic or spasmolytic agents. Osmotic diuresis amounting to 7 ml of urine output per milliliter of angiographic dye is an important consideration, since the average study may promote urine output as high as 500 ml. This volume should be replaced by intravenous fluid. As there is a possibility of urinary retention, the urinary output should be monitored and a urinary catheter inserted if indicated.

PREOPERATIVE CARE

Preoperative care of patients with injured extremities involves four major areas of concern: (1) total physiologic support, (2) immediate wound management, (3) antimicrobial prophylaxis, including tetanus, and (4) information for the patient. Total physiologic support is directly related to care priorities established in the primary and secondary surveys of the multiply injured patient. The extremities may initially have a low priority, but should not be neglected.

The timing of wound management depends on the nature of the injury, which dictates whether surgery should be immediate or delayed. Untidy wounds are best treated by generous normal saline irrigation and sterile dressings with appropriate splints. Antimicrobial prophylaxis includes the use of tetanus toxoid and tetanus immune globulin (TAT). Patients immunized more than 5 years previously should receive 0.5 ml of adsorbed tetanus toxoid. Individuals who have not been adequately immunized and those in whom the immunization history is unknown should receive 0.5 ml of adsorbed toxoid for the non-tetanus-prone wound; for tetanus-prone wounds, they should receive 250 units or more of human TAT at different injection sites. Antibiotic prophylaxis is most useful for wounds that (1) are associated with fractures, (2) include tendon divisions, and (3) disrupt joint capsules. First-generation cephalosporins are generally used for this purpose. Cultures should be taken of all open fractures and heavily contaminated wounds prior to the initiation of antibiotic therapy.

Adequate patient information is perhaps the most important element of preoperative care. The patient must understand that a period of rehabilitation may be required. If communication breaks down in the beginning, the best surgical efforts may be thwarted. A discussion of the extent of injury is often enhanced by showing the patient his roentgenograms, drawing simple diagrams, and obtaining an inclusive consent. The patient with multiple injuries of the extremities should be told of the possible need for vein grafts to repair arteries, tendon grafts to replace segmental losses, and nerve grafts. An estimate of the period of extremity immobilization should also be discussed. Once the consent is obtained, the patient should be medicated appropriately for pain after consultation with the anesthesiologist. Close family members should be included in these discussions whenever possible, since a great deal of assistance may be required in the activities of daily living after major limb compromise.

SPECIFIC TREATMENT

Injuries to be addressed are breaks in soft tissue cover, vascular injury, peripheral nerve problems, and musculotendinous trauma.

Disruption of Soft Tissue Cover

The functions of extremity soft tissue cover include (1) sensibility via specialized micro-end organs of the nervous system, (2) tissue homeostasis by way of venous and lymphatic outflow channels, (3) insulation and heat exchange, and

(4) simple protection. The value of vital, durable cover is greatest in areas of major vascularity and in the hand, where there is a high density of covering, gliding, and skeletal structures. Therefore, the seriousness of soft tissue disruption is governed by location and coincidence with the division of associated structures. The spectrum of soft tissue disruption runs from simple abrasion to complete degloving. Restoration of surface continuity for cosmesis must not proceed at the expense of overall function.

Abrasions and tatooing injuries are best treated by adequate debridement. This may require proximal field blocks in order to scrub away loosely embedded particulate matter and is followed by the application of nonadhering gauze dressings. Immobilization of the part is generally unnecessary in this circumstance. Full healing without skin grafting is expected. Tidy incised wounds involving skin and fat without major sensory nerve division do not require prophylactic antibiotics and may be approximated by a minimal number of interrupted simple or vertical mattress sutures. Subcutaneous and subcuticular sutures are avoided on the extremities, since they result in a higher incidence of wound sepsis which may impair the gliding of underlying musculotendinous units. The treatment of flap-type injuries depends on whether the base of the flap is proximal or distal. Proximally based flaps have a random pattern of distribution, and if the length is greater than one and one-half to two times the width, there is only a marginal chance of flap survival. Perfusion of distally based flaps is generally estimated by visual inspection of color, but marginal flaps may be examined by Wood's lamp following peripheral venous injection of sodium fluorescein.

A newly created device, the digital dermofluorometer, has proved useful as it gives an actual numeric readout of tissue fluorescence following peripheral injection of 1 to 2 mg per kilogram of sodium fluorescein. Nonviable flaps should be debrided back to bleeding tissue or tissue with adequate fluorescence. Closure with a minimal number of simple interrupted sutures may be attempted only if the perimeter of the proximal wound edge can be mobilized safely. The alternatives are to defat the distal portion of the flap and create a full-thickness skin graft or to debride the full thickness of the nonviable portion and close the gap immediately, or in a delayed fashion, with split-thickness skin. Secure coverage over tendons and major vascular structues is vital. Local, pedicle, or free-flap coverage of these structures is preferable if the skin is only marginally viable.

Degloving injury refers to the loss of skin and fat down to the fascia, and the seriousness of this problem is dependent on the location. The degloved tissue, when present, is often of poor quality, since fasciocutaneous circulation has been disrupted. Full-thickness losses overlying muscle bellies proximal to the wrist and ankle are well tolerated and are best treated by initial debridement followed by moist dressings over a period of several days until early granulations appear. At this time, split-thickness skin grafts may be applied. It is important to guard against premature resurfacing of these regions, since a failed attempt with even a brief period of immobilization can impair ultimate functional recovery. It is better to encourage full range of motion of an extremity that has suffered a proximal degloving injury than to tie up the part with extravagant early restoration of surface continuity.

Degloving injuries distal to the wrist present special problems. Fingertip tissue losses can be treated in one of three ways:

1. Defects measuring 1 cm square may be left open and will heal within 8 weeks with minimal residual impairment.
2. Split-thickness skin grafting from the proximal upper or lower extremity provides immediate simple coverage for tip injuries, including those in which bone is involved. Grafts contract at a rate of 40 to 50 percent within 8 weeks, leaving minimal disability.
3. Flap procedures, including axial V-Y advancement (Kutler), or palmar surface V-Y advancement (Kleinert), or cross-finger pedicle tissues may be helpful, but the technical difficulty of the V-Y advancement flap procedure and donor as well as the recipient site stiffness with the cross-finger flap procedure are significant drawbacks. The majority of patients therefore benefit from simple split-thickness coverage of these wounds.

Major finger-degloving injuries in which minimal skin bridges remain at the base of the finger are best treated by amputation in most cases. A small fraction of these are amenable to microvascular anastomosis provided neurovascular bundles have not been significantly crushed. The "red line sign" refers to red streaks over the distribution of the digital arteries, reflecting major crush and breakdown of distal vascular integrity, with subsequent extravasation of blood into tissues. The presence of this sign is an absolute contraindication to microvascular repair. In the absence of crush, microvascular repair may be attempted provided suitable veins and arteries are present in the distal tissues. Volar forearm vein grafts and antebrachial cutaneous sensory nerve grafts are useful in such procedures as primary anastomosis without grafting is seldom secure. Degloved thumbs pose a more serious problem, as the thumb constitutes 40 percent of the value of the hand, according to disability ratings. Debridement, followed by microvascular repair or abdominal pedicle flap, should be considered as part of a major thrust to salvage the thumb. Palmar hand degloving wounds may cause substantial disruption of neurovascular structures. Occasionally, microvascular jump grafts are run from the intact portions of the vascular arch to the distal vessels of the fingers. Time need not be wasted in adding nerve grafting during such salvage procedures since this can be accomplished later in the patient's course of treatment. Often, wounds are not immediately repaired, but are left open without any biologic coverage. In this case, moist dressings are applied, and some minimal active motion is encouraged within a day or two following injury. Split-thickness skin grafts, abdominal pedicles, or free flaps are applied 2 to 7 days after the initial injury. It has been found that supervised early motion of hands with open wounds often provides the best chance of functional recovery.

Dorsal degloving injuries of the hand in which the paratenon is intact are simply treated by debridement and subsequent split-thickness skin grafting. When tendons are exposed or disrupted, extensor function depends on the presence of subcutaneous fat to permit glide. Therefore, abdominal pedicle or groin flaps are preferred. Early granulations must be present on the tendons before such reconstructions are attempted. Dorsal foot degloving injuries require debridement and subsequent split- or full-thickness skin graft coverage. Subsequent reconstruction of the toe extensors is seldom of functional importance.

Vascular Injuries

A list of arterial injuries ranging from most critical to least critical, as determined by the incidence of distal gangrene, is as follows: (1) femoral artery, (2) popliteal artery, (3) combination of anterior and posterior tibial arteries, (4) brachial artery proximal to profunda brachial, (5) superficial femoral artery, (6) iliac artery, (7) axillary artery, (8) brachial artery distal to the profunda brachial. Ligation of the common femoral artery results in a 70 to 80 percent incidence of distal gangrene, and ligation of the brachial artery distal to the profunda results in a 10 to 15 percent incidence of distal gangrene. Ligation of either the radial or ulnar artery results in a 1 to 2 percent incidence of distal gangrene, and ligation of both results in gangrene in 10 to 30 percent of cases. Venous injuries are coincident in 60 percent or more of cases of arterial disruption and should be repaired when possible. Popliteal venous injuries pose the greatest threat to the distal extremity if left unrepaired. Preoperative care of the patient with arterial injury includes rapid control of external bleeding, resuscitation from shock, adequate imaging of the artery and associated arteriovenous fistula, minimizing the time lag from injury to repair, and obtaining a signed consent which includes the possibility of vascular grafting.

Technical considerations common to all vascular repairs include the following: (1) incision planning, (2) proximal and distal control of blood vessels, (3) irrigation of the wound, (4) debridement, (5) repair, and (6) soft tissue coverage.

Incision Planning. Skin preparation and draping must include the entire extremity and, in many cases expose the surface of another limb for harvest of autogenous graft material. Whenever possible, a well-padded, pretested tourniquet should be applied to the proximal aspect of the injured extremity and left uninflated. This permits immediate control if unexpected major hemorrhage occurs; it also allows a dry field for repair of nerves and musculotendinous structures. Incisions generally run over and parallel to the course of the underlying vessels to be repaired, and they cross joint creases at an angle of 45 degrees or less to the transverse axis, in order to avoid scar contracture. The direction of an incision is also influenced by the need to temporarily divide major muscular structures. Such is the case with axillary artery repair, which is facilitated by division of one or both pectoralis muscle tendons near their origins.

Control of Hemorrhage. Proximal and distal control of hemorrhage is seldom gained by application of clamps through the original wound. Temporary control of major hemorrhage is gained in the operating room by direct finger pressure while the extremity is being prepped and draped, inflation of a 5 ml or 30 ml capacity balloon-tipped Foley catheter within the wound, or temporary tightening of a proximally placed tourniquet while the incision is being made. Proximal control is gained first as the operating surgeon works from known to unknown regions and isolates vessels in uninjured tissues. Silastic tubing should be used to encircle vessels whenever possible since it is less traumatic than the application of clamps. When clamps are needed, they should be applied with minimal force to avoid crushing the vessels. Back bleeding should be noted prior to securing distal control. If there is none present, the extremity should be milked in the direction of the wound by pressure over the distribution of the injured vessel. Often, this releases clots, thereby increasing bleeding. Back bleeding only confirms patency of the nearest collateral branches into a vessel and does not indicate that the distal vascular tree is clot-free. Therefore, several gentle passes of a Fogarty catheter of the correct size are strongly recommended to remove clots. Heparinized saline may then be injected into the distal end of the vessel before the Silastic loop or clamp is applied. Collateral vessels should be spared whenever possible, and these are occluded by temporary application of silver clips.

Irrigation of the Wound. The goal of irrigation is to remove clots and to debride. Once the surrounding structures have been cleared, the exposed lumina of the vessels are cleansed to allow direct inspection of vessel walls and determination of additional intimal damage. Debridement is then carried out to freshen the surrounding tissues as well as the vascular wounds themselves. Tidy, incised arterial and venous wounds need not be debrided. However, untidy wounds and blast injuries, in particular, often require careful excision of vascular segments. Contused arterial segments are sometimes challenging and require debridement back to the point where subintimal hemorrhage is no longer noted.

Vessel Repair. The repair itself consists of end-to-end anastomosis, lateral repair, vein patch, or interposition of a vascular graft. Useful suture materials include Teflon, Dacron, nylon, polypropylene and silk. The suture technique itself may be running or interrupted. Lateral repair of large vessels is usually accomplished by running sutures. However, this technique is imprecise with smaller-caliber vessels. I generally favor an interrupted technique in end-to-end anastomosis, consisting of anterior and posterior stay sutures, which are placed 180 degrees apart and held in various positions in order to rotate the vessel for subsequent placement of the remaining interrupted sutures. The final two or three sutures in the smaller-caliber vessel may be laid in and tied subsequently, to permit continuous visualization of the lumen and avoid capturing the back wall with the passage of the needle. This also facilitates assessment of back bleeding, which should always be checked before the final suture is tied. Pulses should return immediately in the distal extremity after clamps or vessel loops are removed. Absence of distal pulses following repair must be investigated by intraoperative arteriogram. When repairs have been performed distal to the wrist and ankle, perfusion is assessed by color, capillary fill, Doppler, and digital dermofluorometry.

Vascular grafts are sometimes needed when end-to-end anastomosis is not possible without undue tension. The saphenous vein is the best source for such a graft and should be taken from the contralateral extremity for leg and thigh repairs. This is important so that additional incisions in a wounded part can be avoided, and potentially important venous outflow of the affected limb is not compromised. The upper extremity cephalic vein is also useful as a graft source, but its relatively smaller caliber limits its usefulness in the proximal thigh or arm. If suitable graft sites are not available, polytetrafluoroethylene (Gortex) is useful, provided adequate muscular soft tissue cover is available. Synthetic grafts are anastomosed with polypropylene suture. Small grafts are sometimes used in palmar and digital wounds of the hand. These may be harvested from the volar forearm or the foot dorsum. Optical loupe magnification, 2 to 6×, is used for repairs in the arm between the elbow and wrist, and in the leg between the knee and ankle. A microscope is used for more distal repairs. Suture caliber at the wrist level is 6–0 or 8–0 nylon; in the palm, 8–0 to 9–0 nylon; and in the digits, 10–0 nylon. The vessels are held by microvascular clamps, and repairs are performed with specially ground jeweler's forceps, which have silicon-coated handles to permit rotation of the instruments between the surgeon's fingers. Patency of anastomoses is tested by applying both pairs of forceps to the distal artery just beyond the anastomosis, milking out the blood from the vessel with one forceps, then releasing the proximal one while the distal forceps occludes the lumen. A patent vessel should instantly fill and be seen to pulsate.

Soft Tissue Coverage. Soft tissue coverage is vital to the survival of vessels that have been exposed and injured by trauma. The understanding of vascular anatomy as it relates to muscle flaps, myocutaneous flaps, and fasciocutaneous flaps has increased tremendously in recent years. This has promoted the acceptability of synthetic graft materials for use in the extremities.

Rectus abdominis muscle flaps are useful in proximal thigh disruptions of the femoral vessels. Similarly, pectoralis major muscle flaps can be used to cover axillary and brachial artery injuries when blast injuries have compromised cover by local muscles. Muscular coverage of vascular repairs allows the surgeon to pack open the soft tissues for delayed primary closure by flap approximation or split-thickness skin graft coverage.

Postoperative Care. Postoperative care following vascular repairs depends on the composite nature of the extremity injury. A period of immobilization for arteriorrhaphy and venorrhaphy alone should be minimal, and certainly no more than a few days. Substantial muscular repairs in conjunction with vascular reconstruction require 1 to 2 weeks of immobolization if proximal to the elbow and knee; 2 to 3 weeks of immobolization if between wrist and elbow or ankle and knee; and 3 to 4 weeks when tendon and nerve injuries distal to the wrist are repaired in addition. Low-molecular-weight dextran is sometimes useful when significant devitalization of structures surrounding the repaired vessel has occurred and poses some threat to the distal microcirculation. However, in most cases, adequate hydration is sufficient to maintain patency of vascular repairs.

COMPARTMENT SYNDROME

Upper and lower extremity fasciotomies may be important adjuncts to vascular reconstruction. They are performed for the relief of compartment syndrome and are effective only if performed early. Compartment syndrome occurs as a result of fluid extravasation from capillaries consequent to refilling after a period of ischemia, and this causes an obstruction of venous return within tight fascial compartments. A vicious cycle is then begun and can only be relieved early, before myonecrosis occurs, by opening of the affected compartments. Generally acknowledged circumstances in which fasciotomy should be seriously considered are (1) prolonged hypotension, (2) delay of more than 6 hours between injury and repair, (3) crush injuries with massive soft tissue trauma, (4) massive edema, and (5) combined arterial and venous injuries. Clinical indicators of compartment syndrome in the upper extremity are numbness and tingling (particularly along the nerve distribution), pain on passive motion of the fingers and thumb, and an increased flexion attitude of wrist and fingers due to flexor spasm. In the lower extremity, the first nerve to suffer ischemia is the deep peroneal, which supplies the dorsal web space between the great toe and second toe. Pain on passive motion of the ankle and, particularly, the great toe may also be present. Compartment pressures are best measured by connecting a wick catheter to a standard pressure transducer and inserting it into the appropriate muscle compartments. Fasciotomy should be seriously considered when pressures are between 30 and 40 mm Hg, and should definitely be performed when pressures exceed 40 mm Hg in the forearm and leg.

Upper extremity fasciotomy requires four incisions:

1. A lazy S-shaped incision, which extends from the proximal palmar ulnar forearm, gently curves across to the radial palmar forearm, returns to the ulnar side, and then extends into the mid-palm just ulnar to the thenar crease. This incision allows the freeing of superficial and deep flexor wads and decompresses the median nerve by carpal tunnel release.
2. A dorsal, linear, longitudinal forearm incision is made between the mobile extensor wad and the extensor digitorum communis muscle bellies. These are two separate compartments which must be opened individually.
3. and 4. Two linear, longitudinal, hand dorsum incisions are carried over the second and fourth metacarpals, and the extensor tendons are retracted, allowing access to the dorsal and volar interosseous compartments which are separate. These compartments are opened by longitudinal slits. Dorsal inci-

sions can generally be closed primarily, and delayed primary closure, with or without skin grafting, is required for the volar surface incision.

Lower extremity fasciotomies must decompress the anterior and lateral compartments as well as the superficial and deep posterior compartments. A single incision opens the anterior and lateral compartments, and a posteromedial incision permits release of the posterior compartments. Primary closures are occasionally possible here, but more often delayed closures are required. A high level of clinical suspicion and the means for monitoring pressure are the keys to avoiding tissue necrosis from compartment syndrome.

PERIPHERAL NERVE PROBLEMS

Injuries to peripheral nerves may result in neuropraxia with eventual complete return of function, in severe crush without hope of functional return, in partial disruptions, or in complete nerve divisions. Careful sensorimotor testing is the first step in planning treatment. Accurate diagnosis depends on a knowledge of normal and anomalous patterns of upper and lower extremity innervation. Timing of repair is then determined by (1) the nature of the wound and wounding agent, (2) relative sensorimotor importance of the nerve division(s) to the patient's extremity function, and (3) the availability of experienced surgeons and proper equipment. Tidy incised wounds in which nerves have been divided should be explored, and repairs should be performed as soon as conveniently possible. When there are tendon divisions at the wrist level, repairs should be undertaken within a day or two because of the great tendency of the flexor and extensor tendons to retract well up into the forearm. Another strong argument for repairing without delay is the ease with which freshly divided nerve ends can be accurately coapted. Within several days of injury, wallerian degeneration reduces the diameter of the distal nerve stump. Meanwhile, the proximal nerve end begins its axonal budding and consequently increases in caliber. Budding also distorts the normally crisp definition of fascicular bundles in the proximal nerve stump. Although loupe magnification, 3.5 to 6×, is generally sufficient for nerve repair, a delay in repair may require use of a microscope to accurately join the differing diameters of the two ends. Repairs should not be performed when total hand function might be compromised, as in the case of digital nerve divisions proximal to nonpinch and nonprotective finger territories in the hand of an arthritic.

Immediate repairs are contraindicated in the presence of untidy wounds such as blast and crush injuries. When nerve ends are visible in such wounds, they should be tagged with nylon sutures and secured into the surrounding tissue, in as close an apposition as possible. Repairs may be accomplished weeks or months later, after the primary wounds have healed. The actual zone of injury in a nerve that has been divided by a blast injury may not become apparent for several days, and premature repair would fail if a devitalized segment were included. Sensory nerve repair can yield good results with delay of up to 2 years between injury and nerve repair. However, motor nerves depend on viable motor end-plates for functional return, and after 12 to 18 months, irreversible loss of neuromuscular junctions can occur, making repair a futile exercise.

The relative importance of the sensory and motor functions of divided nerves in the periphery must be considered before repair is begun. The most important sensory nerve of the hand is the median nerve, which has been referred to as the "eye of the hand" because it innervates the pinch surfaces of the thumb, index, and long fingers, thus governing tactile sensation for the manipulation of objects. The "eye" of the foot is the posterior tibial nerve, which innervates the entire plantar surface, including the heel, by way of its calcaneal, lateral plantar, and medial plantar branches. Therefore priority should be given to posterior tibial nerve repair in an incised ankle wound associated with plantar hypesthesia. Priorities for digital nerve repair in the hand relate to protective borders and pinch surfaces. The border nerves are the thumb radial digital, index radial digital, ring ulnar digital, and little finger ulnar digital nerves. Pinch nerves of importance are the thumb ulnar digital, index radial digital, and long finger radial digital nerves. Digital nerves of lower priority are the index ulnar digital, long ulnar digital, ring radial digital, and little finger radial digital nerves. Because repair of peripheral nerves requires 3 weeks of immobilization for healing, the financial burden of this lost working time may not justify the repair of the lesser nerves if they are not essential to a patient's livelihood or quality of life.

Priority assignment to the repairs of upper extremity motor nerves is difficult and depends on which nerves are injured and at what level. Nerve divisions above the level of the elbow often require subsequent tendon transfers. Motor nerves should be repaired in this region, but there is less than 50 percent chance of regaining useful motor function. The prognosis, from best to worst, following motor nerve repair as follows: radial, medial, and ulnar. Children may regenerate motor nerves at a remarkable rate and therefore should be simply observed following repair for at least 6 months. However, adults often benefit from tendon transfers within 3 months of nerve repair (to be discussed).

Lower extremity motor nerve divisions cause a disturbance of stability against gravity, as opposed to the dexterity and range of motion compromised by upper extremity motor divisions. Femoral nerve division causes the least disturbance, provided strong hip extensors are present. Walking up stairs is difficult for these patients because of loss of quadriceps function. As common peroneal palsy causes foot drop, primary nerve repair is indicated whenever possible, even though subsequent tendon transfers and orthoses may be required. Similarly, divided tibial nerves should be repaired whenever possible, notwithstanding the possibility of subsequent reconstructive procedures.

Operative Techniques

Operative techniques in peripheral nerve repair have been a subject of recent controversy. Claims of superiority of one type of nerve repair over another should be cautiously considered, since our knowledge of the basic physiology of nerve healing lags behind the capabilities of microtechnique. The surgeon should be experienced in microsurgery and flexible in his operative approach. Tourniquet control is essential for repairs at or distal to the elbow and knee. Well-padded, pretested arm tourniquets are inflated to 250 mm Hg for a maximum of 2 hours, with an interval of 15 minues between inflations if more time is needed. Thigh tourniquets are inflated to 300 mm Hg. A minimum of $2\times$ optical loupe magnification is used for the anatomic exposure of peripheral nerves. Exposures are generous, but mobilization of the nerve is minimal, particularly in the case of tidy transections. In the case of untidy transections, such as blast and crush-avulsion injuries, it is best not to attempt primary repair. Delayed treatment is facilitated by tagging the nerve ends with nylon sutures and sewing them into the neighboring muscle or fascia, with the ends in close approximation. These tag sutures are cut 1 cm long for easy retrieval. Fresh, tidy divisions of peripheral nerves without segmental loss seldom require mobilization greater than 2 cm of each stump. Motor nerves are tested intraoperatively by a disposable nerve stimulator set at 0.5 to 2 milliamps of current. Repair of large peripheral nerves begins with inspection of the posterior wall of the stumps and alignment of the longitudinal vasa nervorum. Three posterior wall 6–0 nylon epineural sutures are then placed 60 degrees apart and are serially tied after alignment is rechecked. The ends are left long so that these may act as stay sutures. This provides an excellent display of the fascicular bundles when the nerve is viewed from the anterior side. If the fascicular bundles are well contained within the epineural envelope, loupe magnification (3.5 to 6×) is used for the remaining repair, but if the bundles are splayed, the microscope is brought into the field. In the former case, epineural repair continues with interrupted 9–0 nylon sutures, the first of which rejoins the anterior vasa nervorum. When the microscope is used for splayed fascicular bundles, 10–0 nylon intraneural sutures are used to coapt the fascicular bundles, but no additional dissection is performed to allow individual fascicular repairs. I believe that each additional bit of dissection causes devascularization of the nerve and provides anatomic juncture at the expense of microcirculation of the nerve and provides anatomic juncture at the expense of microcirculation. When fascicular bundles are repaired, under the microscope, no more than two 10–0 nylon sutues are used per bundle. Partial nerve divisions occasionally cause difficulty because the traction of the semi-divided nerve stumps may cause buckling of the intact portion of nerves when they are brought together. Minimal buckling is acceptable; however, significant nerve distortion, as seen in injuries that are 1 to 2 weeks old, is best avoided by interposition of a graft. Favored sites for harvesting nerve grafts are the medial and lateral antebrachial cutaneous sensory nerve of the proximal forearm and the sural nerve of the leg. Fascicular groups are matched for size, and segments are interposed with 10–0 nylon under the microscope.

The most important adjunctive procedures following nerve repair are those that anticipate obstacles to regeneration. Ulnar nerve division, just proximal to or within the cubital tunnel, is benefited by cubital tunnel release. The next point of entrapment for the ulnar nerve is the loge of Guyon at the wrist, and ulnar divisions just proximal to or within the loge are accompanied by release of this compartment. The median nerve is often divided at the wrist, and divisions at the proximal lip of the carpal tunnel are accompanied by carpal tunnel release. Similarly, the radial nerve passes beneath the supinator muscle at the arcade of Frohse, and nerve divisions just proximal to or beneath the arcade require arcade release. Such considerations reduce the uncertainty of follow-up by eliminating questions of entrapment as a cause of failed sensorimotor return after repair.

Postoperative Follow-up

Follow-up of peripheral nerve injuries is concerned with reestablishment of sensibility and evaluation of results. Following 3 weeks of immobilization for nerve healing, the first priority is to regain full range of motion of all joints. During this period, the insensible parts of the body must be protected from accidental thermal, crush, and incising injuries. Smokers are particularly prone to burns when they lack sensation in their index and middle fingers. Patients should be told that regeneration is slow and steady, often involving a wide range of dysesthetic sensations, including "pins and needles," cold intolerance, and occasional pain. Cutaneous sensibility is improved by instructing the patient to practice reaching into a paper bag full of objects of varying shapes and textures and identifying them without looking at them. Sensory recovery should be graded and reported in a standard manner. The system in widespread use is S_0 through S_4 when:

S_0 = absence of sensibility in the autonomous area;
S_1 = recovery of deep cutaneous pain sensibility within the autonomous area of the nerve;
S_2 = return of some degree of superficial cutaneous pain and tactile sensibility within the autonomous area;
S_{2+} = stage two, but with permanent paresthesia;
S_3 = return of superficial cutaneous pain and tactile sensibility throughout the autonomous area with disappearance of any previous over-response;
S_{3+} = stage 3, with some recovery of two-point discrimination in the autonomous area; and S_4 = complete recovery.

Good sensory return is considered to be an S_3 or greater, and this can reasonably be expected in 70 percent of patients under the age of 40. Good fingertip two-point discrimination following neurorrhaphy is 10 mm or less.

Motor recovery is graded on the basis of M_0 through M_5 when:

M_0 = no contraction (complete paralysis);
M_1 = flicker of contraction;

M_2 = contraction only with gravity eliminated;
M_3 = contraction against gravity;
M_4 = contraction against gravity and some resistance;
M_5 = contraction against powerful resistance, and normal power.

Good results in this regard refer to patients with M_4 to M_5 ratings and may be reasonably expected in 40 to 50 percent of patients under the age of 40. The importance of long-term follow-up by the same examiner cannot be overemphasized, and evaluation should not be considered final before 2 to 5 years have passed. During this period, nerve conduction studies are occasionally indicated for apparent failure of regeneration.

Tendon Transfers

Finally, mention should be made of employing early tendon transfers as internal splints, following peripheral motor nerve divisions. The goal of such early tendon transfers is to improve overall hand function by avoiding external splinting devices. The most successful internal splint is the anastomosis of the median innervated pronator teres to the extensor carpi radialis brevis and longus for radial nerve palsy. This acts as a dynamic internal cock-up splint, which allows a more efficient use of the flexors for grasp. I often perform this transfer at the time of radial neurorrhaphy. Low median nerve palsies cause a deficit in thumb pronation and opposition. This can be remedied within 3 to 4 months of injury, if no function is returning to the abductor pollicis brevis, by some form of "opponensplasty" as an internal splint to overcome the supinating forces of the extrinsic thumb extensor and the abductor pollicis longus.

Ulnar claw hand can be reconstructed 3 to 4 months following nerve division, with subsequent improvement in power grip, by extending the extensor carporadialis longus via grafts that pass proximal and volar to the intermetacarpal ligaments and enter the proximal phalanges of the ring and little fingers as dynamic intrinsic transfers.

MUSCULOTENDINOUS TRAUMA REPAIR

Repair of divided muscles and tendons makes special demands on the surgeon's judgment and technical skills. The challenge of restoring glide within a bed of injured tissue increases as the location of wounds proceeds from axilla to fingertip and from groin to toe. This discussion considers the nature and level of injury as related to the timing of repairs, techniques of repair, postoperative care, rehabilitation, and evaluation of results. Tidy incised wounds of less than 6 hours duration, which merely open the superficial fascia over muscle bellies proximal to the midforearm and ankle, may be managed in the emergency room. Such wounds are copiously irrigated with a balanced salt solution, the fascial layer is longitudinally opened in a proximal and distal direction, and the skin is closed. The fascia is not closed in these wounds lest a compartment syndrome develop. Skin edges are coapted with interrupted nylon or Prolene vertical or horizontal mattress sutures. Subcutaneous sutures are avoided because of the possibility of reaction or impairment of the glide of underlying muscles. Deeply incised tidy wounds at the same levels are managed in the operating room. A proximal tourniquet is applied whenever possible as it is of enormous benefit in achieving identification and subsequent anatomic reapproximation of the deep fascial envelopes of divided muscles. Pure muscle units are repaired with 3-0 or 4-0 polydioxanone sutures (PDS), which are placed as horizontal mattress sutures; all the sutures are laid in before any are tied. The laying-in technique avoids tearing of muscle bundles. Serial tying of these sutures is facilitated by the assistant who snugs down the knot as the operating surgeon ties his suture. Repair proceeds from the depths of the wound to the surface, and the superficial fascia is left open. Again, skin edges are coapted with nylon or Prolene, and subcutaneous sutures are avoided because they encourage reaction and ultimately impair the gliding of underlying muscles. Musculotendinous junctions in the forearm and leg have a diminished local vascular supply available for healing following repair. For this reason, nonabsorbable monofilament sutures, such as nylon or Prolene, are used for repair to provide a longer period of tensile strength during the healing phase. Horizontal mattress sutures are used, and knots are buried within the substance of the juncture. Timing of muscle belly and musculotendinous junction repairs is important because of the extreme retraction units that occurs after 24 to 48 hours. Beyond this interval, anatomic repair is extremely difficult. On occasions when delay is necessary, it is best to irrigate the wound and coapt the skin edges with interrupted sutures to avoid desiccation of the muscle bellies.

Untidy wounds of muscle bellies and musculotendinous junctions should not receive primary repair. Such wounds are irrigated, debrided generously, and packed open with sterile dressings. The patient is given prophylactic cephalosporin and is returned to the operating room 2 to 5 days after admission for delayed primary closure only if the severed units are critical to function. Skin grafts are applied for coverage.

Timing the repair of tidy, upper extremity, flexor tendon divisions depends on the level of injury. Between the distal third of the forearm and the midpalm, the tendons are not tethered proximally and retract a significant distance immediately following division. With each passing day, tension-free repair becomes increasingly difficult. Therefore, tenorrhaphy should be performed within 3 days, and certainly within one week. Immediate irrigation and skin closure of the fresh wound is required if delay is anticipated. Slash wounds of the wrist with multiple tendon divisions are included in this category. The technique is as follows:

1. A well-padded, pretested tourniquet is applied to the upper extremity, and the arm is abducted onto two arm boards.
2. The extremity is painted with povidone-iodine solution and draped in the usual manner.
3. Circumferential pressure is applied as the tourniquet pressure is elevated to 250 mm Hg. The wound is irrigated free of clots with normal saline.
4. An incision is extended distally as a formal carpal tunnel release.
5. An ulnar or radial border longitudinal proximal extension is made to raise a flap for the retrieval of proximal stumps.
6. Proximal stumps of deep and then superficial flexors are retrieved by following the clots proximally and milking the forearm to deliver these structures into the wound. As each stump is delivered, it is grasped with toothed Bishop-Harmon forceps and held gently as an anterior-to-posterior stay suture is passed through the stump 1 cm from the cut end. Small hemostats are applied to the individual stay sutures to follow the proximal stumps. Next, the distal stumps are identified with ease since the carpal tunnel has been opened, and the ends are similarly tagged. Each pair of hemostats is then held together by a towel clip, and the system of identification is therefore complete.

All flexors are repaired in the wrists of children when the divisions are tidy. Priorities of repair in adult wrists are (1) all of the profundus tendons, (2) the flexor pollicis longus, and (3) the flexor digitorum superficialis to the index. Our policy has been to repair all tendons, even in adults when the divisions are tidy, with the understanding that the ultimate independence of the profundus and superficialis functions is variable. Repairs proceed from one side of the wrist to the other, starting with the profundus tendons. Sutures of 4–0 nylon are used for tenorrhaphy by the modified Kessler technique, in which the knot is intratendinous. The flexor pollicis longus and the superficial flexors are next repaired. Wrist flexors are generally the last structures repaired, and 3–0 nylon sutures are used for these. The skin is closed with interrupted horizontal mattress sutures of 5–0 nylon, and a short arm splint or circumferential plaster dressing with foam padding is applied, holding the wrist at 35 degrees flexion. The elbow is immobilized at 90 degrees in a long arm cast if wrist flexors have been divided.

Untidy injuries of the wrist are best treated by initial debridement and passage of simple 4–0 nylon sutures through proximal and distal stumps of the profundus tendons, the flexor pollicis longus, the index superficialis, and the radial wrist flexor. These sutures should be left long for easy identification, and the tendon ends should be positioned within less than 1 cm of each other. Continuously moist dressings are applied, and definitive repairs are made within 3 to 7 days. Reconstruction by simplification is the rule in such injuries.

Tidy wounds that divide the flexor tendons between the level of the carpal tunnel and the entry to the fibro-osseous sheath (first annular pulley) are straightforward and, provided the skin has been closed, can be repaired within 1 to 3 weeks with good results. The proximal profundus tendon is easily located because the radial side origin of the lumbrical muscle prevents proximal retraction. Similarly, the divided superficialis is easily found because it has a filmy yolk around the profundus tendon. Modified Kessler suture technique is used for tenorrhaphy of these structures. Lumbrical muscles are repaired with horizontal mattress sutures when they have been divided.

Zone II "no man's land" refers to the region between the distal third of the palm and the midportion of the midphalanx, in which the superficialis and profundus tendons travel close together in the fibro-osseous sheath. Good results can be achieved following meticulous repair of both tendons if the divisions are tidy and the patient is under age 40. Best results occur when such repairs are done within one week of the injury. The technique of zone II flexor tendon repair involves extension of the wound by a palmar zig-zag (Bruner) incision, if the laceration is oblique, or an ulnar border axial incision, if the palmar laceration is transverse. A radial border axial incision is used for the little finger. Proximal retraction of stumps requires a longitudinal distal third of the palm incision just proximal to the first annular pulley. Proximal stumps are then retrieved by passage of No. 5 pediatric feeding catheters from the original wound out through the proximal palmar counter-incision. These are sutured separately to the superficialis and profundus tendons, and the tendons are then drawn sequentially out through the original wound. When annular pulleys must be opened, they are flapped to the radial or ulnar side of the sheath and subsequently repaired with interrupted 6–0 nylon suture following tenorrhaphy. Tendon repairs are performed with 4–0 nylon modified Kessler sutures to the profundus and 5–0 nylon modified Kessler or horizontal mattress sutures to each of the radial and ulnar slips of the superficialis tendons. A running 6–0 nylon suture is then carried 270 degrees around the anterolateral aspect of the profundus repair to smooth it for improved glide. The flexor sheath is repaired, and the tendon glide is checked by passive finger motion. Skin edges are coapted with interrupted 5–0 nylon sutures, and short arm split or circumferential plaster is applied with the wrist in 35 degrees of flexion with the thumb excluded.

Only the profundus is vulnerable distal to the midportion of the middle phalanx (zone I). Standard tenorrhaphy with intratendinous 4–0 nylon and anterior basting suture of 6–0 nylon are performed if the distal stump is adequate. Otherwise, a 4–0 suture is passed through the proximal stump, run out through the distal pad beyond the fingernail, and tied over a foam-padded button. Untidy divisions of flexors within the digital sheath and beyond are not discussed in this chapter.

Upper extremity extensor tendon divisions follow similar principles of timing, out to the distal third of the hand dorsum. Repair as early as possible is favored in this region because of the tendency of proximal stumps to retract upward into the forearm. The extensor/retinaculum consists of six dorsal compartments and, when tendons are divided within these, retrieval is facilitated by the pediatric feeding catheter technique. If repaired tendons do not glide well through their compartments, they should be redone outside the tunnel in the subcutaneous position. Bow-stringing will be visible, but function is good in this circumstance. Juncturae tendinum (conexus intertendineus), which tether one tendon to another, prevent proximal retraction of extensor tendons divided beyond the distal third of the hand dorsum. Horizontal mattress sutures are used for flat tendons in this region, and modified Kessler sutures are used for thicker tendons. Distal to the metacarpophalangeal (MP) joints, the tendon flattens to act as an extensor hood, and paired horizontal mattress sutures of clear 5–0 nylon are used for repair. Black sutures may show through the skin in fair individuals and are therefore avoided. The terminal extensor tendon over the distal interphalangeal (DIP) joint, if cleanly incised, is repaired with 6–0 nylon paired horizontal mattress sutures or simply splinted across the joint for 6 weeks. Untidy divisions proximal to the proximal interphalangeal (PIP) joints may be repaired in a delayed fashion, for as long as 1 week, as long as skin covering is adequate. Untidy PIP joint divisions are splinted for 6 weeks to avoid butonierre deformity, and untidy tendon divisions at the DIP joint level are splinted for 6 to 8 weeks to avoid mallet deformity. Immobilization of extensor tendons involves wrist extension at 70 degrees and metacarpophalangeal joint flexion at 45 degrees, so that the rays of the fingers and dorsal forearm are parallel. PIP and DIP joints are held in 20 degrees of flexion for tendon divisions proximal to the MP joints; they are kept as straight as possible if divisions are distal to the MP joints. Repair of flexor and extensor tendons of the foot is not discussed here, but general techniques are similar.

Postoperative Care

Postoperative care of muscle and tendon divisions requires close attention to elevation of the injured part. If edema is allowed to occur by dependency, results are invariably poor. The form and duration of immobilization is as follows:

1. Immobilization of the muscle proximal to the elbow requires 1 week in a sling.
2. For repair between the elbow and the distal third of the forearm, 2 weeks in a long- or short-arm splint are sufficient.
3. Thumb and finger flexors are immobilized in a short-arm splint or circumferential plaster dressing for 3 weeks.
4. Four weeks are required if wrist flexors are involved, and long-arm immobilization is recommended to avoid disruption of the lateral-based structures by pronation and supination.
5. Short-arm immobilization is adequate for both wrist extensors and extensors of the thumb and fingers and should be continued for a 4-week period. The extra week is added to allow some additional tensile strength, since the overwhelming power of the flexor tendons can easily disrupt an extensor tenorrhaphy after 3 weeks.

Rehabilitation

Rehabilitation is usually carried out by the patient, without formal physical therapy, under the surgeon's continual guidance and close supervision. First, the elbow and wrist are mobilized, then hand rehabilitation is effected by having the patient squeeze a sponge in warm water 3 or 4 times a day for 5 minutes. Three office visits per week are not unusual for the first 2 weeks after cast removal. Functional return after flexor tenorrhaphies is assessed by angle measurements of all involved joints in flexion and in extension, with calculation of range of motion and the differences between hands. Grip and pinch strength are measured at regular intervals when appropriate. Angle measurements are supplemented by the patient's ability to straighten his fingers to the plane of a table when the hand is resting supine, and the distance by which the flexed finger(s) fail(s) to touch the proximal, mid, and distal palm. This is measured in centimeters. Steady recovery may continue for as long as 2 years; therefore, great optimism must be projected to the patient.

REPLANTATION

Replantation of amputated parts requires careful patient selection. Enthusiasm for widespread application of these expensive surgical techniques should be tempered by a careful history of the mechanism of injury, close scrutiny of the amputated part, and an overview of the patient's total hand requirements. A recent survey of nearly 200 surgeons worldwide, who had lost one or more of their own digits which were not replanted, revealed that more than 95 percent of these individuals continued to work and claimed no significant disability.

Poor candidates for replantation include (1) drug or alcohol-dependent individuals, (2) transients, who are not likely to maintain the close follow-up required, (3) unemployed individuals who are not actively seeking work, (4) patients who have lost single digits, except for the thumb, (5) victims of severe crush injuries, and (6) patients whose medical condition cannot tolerate 4 to 12 hours of anesthesia. The influence of age on outcome following replantation is being reassessed in recent years. However, children and patients under 40 years of age seem to obtain the best results. The best approach to making a decision is a careful review of the patient's needs for total hand function.

All primary care physicians should be aware of the "red line" sign. This refers to red steaks over one or both neurovascular bundles within an amputated part and indicates diffuse blood extravasation caused by severe crush injury to the distal arterial tree. This finding represents an absolute contraindication to replantation as reanastomosis of such vascular segments is doomed to failure. False expectations and costly patient transfers can best be avoided by recognition of the red line sign.

Replantation should be considered for amputations involving (1) multiple digits, (2) the thumb, (3) partial hand (through the palm), (4) wrist or forearm, (5) sharp amputations at or above the elbow, and (6) almost any body part in a child. Once the decision to replant a part has been made, transportation of the patient and part to the appropriate facility should be as rapid as possible. Management of the amputated tissue before replantation consists of wrapping the part in gauze moistened with saline or Ringer's lactate solution, sealing it in a plastic bag, and placing the bag on crushed ice. Parts handled in this way will survive for 12 hours, and occasionally 24 hours, but the best results are obtained with the shortest time intervals. Patient care involves complete physical examination to ensure that 4 to 16 hours of surgery can be well tolerated, placement of an intravenous line to administer antibiotics, tetanus prophylaxis and maintenance of NPO status.

Expectations following replantation include (1) active range of joint motion, approximately 50 percent of normal, (2) nerve recovery comparable to that achieved following repair of isolated peripheral nerve divisions, (3) cold intolerance that generally resolves by 2 years, and (4) an acceptable cosmetic result.

GUNSHOT WOUNDS

Most gunshot wounds seen in civilian practice involve low-velocity missiles, generally ranging from .22 to .38 caliber. Any part of the body may be injured, but priority is given to assessment of the vascular system. Arteriography is performed for wounds that have traversed regions of major blood vessels. It is remarkable how seldom these low-velocity injuries involve tendons and nerves. In most cases, debridement of 1 or 2 mm of devitalized skin and subcutaneous tissue, in addition to fixation of fractures, constitutes sufficient treatment. Vessel, nerve, and/or tendon injuries require exploration. Primary repairs of all three structures are often possible in low-velocity wounds. However, if there is any question as to degree of contamination and viability of structures, it is best to tag nerve and tendon stumps and return several days later for definitive repairs. Delayed primary closure or split-thickness skin grafting is best for the reestablishment of cover following appropriate repairs, provided there is adequate muscle protection over the part.

Wounds caused by high-velocity missiles traveling at speeds greater than 2,000 ft per second uniformly require exploration and debridement. The principles of treatment are similar to those for low-velocity wounds, except that wider debridement is often necessary, and it is uncommon to perform primary nerve and tendon repairs at the first operation. A second-look procedure at 24 to 72 hours is mandatory and, depending on the wound environment, may permit repair of essential tendons and nerves. Abdominal pedicle flaps are useful to provide durable coverage of the hand following major tissue losses, but these should not be performed until 3 to 5 days after the injury to permit improvement of tissue equilibrium.

High-velocity gunshot wounds to the hand require prolonged hospitalization, with early range of motion of the fingers whenever possible, supervised by the surgeon and physical therapist. As pain is often a limiting factor in mobilization, peripheral nerve blocks are often helpful for patients receiving physiotherapy.

CRUSH INJURIES

Crush injuries may be open or closed. Open wounds have a greater potential for bacterial contamination than closed ones, but there is a risk of local myonecrosis and compartment syndrome with both. Additionally, myoglobinuria may occur and should be treated by alkalinization of urine and promotion of osmotic diuresis in order to spare the kidneys. One to 2 ampules (50 to 100 mEq) sodium bicarbonate and 12.5 g of sodium mannitol are added to each liter of 5 percent dextrose in water, and the solution is administered at a rate of 200 ml per hour until brisk diuresis is obtained; the rate is then reduced to 100 ml per hour. The urine is tested frequently for the presence of myoglobin.

INJECTION INJURIES

These injuries call for special mention since they pose a great threat to the hand and are often treated inadequately, after too long a delay. High-pressure grease and paint guns are the most common cause of injury, and the site of injury is often the pad of the thumb or index finger, or the palm. The injected substance passes rapidly through the subcutaneous tissue and enters the flexor tendon sheath. From there, it passes into one or more of the deep spaces of the hand. The thumb and index finger conduct substances into the thenar space, and the long ring and little fingers conduct injected material into the midpalmar space. These two spaces may communicate with each other, and they also refer material proximally into Parona's space. All three spaces are deep to the profundus tendons. Proper treatment involves emergency debridement within 2 hours, consisting of (1) opening of the fingers along nonpinch, nonprotective border surfaces, (2) dorsal thumb web incision to debride the thenar space, and (3) midpalmar incision to open the midpalmar space. The midpalmar incision is often extended proximally to allow carpal tunnel release. Failure to perform adequate wide debridement immediately results in necrosis and gangrene. Plain roentgenograms are useful in evaluating this injury; they reveal the spread of paint which is radiopaque or changes in tissue planes by the spread of grease which is radiolucent. Second-look operations within 24 to 28 hours are sometimes required.

POSTOPERATIVE CARE AND REHABILITATION

The mainstays of postoperative care for the patient with extremity injury are (1) steady psychological support, (2) comfortable dressings which support the injured part in an appropriate position, (3) elevation of the injured extremity when appropriate, particularly in the case of the hand, which should be kept above the level of the heart by the use of pillows or a tubular stockinette tied around the trunk, run up over the arm and hand, and secured to an IV pole (this latter means of elevated immobilization is safe only when the elbow is well supported), and (4) appropriately timed wound inspections which are coordinated with analgesia.

Physiotherapy is often helpful, but also expensive, and should never supplant the surgeon's responsibility for teaching the patient a series of graded exercises and setting realistic goals that include a time-frame for the patient's return to work. Reeducation of the nondominant hand is beneficial for patients who face a long care sequence or who are likely to be left with significant permanent disability. The best results following complex injuries are gained in motivated patients who understand precisely what is expected of them at each stage of recovery. Daily visits to the office during the early post-hospital phase are required, and the patient should be encouraged to call at any time if any questions arise. In contrast to the automaticity with which injured internal organs are reintegrated into the patient's total function, the injured hand requires great expenditure of physical and emotional energy by all involved to return to productive activity.

The annual cost of disability from hand and upper extremity injuries is approximately 30 billion dollars in the United States, three times more than the annual cost of head injuries. Cost containment is best achieved by (1) early assessment of the individual patient's "functional extremity" needs, (2) appropriate timing of interventions, (3) single team management of soft tissue cover, neurovascular structures, and musculotendinous units, (4) close personal follow-up with appropriate guidance and goal setting, and (5) physiotherapy, when needed, with emphasis on a proper balance of exercise, elevation, and rest. Numerous expensive adjunctive therapies are currently available and, in our experience, find a limited place in the care of most patients with extremity injury.

SPECIAL TYPES OF INJURY

FRACTURES

PETER G. TRAFTON, M.D., F.A.C.S.

The purpose of this chapter is to alert the general surgeon to recent advances in the management of musculoskeletal trauma. Emphasis is on therapeutic decisions that must be made during the early period after injury. It is my belief that knowledgeable, aggressive, early management of the trauma patient's musculoskeletal injuries will contribute significantly to his overall care, and to his ultimate rehabilitation. This is not a "how-to-do-it," but a plea for immediate collaboration with an experienced orthopaedic traumatologist. The care of musculoskeletal injuries can be dealt with only briefly and arbitrarily in a chapter like this. Several alternative treatments exist for most fractures. Controversy is unavoidable.

Skeletal injuries cannot be managed safely in isolation. The treating physician must always think beyond the broken bone and include in his assessment the associated soft tissue trauma, the status of the rest of the injured limb, and the whole affected patient—his other injuries, his age and anticipated activity level, his pre-existing musculoskeletal resources, and his ability to contribute to a rehabilitation program. The choice of management for fractures and joint injuries may depend on whether an injury is isolated or is one of several problems affecting a multiply traumatized patient. Treatment is also affected by the resources available to the surgeon. In the absence of a well-stocked operating room, effective roentgenographic monitoring, and an experienced team, modern techniques of internal fixation are likely to come to grief. The advice offered in a book must always be interpreted carefully in the light of the responsible surgeon's experience. Finally, no book is a substitute for consultation, which may be invaluable for appropriate management of trauma to the musculoskeletal system.

EARLY CARE OF MUSCULOSKELETAL INJURY

Injuries of the musculoskeletal system may appear dramatic, but rarely pose immediate threats to life or even limb. As described in the section on Emergency

Room Care, initial attention is directed toward the patient's resuscitation. During these efforts, one must heed the possibility of an unstable fracture or dislocation of the spine, especially in the neck. History and physical examination, if possible, are rarely adequate to exclude such injuries. Roentgenograms are essential, beginning with a cross-table lateral film that shows the entire cervical spine, down to T1. Such a film is mandatory for all patients with head or face injuries, unconsciousness, neck pain, or abnormal neurologic findings. Most unstable cervical spine injuries are evident on this x-ray study, but its normality does not guarantee a stable spine.

If manipulation of the head or neck is necessary before roentgenograms are obtained, it should be done in a way that minimizes the risk of damage to the spinal cord. Flexion, hyperextension, and rotation of the neck away from the midline must be avoided. Gentle (5 to 7 lb) traction on the head applied with hands or a cervical halter will stabilize the neck. If the head is adequately supported, the patient may be rolled "like a log," to permit examination of the back. A patient who is alert enough to be moving his head and neck spontaneously has little risk of injuring himself. Poorly tolerated restraints add little protection. The patient with a painful neck and an acute unstable injury usually appreciates immobilization with sandbags taped together over the forehead, or traction by means of a head halter or tongs.

In an acutely injured patient, the thoracic and lumbar spine and the pelvis cannot adequately be evaluated by physical examination alone. If the injury is due to a significant fall, a vehicular accident, or other high-energy trauma, and if the patient is unable to deny pain in back and pelvis and cannot demonstrate normal active motion of back and legs, AP and lateral roentgenograms of the entire spine and an AP film of the pelvis must be obtained. However, these studies should not interrupt more urgent early evaluation and treatment. Until they have been obtained and reviewed, spine precautions are followed.

Extremity injuries may be obvious or occult. Initial care of obvious injuries includes control of bleeding with pressure dressings, splinting unstable injuries in an acceptable position, and urgent identification and treatment of arterial occlusion.

Once resuscitation is under way and the patient is responding, a thorough and systematic search must be made for more occult injuries. Inspect all skin surfaces, from digits to trunk, for deformity, swelling, ecchymosis, and laceration. Skin abrasions are significant. If in the region of a musculoskeletal injury, they require that any needed operation be done promptly or else delayed until the abrasion heals. Palpate each bone and joint for swelling, deformity, and tenderness (if the patient is responsive). Stress each bone to confirm stability. Move each joint to demonstrate normal range of motion and absence of abnormal motion. When emergency surgery is a part of the resuscitation or early care of a trauma patient, extremity examination should always be completed before terminating the anesthetic. Confirm presence of peripheral pulses. Obtain roentgenograms of all abnormal areas.

When the patient is conscious and able to cooperate, active voluntary motion of each joint must be assessed to check motor nerve and myotendinous integrity. Check sensation in the isolated sensory area of each major peripheral nerve. For critically ill patients who are unable initially to cooperate, completion of this evaluation may take several days. Such follow-through is mandatory to avoid the embarrassment of missing injuries. Resuscitation of the multiply injured patient necessarily places diagnosis and treatment of musculoskeletal conditions at a relatively low priority. Many injuries are not initially appreciated. Repeated examinations during the early recovery period are frequently rewarded by the discovery of additional diagnoses in time for effective treatment.

OPEN FRACTURES

Classification

Open fractures require special attention to minimize the risks of clostridial and pyogenic infection. Treatment is guided by classification of the severity of injury, primarily according to the extent of soft tissue trauma and level of contamination. It is important to consider the entire soft tissue wound instead of just the skin opening. In severe crush injuries, small lacerations may overlie extensively contused or necrotic soft tissues.

Grade I	Small wounds caused by low-velocity trauma, with minimal contamination and soft tissue damage, e.g., skin laceration by a bone end or a low-velocity gunshot wound.
Grade II	Wounds extensive in length and width, but with little or no avascular or devitalized soft tissue and relatively little foreign material.
Grade III	Moderate or massive wounds with considerable devitalized soft tissue, foreign material, or both. Extensive wounds without significant periosteal stripping may technically fall into this type, but generally fare much better than those with marked devascularization of bone and destruction of overlying soft tissue. When these wounds are associated with an arterial injury that requires repair, the risk of wound infection rises steeply.

Identification of an open fracture is the first step of early management. Although usually obvious, open fractures occasionally are not appreciated because of incomplete examination. Posterior surfaces must be checked. Seemingly superficial wounds may communicate with underlying bone or joint injuries. Whenever the pelvis is fractured, perineal, vaginal, and rectal lacerations should be ruled out. Neurovascular status, myotendinous function, and the possibility of multiple injuries must be checked. When totally satisfactory examination and treatment of a wound near a fracture cannot be carried out in the emergency ward, assume that the fracture is open, and proceed to the operating room where adequate anesthesia, assistance, hemostasis, and lighting usually confirm suspicions and facilitate treatment.

Once an injured limb has been examined, control of bleeding is achieved with sterile compression dressings, and a splint is applied before transportation to the radiology department or the operating suite. If a patient arrives with a well-described open fracture already covered, the dressing should be removed only in the operating room.

Roentgenograms of injured or suspect areas are essential for evaluating the trauma patient. Unfortunately, the quality of emergency studies is variable, and it is risky for the patient to languish, poorly monitored, in the radiology department. The responsible surgeon must be prepared at any moment to conclude that the films already obtained are the best possible and that the patient should proceed to surgery. Chest and cervical spine films are of highest priority. Those of extremities are necessary for a complete evaluation. Without adequate x-ray study, the fracture surgeon operates at his peril. For example, views centered on joint rather than the diaphysis may be needed to define fully an intra-articular injury. Of course, such films may be obtained in the operating room once the patient's condition has been stabilized.

Management of the Open Fracture

I strongly believe that each open fracture should be cared for in a well-prepared operating room, with adequate anesthesia, as soon as is safely possible.

Immediate Wound Care

The basic aspects of surgical wound care have changed little since their description by Desault in the late eighteenth century. Effective medical adjuncts are more recent. Tetanus prophylaxis is administered immediately. I urge the use of an appropriate intravenous antibiotic promptly on the diagnosis of an open fracture. The value of this *adjunct* to surgical treatment has been shown by several comparative studies. We currently use 1 g intravenous cefazolin every 6 hours, beginning in the emergency ward and continuing through the first 48 hours after injury, whether or not the wound is left open. Depending on the source and extent of contamination, aminoglycosides for better gram-negative coverage and/or penicillin for anaerobic organisms might appropriately be added to the initial antibiotic regimen. Alternative antibiotics are required for allergic patients.

The properly evaluated patient is brought to the operating room as soon as team and equipment are assembled. Adequate anesthesia is induced, and following or concurrent with higher-priority surgical treatment, definitive care of the open fracture is begun.

This starts with a careful reassessment of the injured limb—an examination under anesthesia. Is salvage warranted or must primary amputation be considered? If amputation appears to be a possibility, I attempt to discuss this with the patient pre-operatively in the emergency ward.

A pneumatic tourniquet is applied, but inflated only if necessary, to control bleeding or to assess tissue viability with postischemic hyperemia. In principle, the cleansing of an injured limb should not be allowed to contaminate further the wound of an open fracture. However, in practice it is hard to scrub the limb adequately while a sterile occlusive dressing is kept over the usual wound. Most detergents and soaps are injurious to tissue. Therefore, avoid the wound itself with scrub solution. The scrub is done with the limb lying on a sterile waterproof disposable drape, which is replaced twice during the 10-minute wash. Detergent suds are rinsed and the skin is dried with sterile towels. Then the entire limb, including the wound, is painted with iodophor antiseptic solution, and new waterproof sterile drapes are applied.

Irrigation and Debridement

Next irrigation and debridement are performed. It is often necessary to enlarge the wound to permit adequate inspection and cleansing. This should be carefully planned so as not to devitalize skin flaps or interrupt superficial veins, which might be essential for blood return. If possible, incisions should avoid contused skin and preserve a healthy flap of tissue to cover the fracture site and any implanted internal fixation device. With sufficient exposure, all foreign material and dead or questionable tissue are removed, while sparing nerves, major vessels, and as much bone as possible. Small free fragments of cortical bone are discarded. Grossly contaminated bone surfaces are removed with rongeur or curette. All joints that have been penetrated are opened and inspected for debris including osteochondral fragments. We leave questionably viable skin, which can readily be assessed during the days following injury. Subcutaneous fat, fascia, and injured muscle are aggressively removed if dead or dirty, although it is important not to undermine excessively a viable skin flap. Contractility, consistency, and especially the presence of bleeding from small intrinsic vessels are more helpful than color as indicators of muscle viability.

A pulsatile irrigation system enhances cleansing of injured tissue. This generally permits use of less than the 10 or more liters of irrigant previously recommended. I use at least 5 L of normal saline or Ringer's solution for the average grade II open fracture. I use 0.2 percent kanamycin solution as a final antibiotic rinse (2 g kanamycin in 1 L, with 2 ampules of sodium bicarbonate to ensure an alkaline solution).

During debridement, decisions must be made about two other aspects of care for the injured limb: fracture stabilization and wound closure. Complications arising from either of these controversial areas can considerably increase the patient's period of disability and can jeopardize the eventual result. Avoidance of grief is perhaps best achieved by the surgeon's use of techniques with which he is thoroughly familiar and for which he is completely equipped. Adequate fracture stabilization is important, and external or internal fixation may both reduce the risk of infection and facilitate overall management. Meticulous wound toilet and *delayed* primary closure are essential if internal fixation is used and in all grade II and grade III open wounds.

Reduction and Fixation

Whereas articular surface fractures should be reduced anatomically, extra-articular fractures generally require only adequate restoration of angular and rotational alignment, with preservation of length. How to stabilize an open fracture remains controversial. Traction, plaster cast, external skeletal fixation, and the several forms of internal fixation are all useful, individually and in combination. The problems that must be solved anew for each fracture patient are: (1) how much stability is necessary, or even possible? (2) what is the most beneficial and least hazardous way of obtaining that stability? No direct comparative studies document the unequivocal superiority of one form of stabilization over another.

For certain injuries and certain patients *internal fixation* may yield improved results. Therefore, this seems indicated selectively. Patients with intra-articular fractures, multiple injuries, segmental fractures, acute spinal cord injuries, and some with significant bone loss are prime candidates. Those with severe soft tissue wounds over fractures that can be stabilized better with internal than external fixation (e.g., ankle fractures, some radius shaft fractures, and proximal femur fractures) are also more easily managed this way, although infection is risked. This use of internal fixation should be recognized as an attempt at salvage of a limb that might otherwise be amputated. Primary internal fixation of fractures adjacent to arterial anastomoses is not necessary to protect the vascular repair.

External skeletal fixation must be coordinated carefully with wound management and bone grafting. It offers a powerful and adaptable technique for stabilizing open fractures without additional exposure or devascularization of bone and without the encumbrance of plaster casts or traction. If delayed wound closure or the use of a muscle pedicle or myocutaneous flap is anticipated, an external skeletal frame is preferable to pins and plaster, but familiarity with the technique and the specific device is necessary to avoid complications. Whenever possible, I prefer to use half pins inserted through the subcutaneous surface of a bone. External skeletal fixation is especially applicable to unstable open fractures of the pelvis, which have a mortality rate of up to 50 percent. External fixation devices can also maintain fixed traction across an injured joint, thus permitting mobilization of a patient who might not tolerate recumbency.

Skeletal traction often provides a safe provisional or definitive means to stabilize open fractures for the patient with an isolated injury. Variations on traditional traction techniques can be valuable for the management of open fractures. *Plaster casts* are satisfactory for some less severe open fractures. Military surgeons have popularized open wound treatment under plaster. Functional use of the limb is stressed. Wounds can be closed later through a window or with a cast change, or they can be left open until they heal. However, it is difficult and unpleasant to manage large soft tissue wounds this way in a civilian orthopaedic practice. Early coverage with split-thickness skin is appreciated by patients with large granulating wounds.

Wound Coverage

The questions of whether, when, and how to close an open fracture wound are as controversial as the question of stabilization. Once again, comparative clinical trials do not exist to guide us. Skin closure is dangerous when a wound is contaminated. When host defenses are further compromised by the implantation of foreign material, primary suture seems even more risky, and failure is nearly assured if skin tension is produced by the closure.

It is easy to say that the early goal of open fracture care is to convert the initially contaminated open wound into a clean closed one. Several techniques are advocated for this, ranging from leaving the wound open until it heals secondarily to primary closure with any of a variety of plastic surgical procedures, if simple suture is not possible. While military surgeons maintain their hard-learned tradition of open wound management, a number of civilian traumatologists have presented examples of early closure techniques, which are said to promote wound healing and even fracture union. Several types of pedicle flap may be used: skin and subcutaneous tissue, muscle alone, or muscle with overlying subcutaneous tissue and skin. More recently, one or othe other of the two last-mentioned flaps has been done ''free,'' with microvascular anastomoses to local vessels. It appears that such procedures are most successful if carried out a few days after injury or postponed for a number of weeks, until the period of delayed reconstruction. Split-thickness skin graft can be used to cover healthy wound tissue at any time, although it is unsatisfactory over exposed blood vessels, tendons, and bare cortical bone. The multiple perforations produced by a meshing device minimize fluid accumulation under split-thickness grafts.

It is entirely possible to manage most severe open fractures without the use of elaborate plastic surgical procedures. Open fractures heal successfully in spite of bone and hardware remaining exposed for periods of several months or more.

COMPARTMENT SYNDROME

A variety of injuries can cause progressive elevation of tissue pressure within the confines of "compartments" formed by the normal fascial envelopes around groups of skeletal muscles. Once compartment pressure is elevated sufficiently to block microvascular perfusion, muscle and nerve ischemia leads to necrosis of the involved tissue. Eventually the pressure recedes to normal levels, leaving behind dead muscle and nerve, the cause of Volkmann's contracture.

The key to effective treatment is early diagnosis. This requires suspicion of compartment syndrome whenever an extremity sustains a crushing or severely contusing injury, with or without a fracture. Conscious patients with compartment syndrome develop pain and firm swelling of the entire involved compartment, and they soon lose function of the muscles and nerves that lie within it. Pulses and skin perfusion are often normal.

At least every 2 hours, patients with significant extremity injuries must be monitored for inordinate pain and for loss of sensation or motor function distal to the area of injury. Release of any constricting bandage or cast is the essential first step in treatment of a suspected compartment syndrome, to permit examination and to allow maximal elasticity of the involved compartment. This may reduce pressure sufficiently to restore tissue perfusion and prevent necrosis. If the patient is unconscious or has an associated nerve injury that prevents clinical assessment, compartment pressures are measured with a commercially available wick catheter (or "slit-wick," made from polyethylene tubing with the terminal end slit about 1 mm longitudinally in several places). This is connected to a sterile strain gauge of the type used for monitoring intra-arterial pressure and is introduced through a large-bore needle into the suspected compartment. A satisfactory measurement system responds promptly to manual pressure on the compartment and falls to a reproducible level soon after such external compression is released. It is important to measure the pressure in *each* compartment of the involved area. For the leg, this means anterior, peroneal, deep posterior, and superficial posterior spaces. In the forearm, both flexor and extensor groups should be assessed at multiple sites.

If neuromuscular findings are perfectly normal, a patient with elevated pressure may be monitored clinically or by repeated pressure measurements. If sensation or contractility is impaired, or if they are unassessable and the compartmental pressure is over 30 or 40 mm Hg, fasciotomy is required. All involved compartments must be released. For the leg, I use two incisions: one, which is anterolateral with identification and preservation of the superficial peroneal nerve, for release of anterior and peroneal compartments; the other, which is just posterior to the medial tibial shaft, for release of the deep and superficial compartments. Skin incisions 8 to 10 cm long should permit adequate decompression with minimal tissue damage, with longer fasciotomies using partially opened scissors as a fasciotome. Usually the skin is left open for delayed closure by suture or split-thickness graft. If an associated fracture is present, fixing it at the time of fasciotomy simplifies wound management. Either external or internal skeletal fixation may be used, depending on fracture configuration and the degree of additional soft tissue dissection required.

Forearm compartment syndromes may involve anterior (flexor) or posterior (extensor) muscles and may require release of the intrinsic fascia of each involved muscle. An extensive surgical approach is required, such as McConnell's combined exposure of the median and ulnar nerves, as portrayed by A.K. Henry.

Compartment syndromes that are recognized after necrosis is far advanced are probably best left closed rather than treated with fasciotomy because of their significant risk of infection and the lack of potential benefit from decompressing dead tissue.

FRACTURE AND DISLOCATION OF THE SPINE

Initial and subsequent evaluations must deal with two fairly separate issues. The first is the status of the neural elements: spinal cord and nerve roots (see section on *Neurologic Injury*). The second area of concern is structural damage to the spine. An injury may involve bone, ligaments, or both. Spine injuries may be stable or unstable. Unstable injuries risk early neurologic damage and/or subsequent mechanical failure with excessive mobility or progressive deformity, either of which might cause late neurologic damage or pain.

Principles of Treatment

The principles that guide treatment of spine injuries are:

1. Consider all injured spines unstable until assessment is complete.
2. Identify unstable injuries and treat them so as to minimize the risk of neurologic damage and persisting instability.
3. Identify and carefully follow neurologic deficits. Provide treatment that maximizes the potential for neurologic recovery and facilitates rehabilitation of the patient.
4. Generally speaking, correction of spinal deformity is essential to prevent further mechanical damage to an injured spinal cord. Debridement of the spinal canal anterior to the neural elements may also be required to eliminate continuing compression and promote maximal recovery of an incomplete injury to cord or roots. Laminectomy is of no benefit.
5. If a cord injury is neurologically "complete," attention should be directed toward achievement of a stable well-aligned spine, rather than toward decompression of the neural elements, since no currently available treatment improves neurologic recovery in these patients.

6. Patients with significant spine and cord injuries should be transferred to a spinal cord injury center as soon as this can be done safely, preferably within the first 2 days.

Dislocation or significant angulation can usually be improved by longitudinal traction, which also splints the injured area, minimizing motion that might further damage the cord. If traction is not successful within several hours, open reduction should be considered promptly. After correction of angulation and displacement evident on AP or lateral films, persisting canal compromise anterior to the cord may be caused by retropulsion of vertebral body bone fragments. These are clearly demonstrated by CT scans. Removing significant neural canal fragments might improve neurologic recovery in patients with incomplete injuries, but the optimal timing for such procedures is not yet established. Many patients do recover function in spite of such fragments in the neural canal. This is consistent with the belief that neural injury is due primarily to crushing and contusing sustained at the moment of impact, when deformation is greatest. The initial films do not show this maximal deformity, but reveal instead the final resting position of bone fragments and spine once all injury forces have dissipated. Removal of bone fragments from the neural canal has not been shown to restore function after *complete* cord injuries.

Cervical Spine

Stabilization

Patients with potentially unstable cervical spine injuries should be transported with the head secured to a spine board. In the emergency room, bilateral sandbags, joined by a strip of 3-inch wide cloth adhesive tape over the forehead, provide the most secure stabilization of the neck. Skeletal traction should be instituted immediately if a cervical cord injury is present, or if an unstable fracture is evident on x-ray examination (angulation greater than 11 degrees or displacement over 3.5 mm at a single level on the lateral roentgenogram). Five pounds of traction is sufficient to immobilize most injuries in the upper cervical spine, progressing to 10 to 15 lbs for lower cervical injuries. Significantly greater traction, increased in stages with careful radiologic and neurologic monitoring, may be required to reduce a fracture or dislocation. Alignment must be monitored with roentgenograms, with special attention to the possibility of overdistraction of upper cervical injuries and to loss of alignment with postural changes.

Gardner-Wells tongs can readily be applied in the Emergency Room by a single surgeon without significant assistance. No shaving is needed. Hair and scalp are soaked with iodophor solution, and the tongs are applied according to the attached instructions with the pines centered over the auditory meati, below the maximal circumference of the head. Lidocaine (1%) anesthesia is first injected into the scalp and down to the skull in the appropriate sites. Once the tongs are secure, traction is applied with a rope through a pulley attached to the head of the bed or stretcher. If this is unavailable, the rope is merely passed over the rail at the top of the stretcher.

Although its application is more complicated, the cranial halo is a most valuable device for skull traction, as it can be used not only for traction, but also to provide immobilization by attachment to a plastic vest or plaster body jacket. This technique provides the most secure external support available for cervical spine injuries and may permit early sitting and ambulation. However, it does not maintain fixed traction. Alignment that requires traction or recumbency can be lost in a halo-vest. For cervical spine injuries, it is important to choose a model of halo-vest that permits unobstructed lateral roentgenograms of the entire neck so that alignment of the injury can be easily monitored.

Injuries of the upper cervical spine may be extremely unstable and threaten the medullary respiratory and circulatory centers. Forceful traction may cause additional neural injuries. Patients resuscitated at the scene of injury may have *occipitoatlantal dislocations*, with subtle radiologic signs. Halo-vest immobilization should be applied as soon as possible, and careful radiologic monitoring is needed to identify displacement that may occur even with this support. Arthrodesis will be required, but probably offers little additional early stabilization.

Burst fractures of the atlas (Jefferson fractures) may disrupt the transverse atlantal ligament and remain unstable even after the ring fractures unite. Generally, I prefer halo-vest immobilization for 12 weeks, followed by assessment of stability with flexion-extension roentgenograms in hopes that if C1-C2 instability persists, union of the posterior arch of C1 will permit fusion at this single level rather than to the occiput as well.

Fractures of the odontoid process (dens) are controversial. If they involve the narrow waist (sometimes called "base") of the dens and are displaced, the incidence of nonunion is significant; thus early C1-C2 fusion is often advised. If an anatomic reduction is achieved and maintained with 12 weeks of halo-vest or halo-body-cast immobilization, a trial of nonoperative treatment seems reasonable, deferring arthrodesis until failure to unite is demonstrated. Fractures of the true base of the dens, which involve significant amounts of the cancellous bone of the C2 vertebral body, usually unite during the 12 weeks of halo-vest or cast immobilization. *Fractures of the pedicles of C2* (Hangman's fractures) unite reliably with similar treatment.

Fractures and dislocations of the lower cervical spine usually can be satisfactorily reduced in traction and maintained in alignment until bone and ligament healing are secure enough to provide stability, which must be proved by flexion-extension roentgenograms following removal of immobilization and restoration of normal neck mobility. Halo-vest treatment with fairly early patient mobilization may be possible. Open reduction may be required, particularly with incomplete posterior ligament disruptions and a unilateral jumped facet joint.

A posterior approach provides direct access to the fracture and permits local posterior fusion once reduction is achieved. Even grossly unstable fractures usually become stable after healing. If the injury is predominantly ligamentous, late instability is more likely, and early arthrodesis deserves consideration to prevent this possibility with the attendant need for arthrodesis and continued restriction of activity while it heals.

Thoracolumbar Spine

Associated thoracoabdominal and extremity injuries may be present and may require immediate treatment. Since physical examination may not reveal the presence or degree of injury to the spine, good-quality roentgenograms, carefully interpreted, are mandatory. Injuries range from stable wedge compression fractures, through bursting vertebral body fractures with more or less ligamentous disruption, to fracture dislocations that are grossly unstable. Such dislocations may appear deceptively well aligned on a single roentgenographic projection.

Significant instability is present in thoracolumbar spine injuries if the anterior portion of the vertebral column is so disrupted that it is unlikely to be able to support the compressive load of body weight, or if the posterior complex of bone and ligaments is unlikely to sustain the tensile loads that will be placed upon it by normal forward flexion. Instability clearly comes in varying degrees, rather than "all or none."

Surgical treatment for thoracolumbar spine injuries is controversial. Unreduced fracture dislocations and marked angular deformity are strong indications. If a neurologic deficit is present, surgery is easier to justify, especially to maximize cauda equina recovery if the neural canal is compromised, as well as to facilitate rehabilitation, to prevent late deformity that may interfere with wheel-chair sitting, and possibly to decrease the risk of late pain. Most thoracolumbar fractures become stable in 3 months. If no neurologic deficit exists, surgery may only provide mobilization a few weeks earlier.

The gross instability of a *fracture-dislocation* mandates anatomic reduction of the vertebral column and maintenance of alignment during healing. Initially, I attempt this with halo-tibial traction, applied as soon as possible. For adults, 15 to 20 lbs is applied to the halo and a similar weight to each tibia, with careful attention to ensure that traction attachments do not press against insensible skin. Halo-tibial traction is usually best managed on a turning frame, on which the patient can be anesthetized and undergo operation without additional traumatic transfers. This traction technique provisionally stabilizes the thoracolumbar spine during emergency treatment of associated injuries, which are disturbingly frequent in our patients.

The need for halo-tibial traction can usually be judged from AP and lateral roentgenograms. A detailed demonstration of the injured area and of residual deformity is best provided by a CT scan, which I prefer to obtain with the patient in traction if marked instability is present. Although the routine transaxial views clearly show retropulsed body fragments, the scout view or appropriately chosen computer-reconstructed views may be needed to demonstrate angulation and displacement or posterior element injuries. Routine myelography does not appear to be helpful.

When displaced thoracolumbar injuries are initially treated with halo-tibial traction, alignment is usually fairly well achieved. The improved alignment and effective splinting facilitate surgery, which is often indicated for patients with highly unstable spines. Posterior open reduction, stabilization with Harrington instruments, and arthrodesis should generally be performed as soon as the patient's overall condition permits and appropriate personnel and equipment are available.

Postoperatively, halo-tibial traction is discontinued. When wounds are healing, ileus is resolved, and sufficient stability is present, the patient may get up in a plaster or molded plastic body jacket.

Interest is growing in anterior, retroperitoneal, or transthoracic surgery for thoracolumbar spine injuries. These are major procedures, often associated with significant blood loss in acute injuries. Anterior approaches provide excellent access for decompressing the anterior portion of the neural canal, but effective and safe anterior stabilization techniques for the traumatized spine are still under development.

Unstable thoracolumbar injuries without marked displacement usually become stable after bone and ligaments have healed—a process that might require 3 or more months. Since external support alone often fails to provide satisfactory immobilization for these injuries, bed rest should also be advised. Individualized treatment is necessary, but I generally plan 6 weeks recumbency, followed by gradually increased ambulation and sitting in a body jacket or cast. Roentgenographic monitoring and eventual confirmation of stability are necessary during recovery.

PELVIC RING INJURY

The pelvic ring consists of the sacrum and both innominate bones with their sacroiliac and pubic symphysis articulations. Disruptions may be caused by (1) sideways compression, (2) anterior forces that tend to open the pelvis like a book, and (3) posterosuperiorly directed shearing forces, typically a fall from a significant height. Although the anterior ring disruption through pubic rami or symphysis pubis tend to be obvious on an AP pelvic film, more careful inspection is necessary to identify the site of posterior injury. Yet such posterior disruption must be present for the ring to be displaced anteriorly. The posterior injury is generally the more significant, and its precise identification is necessary to permit appropriate treatment; 45-degree downshot (pelvic inlet) and 45-degree upshot (tangential) roentgenograms demonstrate displacement clearly. A CT scan shows the posterior lesion especially well, but does not reveal longitudinal displacement. Posterior pelvic ring injuries may involve, singly or in combination, the sacral wing, the ilium, or the sacroiliac joint. The sacroiliac joint can be totally disrupted or merely hinged open on its stout posterior-superior ligaments.

Instability of a pelvic ring injury can be inferred from roentgenograms that show gross displacement. However, even minimally displaced injuries can be significantly unstable. Physical examination is required to evaluate ring stability. Significant instability is present if either or both iliac wings can be moved by manual force applied mediolaterally to the anterior iliac crests.

Pelvic ring injuries pose several problems. Retroperitoneal bleeding from the fracture surfaces and adjacent blood vessels may be life-threatening. Associated abdominal and thoracic injuries are common and often serious. Urologic trauma, especially ruptures of the bladder or posterior urethra, may be present. Neurologic injury, usually involving the sacral nerve roots, also may occur. In addition to the sequelae of these injuries, pelvic deformity and pain may persist to cause permanent disability. Open pelvic fractures have exceptionally high morbidity and mortality.

Initial management of a pelvic ring injury requires hemodynamic monitoring and stabilization, with identification and appropriate treatment of associated injuries. Catheterization, preceded by urethrography if indicated, and a cystogram are routine. If one hemipelvis is displaced proximally, 15 to 30 lbs of skeletal traction should be applied via a Steinmann pin in the tibial tubercle. If done early, this decreases motion at the site of injury and usually restores pelvic symmetry.

External Skeletal Fixation

Unstable pelvic ring fractures usually are treated by early stabilization. The traditional pelvic sling fails to provide this and may increase deformity if medial displacement is possible. A spica cast offers considerable external support, but it is cumbersome and interferes with mobilization of the patient. Internal fixation is advocated by some authors, but it is not always possible or safe. External skeletal fixation permits early, rapid, and minimally invasive stabilization of most unstable pelvic ring injuries. By controlling motion at the site of injury and by restoring the normal close confines of the true pelvis, bleeding may be staunched. Pain relief is often dramatic. Unless posterior disruption is complete with obvious vertical shear displacement, traction is omitted, and early mobilization of the patient may be possible. However, with an anteriorly attached pelvic external fixator, vertical shear injuries can displace. To avoid this, additional protection is generally required, by bed rest and traction on the involved side for several weeks or by posterior internal fixation.

I believe that external pelvic fixation significantly facilitates the management of patients with unstable pelvic ring injuries, and I recommend that it be used whenever examination demonstrates pelvic instability or roentgenograms show significant displacement. The fixator should be applied as early as possible, immediately after any indicated laparotomy, or as soon as initial evaluation is complete and before development of an extensive retroperitoneal hematoma, which it may help to contain.

One must occasionally choose between application of an external fixator and arteriography with embolization to control bleeding associated with pelvic fractures. Studies have shown that less than 10 percent of such patients have significant arterial bleeding that might respond to embolization. Therefore, I would recommend external fixation first because bleeding from fracture and veins often responds to external fixation and volume replacement. If this measure fails to control hemorrhage adequately, arteriography is the next appropriate step, and it is not compromised by the presence of the fixator.

The fixator must be applied in the operating room with sterile preparation and draping. Depending on the ease of demonstrating the iliac crests, the exact insertion site chosen, and the surgeon's experience, pins may be placed percutaneously or with small incisions to permit placement of thumb and index finger on opposite sides of the ilium for precise control of the pins. I prefer at least three (5 mm in diameter) pins, inserted deeply into each ilium. They should not tent the surrounding skin, which may be left open if necessary to avoid this problem. A number of configurations have been proposed for the external frame used to connect the iliac crest pin clusters. It should be as rigid as possible and must not impinge on the abdomen or the skin near the pin insertion sites. Triangular cross-bracing helps to prevent displacement, as does adjustment of the frame to maintain a compressive force across the posterior ring injury, which must be reduced as much as possible at the time of fixator application. Reduction is aided by traction on the involved limb and by the lateral decubitus position, with the surgeon manipulating the pelvis and holding alignment while an assistant tightens the fixator.

In contrast to reports of late pain and disability following significant pelvic ring injuries managed with traditional techniques, external pelvic fixation appears to offer an improved long-term result. In my experience, anatomic reduction of pelvic ring injuries has not always been maintained by external fixation, but significant complications are rare and usually minor.

SHOULDER INJURY

Shoulder trauma may cause neurovascular injuries. A careful physical examination is as necessary as high-quality roentgenograms for complete assessment of the patient with an injured shoulder.

Clavicular Injury

Sternoclavicular Dislocation

Sternoclavicular (SC) dislocations are either posterior or anterior. Although they are not obvious on routine roentgenograms, physical examination demonstrates asymmetry, swelling, and tenderness. Signs of respiratory or vascular compromise may be present in some patients with *posterior sternoclavicular dislocations*. A closed, manipulative reduction is almost always possible, although anesthesia and muscle relaxation may be required. The technique is as follows. Lateral traction is applied to the clavicle by placing a narrow sandbag between the scapulae of the supine patient. Pressure on the anterior aspects of the shoulders produces scapular retraction and distraction of the overriding sternoclavicular joint. Percutaneous manipulation of the clavicle with a stout sterile towel clip may be required. Posterior sternoclavicular dislocations that do not respond to closed manipulation should undergo open reduction, with appropriate thoracic surgical assistance, because associated mediastinal complications are common and may persist if the clavicle remains dislocated. Once reduced, posterior SC dislocations are usually stable. A figure-of-8 dressing is worn for 4 to 6 weeks to prevent shoulder protraction.

Reduction of *anterior sternoclavicular dislocations* is usually easy with forcible retraction of the shoulder, but may be difficult to maintain. However, the complications of internal fixation exceed the problems of a chronic dislocation. Therefore I attempt an initial reduction, but counsel the patient to accept redisplacement of an anterior SC dislocation, deferring resection of the medial end of the clavicle for those few cases that remain symptomatic after several months of rehabilitation.

Clavicle Fracture

Clavicle fractures usually heal unless open reduction is performed. Deformity is common, but while occasionally unsightly, almost never compromises function. A figure-of-8 bandage and sling usually provide enough support to minimize early discomfort and can be discarded as soon as the patient wishes. Efforts should be directed toward early and complete shoulder rehabilitation.

Acromioclavicular Separation

Some authors advocate repair of complete acromioclavicular (AC) separations. I am unimpressed with the functional deficit that results from this injury. Primary surgical repair, with or without reconstruction of the coracoclavicular ligaments, is not free of complications, including failure to achieve the desired result. Therefore, I prefer to accept the anatomic deformity, unless it is severe, and concentrate instead on shoulder rehabilitation, which usually takes only a few weeks. Those few patients who remain symptomatic may be candidates for subperiosteal resection of the distal clavicle, with careful reefing of the local soft tissues to minimize residual prominence.

Shoulder Dislocation

Anterior dislocations are usually obvious by their asymmetry, deformity, and typical anteroposterior (AP) roentgenographic appearance. *Posterior dislocations*, although much less common, are frequently overlooked, perhaps because the deformity is less obvious, but primarily because of overreliance on the AP film, which looks deceptively normal. A crucial physical finding in posterior shoulder dislocation is absence of external rotation of the joint. If external rotation is limited, posterior dislocation must be excluded by an adequate lateral roentgenogram.

Once diagnosed, a shoulder dislocation should be reduced as soon as possible. Many techniques are described. Closed manipulation almost always suffices, but the total muscle relaxation provided by general anesthesia may be required. I usually reduce anterior dislocations of the shoulder by manual traction on the humerus, using countertraction on the chest with a sheet, if needed. Preliminary analgesia and muscle relaxation are valuable aids.

Following reduction, shoulder alignment and integrity are confirmed by adequate AP and lateral roentgenograms, a sling and swath or commercial shoulder immobilizer is applied, and the patient is observed until he is clearly recovered from the effects of medication. The length of immobilization for a first dislocation depends primarily on the age of the patient. Because of their high risk of recurrence, 6 weeks is appropriate for young adults. Older individuals are more at risk of limited motion and should be mobilized sooner (within 3 weeks if over 40), beginning with pendulum exercises, but avoiding external rotation stresses for several weeks after injury. Recurrent dislocations need be immobilized only long enough for comfort. If redislocations are frequent enough to trouble the patient, elective shoulder repair should be advised.

Posterior shoulder dislocations usually can be reduced with traction along the humerus, similar to that for anterior dislocations, after muscle relaxation is adequate. Immobilization after reduction is best done with a wide adhesive tape that surrounds the supracondylar region and is attached to the back so that the elbow cannot move anterior to the coronal plane of the body.

Fracture of the Proximal Humerus

These injuries may be isolated or associated with dislocation. A number of factors influence treatment, including amount of comminution and of displacement, whether or not soft tissue attachments to the humeral head are sufficient to maintain its blood supply, and whether or not bone quality will permit surgical fixation. Dislocations require urgent treatment. When only a fracture is present, temporary mobilization of the multiply injured patient can be obtained by supporting his shoulder with a sling and swath, deferring definitive care until the patient's general condition permits, although delay beyond 7 to 10 days increases the difficulty of surgery and may compromise the result. *Undisplaced fractures of the proximal humerus* usually heal reliably with sling and swath immobilization and proceed rapidly to the rehabilitation phase of treatment. Fortunately, most proximal humeral fractures fall into this category.

Significantly displaced proximal humeral fractures pose greater problems. Neer's four-part classification is helpful, emphasizing the status of soft tissue attachments. The four parts are humeral head, shaft, greater tuberosity, and lesser tuberosity. The tendinous portion of the rotator cuff attaches to the tuberosities. Comminuted fractures and fracture-dislocations of the proximal humerus that separate soft tissue connections from the proximal humerus have a significant risk of avascular necrosis of the isolated humeral head, with resulting pain and limited motion. This risk is probably increased by extensive surgical exposure for open reduction and internal fixation (ORIF).

The ultimate result of a serious shoulder injury is often determined by how soon, and how effectively, the patient is able to begin range-of-motion exercises. Any treatment that requires prolonged immobilization of the arm is likely to result in permanent loss of mobility. When comminution is marked or bone is osteoporotic, internal fixation offers unreliable stability. Avascular necrosis and nonunion may follow extensive stripping of soft tissue attachments in an effort to improve fixation.

Displaced fractures of the tuberosities require ORIF to repair the rotator cuff and prevent impingement on the coracoacromial arch. If the humeral head is detached from the shaft as well, I attempt to fix the fracture as atraumatically as possible, and securely enough to begin passive range-of-motion exercises immediately. If this is impossible, I perform reconstruction arthroplasty promptly, as advised by Neer, replacing the humeral head and reattaching the tuberosities to the shaft below the prosthesis. For two-part displaced humeral neck fractures or three-part fractures with the greater tuberosity still attached to the head, I attempt closed reduction and percutaneous fixation with temporary pins under fluoroscopic control.

Many displaced fractures of the neck of the humerus can also be aligned satisfactorily with skeletal traction, applied to a screw or threaded pin inserted into the olecranon. Care must be taken to avoid the ulnar nerve and the elbow joint and to ensure secure bone fixation. The traction is arranged so that the forearm hangs over the head of the supine patient, supported by an additional fixed sling. Although this technique usually aligns proximal humeral fractures satisfactorily, it requires several weeks of recumbency and may compromise the overall care of the multiply injured patient.

HUMERAL SHAFT FRACTURE

Fractures of the shaft of the humerus can be accompanied by radial nerve palsy. This usually occurs at the time of injury, but may develop subsequently if the injured limb is inadequately splinted and occasionally after manipulative reduction. In my experience, these radial nerve palsies resolve during closed treatment of the humeral shaft fracture.

Almost all humeral shaft fractures are amenable to closed treatment. If the injury is isolated and the patient ambulatory, a light-weight hanging-arm cast or a U-shaped coaptation splint, changed frequently to maintain fit and alignment, provide adequate fracture control during the 3 or 4 weeks required for early consolidation, after which less constricting support may be possible. Difficulties arise when the patient is multiply injured, or must remain recumbent. Gravity no longer helps to keep the fracture reduced. Malunion and perhaps nonunion become more likely. Overhead olecranon traction, as described for proximal humerus fractures, offers a possible solution, but interferes with mobilization and nursing of a multiply injured patient. Intramedullary nailing, with open or closed reduction of the fracture, is the solution for some patients. I prefer small Ender's nails, inserted from either the lateral aspect of the greater tuberosity or from a distal approach just above the olecranon fossa. Open reduction with plate fixation is another alternative. It offers an opportunity to explore the radial nerve (if this is thought to be indicated), to obtain secure rotational control, and to bone graft an extensively comminuted fracture. Because plating of the humeral shaft requires significant stripping of the fracture site, it may hinder bone union. Complication rates are high for multiply injured patients. Yet another alternative for the management of humeral shaft fractures in polytraumatized patients or those with significant soft tissue injuries is external skeletal fixation. Half pins are inserted laterally, taking care to avoid the axillary nerve and posterior humeral circumflex artery proximally and the radial nerve distally. Open pin placement is advisable for safety. Such external fixation is minimally invasive, does not significantly encumber the patient, and usually provides satisfactory fracture control. It is generally my first choice for humeral shaft fractures in multiply injured patients who cannot be treated satisfactorily by nonoperative means, although intramedullary (IM) nailing may permit earlier crutch walking if concomitant lower extremity injuries require this.

ELBOW INJURY

Elbow fractures and dislocations may have associated neurovascular injuries and may cause forearm ischemia due to arterial occlusion, compartment syndrome, or both. Resulting Volkmann's contracture is seriously disabling and should be prevented by careful attention to early diagnosis and appropriate treatment of neuromuscular ischemia. Forearm pain, impaired sensation, and loss of motor function are the important signs of problems. They should not be ascribed to nerve injuries until it is clear that perfusion is adequate. Elbow injuries should be splinted in moderate flexion since forced extension or flexion may compromise the nerves and vessels crossing the joint. No attempt at reduction is appropriate until satisfactory roentgenograms have been obtained. If skin damage is present, the possibility of early operative treatment must be considered because intra-articular elbow fractures frequently do require surgery, and delay may compromise the result.

Elbow dislocations should be reduced promptly, with adequate analgesia and muscle relaxation. An assistant holds the humerus stable while the surgeon exerts manual traction on the forearm with the elbow moderately flexed and corrects medial or lateral displacement as required. Following reduction, stability is assessed by checking range of motion and exerting varus and valgus stress on the extended elbow. If the medial collateral ligament is intact and the joint remains located throughout its range, a long-arm splint is needed briefly. If mobilization can begin within a few days, when the patient is comfortable, recovery is swifter and possibly more complete. If the elbow is unstable, movement must be deferred until soft tissue healing is well under way, usually 3 weeks after injury. Furthermore, there is some risk of early redislocation unless the joint is immobilized in more than 90-degree flexion. A long arm cast or splint actually offers marginal protection for an unstable elbow injury. Increasing flexion and preventing shoulder motion by securing the arm to the chest augments its effectiveness. Before applying any radiopaque splint or cast, postreduction films should be obtained to confirm satisfactory reduction and to check for associated fractures. Any immobilizing device must avoid constriction of the antecubital fossa.

Displaced fractures of the elbow joint are often best treated by surgery. Those of the distal humerus can offer formidable challenges. Postoperative complications, including inability to achieve sufficient fixation for early motion, may lead to a result no better than that achieved by overhead olecranon traction with motion as tolerated in such a device. In the absence of extensive experience with internal fixation of distal humeral fractures, when comminution is extreme or when extensive soft tissue injury is also present, traction deserves serious consideration. If multiple injuries preclude its use, external fixation across the elbow joint may maintain alignment while permitting the patient (but not the elbow) to be mobilized.

Olecranon fractures tend to separate because of the pull of the triceps on the proximal fragment. If displacement occurs, repair is advisable with either ORIF or excision of proximal fragments and triceps reattachment. Olecranon fractures associated with subluxation or dislocation of the elbow joint are much more extensive injuries. The distal humerus has been driven posteriorly through the olecranon: ligaments are disrupted, and there is often marked comminution of the distal olecranon, which may involve the coronoid process. Incongruity of the radiocapitellar joint is evident on the lateral roentgenogram. A radial head fracture may be present. Treatment of these injuries must be directed at restoration of elbow alignment and maintenance of stability during the first few weeks of healing. Internal fixation is often tenuous. Roentgenograms should be monitored to ensure that redisplacement, if it occurs, is identified promptly.

Radial head fractures are painful injuries that usually respond well to early active mobilization. Aspiration of a tense painful elbow hemarthrosis and injection of a local anesthetic provide immediate relief. A splint and sling applied for the first few days should be removed as soon as possible to encourage early movement. Only comminuted displaced radial head fractures are candidates for early excision.

FOREARM FRACTURE

Open reduction and internal fixation (ORIF) with plates and screws is the standard treatment for displaced *fractures of the radius and ulna* in adults. Satisfactory initial immobilization is usually obtainable with a well-padded splint or cast, and unless the fracture is open or ischemia develops, fixation can be done semielectively during the week or so after injury, but becomes progressively more difficult with much further delay.

It is important to assess the elbow and wrist of a patient with a forearm fracture. If a *displaced fracture of either radius or ulna* is present without fracture or plastic deformation of the adjacent forearm bone, there must be damage to the proximal or distal radioulnar joint. With ulnar fractures, dislocation is at the elbow, with displacement of the radial head from the capitellum as well—the so-called Monteggia fracture. Isolated radial shaft fractures may have associated injuries of the distal radioulnar joint—Galeazzi's fracture. Successful treatment of both these injuries reduces the joint disruption as well as the fracture and maintains alignment during healing and mobilization. In adults, ORIF of the diaphyseal fracture and occasionally open joint repair are necessary.

Isolated radial shaft fractures, even without distal radioulnar joint disruption, are poorly controlled with casts, and therefore should generally be repaired. External fixation is an option for severely contaminated wounds. Intramedullary nailing is possible, but not always technically satisfactory. Functional bracing has also been proposed as an alternative when the distal radioulnar joint is intact.

Isolated ulnar shaft fractures may require surgery, but many can be managed nonoperatively if displacement is slight. A long arm cast significantly impedes use of the arm and seems to delay union of ulnar shaft fractures. With minimal immobilization, most of these unite rapidly. For *isolated* fractures of the ulnar shaft, with less than a full diameter's displacement, I apply a long arm splint for the first few days until swelling has receded, and then support the forearm with a snugly molded sleeve of plaster from below the elbow to the wrist. This is applied with the forearm fully supinated. Activity, including wrist and elbow motion, is encouraged, and healing generally occurs within 6 weeks. For more proximal fractures of those with more intrinsic instability, intramedullary nailing with a pre-bent Rush rod often provides satisfactory control. Unless there is a significant comminution, I prefer IM nailing to the more conventional plate fixation, to avoid hardware-related problems and to permit earlier weight-bearing in patients with concomitant leg injuries.

WRIST INJURY

Fractures of the distal radius are the most common injuries in this region, but other less obvious ones may prove equally disabling. Careful examination and thorough interpretation of adequate AP and lateral roentgenograms are essential to distinguish fracture-dislocations from purely metaphyseal injuries and to avoid missing distal radioulnar dislocations, as well as fractures and dislocations of the carpals. Since the initial physical findings of a wrist injury may appear minimal in patients with other serious trauma and because their arms rapidly become encumbered with infusion needles, wrist roentgenograms must be obtained on the slightest suspicion of injury.

Distal radius fractures range greatly in severity. If comminution is marked or either radiocarpal or distal radioulnar articular surfaces are involved, poorer results are likely. Although closed reduction and appropriately molded plaster cast suffice for the less severe cases, pins and plaster, external fixation, or internal fixation might be required to achieve and maintain nearly normal anatomy. Casts applied to severely injured wrists frequently need to be loosened to accommodate swelling. During this period, maintenance of reduction is secondary to preservation of blood flow. If an initial closed reduction proves unstable, it can be followed later by a more extensive procedure. If there is palmar or dorsal displacement of the carpus and an attached fragment of distal radius, ORIF may be necessary.

Carpal dislocations usually involve the lunate and its attachments to radius, capitate, or both. An associated scaphoid fracture may be present or the scapholunate ligaments may be ruptured. Dislocation is best diagnosed on the lateral film of the wrist. A prompt closed reduction is usually successful with fingertrap distraction and manipulation. This should be done as soon as possible to minimize swelling and neurovascular compromise. These are unstable injuries, however, and thus open reduction and internal fixation frequently are needed to maintain alignment, as well as for reduction if closed manipulation fails.

Scapholunate dissociation is indicated by widening of the normal interosseous gap seen on an AP roentgenogram. Early treatment of this frequently missed injury is more successful and simpler than delayed reconstruction.

Carpal fractures without dislocation or persistent displacement should be managed closed initially. A short arm splint alone is sufficient for the first few days. The thumb is included for scaphoid fractures. If reduction is satisfactory, the splint is replaced with a cast once swelling has abated. Displaced carpal fractures, especially of the scaphoid, may require ORIF.

FRACTURE AND JOINT INJURY OF THE HAND

Hand injuries are readily ignored in polytrauma patients. Yet their inadequate early treatment can result in significant permanent disability. Therefore the hands must be carefully evaluated for fractures and joint injuries as well as damage to skin, nerves, blood vessels, and tendons. Stiffness, the most common complication after hand fractures, is best avoided by the early achievement of skeletal stability and prompt range-of-motion exercises. Closed treatment is often possible with isolated injuries. More severe, multiple, or intra-articular fractures may require internal fixation. If external immobilization is employed, it should be in a safe position, with the metacarpophalangeal joints flexed nearly 90 degrees, the interphalangeal joints nearly extended, and the thumb in opposition, anterior to the hand. The fate of the whole hand should not be compromised by ill-advised immobilization to treat a single joint or digit.

Interphalangeal dislocations usually can be reduced closed, but may be unstable and require splinting for a brief period. Dislocations of the finger metacarpophalangeal joints usually require open reduction as do those of the thumb. The metacarpophalangeal joint of the thumb is prone to sprains, especially of its ulnar collateral ligament. If it is unstable, this ligament needs repair. The carpometacarpal joints of the thumb and of the little and ring fingers are unstable after dislocation or fracture-dislocation, injuries that may be difficult to see on routine films. Closed reduction is usually possible, but percutaneous pinning is often needed to maintain it.

HIP INJURY

Acetabular fractures are a major area of interest in orthopaedic traumatology. Traditional reluctance to undertake open reduction and internal fixation is being challenged, but treatment remains controversial. Like pelvic ring fractures, which may also be present, acetabular fractures are usually caused by high-energy trauma and can be accompanied by life-threatening hemorrhage and other serious thoracoabdominal or extremity injuries. The whole patient must not be obscured by concern for the acetabular fracture. The presence of an acetabular injury is generally evident on the routine screening AP film of the pelvis, if not on physical examination. Its precise definition requires 45-degree right and left oblique views of the entire involved innominate bone and is greatly facilitated by CT scans with appropriate parasagittal and paracoronal reconstructions. Physical examination of the ipsilateral knee is essential to exclude ligament injuries.

If the femoral head is dislocated (posteriorly, centrally, or, rarely, anteriorly), a closed reduction is performed as soon as possible. I prefer to do this with the patient under general anesthesia, with adequate muscle relaxation. Skeletal traction is instituted via a pin in the tibial tubercle. Roentgenograhic assessment is then completed. If there is incongruity of the weight-bearing portion of the hip joint, if traction cannot maintain a satisfactory reduction, or if fragments of bone are interposed between the articular surfaces, open reduction and internal fixation are advisable. These procedures require extensive exposure, and there is risk of infection, hemorrhage, and neurovascular injury. An alternative to ORIF is continued traction for the 2 to 3 months generally required for union, followed by total hip arthroplasty if and when the patient's symptoms warrant. If displacement is severe, there can be significant problems associated with anchoring the acetabular component of a total hip prosthesis, a factor that should be considered in the choice of early treatment.

Nonoperative treatment is appropriate for undisplaced acetabular fractures. I prefer traction for those that have an intact weight-bearing articulation or those that occur in older patients who have adequate bone stock for total hip arthroplasty. For others, I advise ORIF by a well-prepared team of experienced surgeons. This should be delayed until the patient's overall condition permits, but it becomes significantly more difficult with time, especially after 2 weeks.

Hip dislocations without acetabular fractures should be reduced as soon and as gently as possible to minimize the risks of avascular necrosis and further damage to the articular surface. If at all possible, I prefer general anesthesia with muscle relaxation, which permits reliable assessment of stability as well. The dislocated hip can be reduced immediately after endotracheal intubation and minimally delays any other necessary procedures. On those rare occasions when closed reduction is unsuccessful, prompt open reduction is required. Postreduction films must confirm anatomic reduction of the femoral head. If there is any sign of incongruity, I obtain a CT scan to search for intra-articular fragments that will require arthrotomy for removal.

If the hip is stable after reduction, rest in 5 lb Buck's traction with the hip extended is advised until the patient is able to control the limb comfortably. At this point, crutch walking is begun, with progressive weight-bearing. If the hip is not stable, several weeks of traction are required before mobilization.

Proximal Femur Fracture

Hip fractures are often the result of a minor fall. They tend to be more severe in the victims of high-energy accidents and, until internally fixed, significantly compromise the patient's mobility. Even in closed injuries, local blood loss may cause shock.

Femoral Neck Fracture

Femoral neck fractures may occur in isolation or together with a fracture of the femoral shaft. Often initially undisplaced, they must be looked for carefully on the pelvic films of every multiply injured patient. Especially in young persons, femoral neck fractures have a high incidence of nonunion and of avascular necrosis of the femoral head. Treatment is surgical, and the hip is protected in splint or traction until the surgical treatment can be carried out. I attempt closed reduction and fixation with multiple pins or cancellous screws inserted under fluoroscopic control. If an adequate closed reduction cannot be obtained, arthrotomy and open reduction, possibly with posterior bone graft, should be performed in those under 50 years; older patients are candidates for hemiarthroplasty.

Intertrochanteric Fracture

Intertrochanteric fractures are also best managed by internal fixation, as soon as possible in multiply injured patients. Union and femoral head survival are rarely problems, but difficulty in nursing the patient in traction for 3 to 4 months and malunion of fractures mobilized earlier can be avoided if internal fixation is used. Modern compression hip-screw devices have proved reliable in our hands. After fixation, the wound should be debrided of traumatized muscle, irrigated copiously, and closed over suction drains to minimize the risk of infection.

Subtrochanteric Fracture

Subtrochanteric fractures must be considered separately because of their association with high-energy trauma and because of their well-recognized incidence of nonunion and fixation failure. These injuries involve the proximal femur from the trochanteric region down to an arbitrary 10 cm below the lesser trochanter. Below this level, intramedullary nailing techniques for femoral shaft fractures are usually reliable. Treatment of a subtrochanteric fracture should be individualized, and the patient must be followed until bone union is secure for failure, when it occurs, often is not seen until 4 to 6 months after injury. Problem subtrochanteric fractures are generally those with medial comminution. Traction may be considered for subtrochanteric fractures in healthy individuals with isolated injuries if a satisfactory alignment is achieved promptly. It is usually followed with a 1½ spica cast or a single abducted spica cast-brace for the several months required to complete healing. Internal fixation generally facilitates early management and is preferable for the multiply injured patient. Several techniques are available. Condylocephalic (Ender) nailing appears attractive, but in my experience often requires opening the fracture site to obtain reduction and to permit passage of the nails into a satisfactory position. The Zickel subtrochanteric nail provides generally good fixation and is stout enough to outlast a delayed union. It is most appropriate for pathologic subtrochanteric fractures in the elderly. Comminution in the trochanteric region increases the difficulty of inserting the Zickel device, and its removal may result in refracture. Therefore its use in younger polytrauma patients is limited.

I think the compression hip screw is the most adaptable device for most of these injuries. It must be used carefully, with achievement of a stable reduction or with supplementary bone graft. I prefer to protect the soft tissue attachments of comminuted fragments and to bypass such a zone with medially placed bone graft rather than attempt a "jig-saw puzzle" reduction. The compression screw is attached securely to intact proximal and distal portions of the femur, bridging the comminuted zone. For more distal injuries, the interlocked femoral nail provides a better solution to the problems of stabilizing subtrochanteric fractures.

FEMORAL SHAFT FRACTURE

These injuries are usually due to significant force. The possibility of associated trauma must always be remembered. A roentgenogram of the pelvis is mandatory so that a fracture or dislocation involving the hip is not missed. Tenderness, swelling, or roentgenograhic abnormalities may indicate injury to the knee. Blood loss into the fracture site may cause shock. The considerable pain of a femoral shaft fracture can be controlled partially by traction-splinting. If operative treatment is not to be carried out within a few hours, skeletal traction should be instituted via a Steinmann pin in the tibial tubercle, or in the distal femur if the knee is injured; 20 to 30 lbs are initially required, depending on the muscularity of the patient.

Although several options are available for the definitive management of femoral shaft fractures, it is becoming clearer that prompt intramedullary nailing is especially beneficial for significantly injured patients. Interlocking nails, with proximal and distal transfixing screws to control length and rotation, extend this technique to nearly all femoral shaft fractures. Complications with this device are less common than with other techniques, which may still be chosen for selected patients.

In multiply injured patients, femur fractures should be fixed securely as soon as possible, preferably during the patient's first anesthetic, since this facilitates patient mobilization and decreases the incidence of respiratory failure. The risk of infection in grade II and grade III open fractures is probably decreased by initial irrigation and debridement, skeletal traction, delayed primary wound closure, and early soft tissue healing. Closed intramedullary nailing is then done 10 to 14 days after the initial injury. Another valuable alternative for femur fractures with severe soft tissue damage is external skeletal fixation with the Wagner "leg-lengthening" device.

KNEE INJURY

Mobility, trustworthy stability, and absence of pain are necessary for normal knee function. To regain these after injury, bone and articular cartilage anatomy, ligament function, and muscle strength must all be restored. Depending on the specific injuries, this may require fracture reduction, ligament and/or tendon repair, repair or excision of a damaged meniscus, and rehabilitation to regain motion, strength, and agility. It must always be remembered that high-energy knee injuries, such as dislocations and badly displaced fractures, may damage the popliteal artery and perhaps necessitate amputation.

Fractures of the distal femur can seriously compromise knee function. If displaced or angulated, they require accurate reduction. ORIF may be necessary. Properly selected fractures can be managed with traction or cast-brace and early motion. If articular surface displacement cannot be corrected, ORIF is indicated if the condition of the patient and soft tissues permits. These procedures may be demanding. I prefer a wide anterolateral exposure and use the 95-degree blade plate, condylar compression screw, or condylar buttress plate depending on the extent of comminution. Bone grafting is advisable for significant comminution, especially of the medial cortical surface.

Patellar fractures that are displaced require repair to restore quadriceps continuity. If the articular surface can be reconstructed, ORIF is done with K-wires and tension band, interfragmentary wiring, or screws. If comminution prevents ORIF, treatment consists of a partial or total patellectomy with repair of the quadriceps mechanism, including torn retinacular expansions.

Meniscus tears may be either peripheral or within the substance of the semilunar fibrocartilage. The former should be reattached. The latter may require partial or possibly total meniscectomy. In the absence of other indications for arthrotomy, treatment can be postponed until it is clear that the patient is symptomatic. Arthroscopy is now the standard means of evaluating and treating meniscal injuries of the knee, as well as evaluating acute hemarthroses.

If *knee dislocation* is present, it should be reduced promptly with axial traction and manipulation as needed. Arteriograms are routinely obtained. *Penetrating injuries* of this superficial joint require arthrotomy for irrigation, removal of retained foreign material, and debridement of any osteochondral fracture fragments.

Obvious *ligamentous instability* usually needs surgical repair. Examination reveals varus or valgus laxity in collateral ligament ruptures. Posterior cruciate ruptures often, but not always, show posterior mobility of tibia on femur. This may be produced by the force of gravity on the flexed knee and should be looked for carefully with the leg in this position. Remember that apparently stable knees with acute post-traumatic hemarthroses usually have sustained a significant injury, most often disruption of the anterior cruciate ligament. Although treatment of such patients is controversial, many advocate early surgical repair or reconstruction of anterior cruciate ligament disruptions in young and active patients.

Fractures of the tibial plateau split off part of the articular surface, depress a portion of it with an impacted fracture of the underlying cancellous bone, or combine these two modes of injury. Depending on the stability of the knee to stress examination in extension and the degree of deformity of the articular surface, treatment may require open reduction, with elevation and bone grafting of any depressed area. Alternatives include traction arranged to permit early motion, cast brace, and plaster cast. For best results, treatment should permit early motion, but weight-bearing is deferred until healing is secure. Extensive surgical exposure is required for mechanically adequate ORIF of severely comminuted proximal tibial fractures. This risks serious wound complications. Delayed or more limited ORIF must be considered when associated soft tissue injury is significant.

FRACTURE OF TIBIA AND FIBULA

These common fractures are frequently open, may have associated nerve or vessel injuries, including compartment syndrome, and vary greatly in severity. The appropriate treatment for an isolated, minimally displaced spiral fracture of the tibia is rarely the best for a transverse, comminuted, grade III open fracture in a multiply injured patient. Occasionally an open tibial fracture is such a severe injury that reconstruction, even if technically possible, will take so long and offer such unpredictable results that the patient might reasonably prefer a below-knee amputation.

Although tibial shaft fracture with intact fibula usually indicates a milder injury, such fractures may have a higher incidence of varus deformity and delayed union. When only the fibula is fractured, it is important to evaluate both knee and ankle carefully, as this generally innocuous fracture may be associated with a collateral ligament injury of either joint.

Many treatments are advocated for tibial shaft fractures. Before a choice is made, the patient, other medical problems, and the extent of injury to the soft tissues must be considered, in addition to the fracture's roentgenographic appearance. Many tibial fractures can be managed adequately in a plaster cast or fracture brace, usually with early weight-bearing. I prefer a long leg (knee flexed 10 to 15 degrees) plaster initially, with subsequent conversion to a so called patellar tendon bearing (PTB) if the fracture is in the distal half or a hinged knee cast-brace if it is more proximal. Healing usually requires about 4 months. Open wounds may be difficult to care for in a cast. Windows and multiple cast changes frequently compromise wound care, fracture alignment, and mobilization of the patient.

for early mobilization, but risks pin wound complications and delayed union. The former can be minimized by using half-pin fixation inserted through the subcutaneous border of the tibia instead of transfixion pins that perforate the leg muscles. Prevention of the latter may require early aggressive bone grafting. Another approach is to discontinue external fixation as soon as the wounds are healed and manage the fracture with external support.

Plate fixation of tibial fractures can be helpful. It offers a reliable way of stabilizing a highly comminuted fracture for wound care and mobilization of the patient. However, weight-bearing must be delayed, and wound complications, including sloughs and infections, are common. Therefore, I generally restrict the use of plates to situations in which a metaphyseal or intra-articular fracture requires anatomic reconstruction or in which an extensive wound is already present (so that further dissection is minimal) and fracture comminution prevents adequate stabilization with external fixation or intramedullary rods.

Intramedullary rodding of suitable tibial shaft fractures is a promising technique. *Unreamed* nails should probably be used for fresh fractures, definitely if the fracture is open. While Lottes's nail is acceptable, I prefer two flexible, unreamed rods (Ender nails), inserted from the medial and lateral surfaces of the proximal metaphysis into corresponding positions inside the cortical bone of the distal metaphysis. Some motion may persist at the fracture, but it is well controlled, and alignment is readily maintained. A splint or cast worn initially can usually be discarded within 6 weeks, and weight-bearing is generally well tolerated early after injury, a major benefit for patients with bilateral injuries or upper extremity problems that preclude crutches. I think complications are less frequent with this fixation technique than with any other for severe tibial shaft fractures, and advocate it whenever skeletal fixation is needed and the fracture is neither too comminuted nor too close to either end of the bone. The appropriate role of interlocked nailing for tibial shaft injuries is still unclear. Although it provides secure fixation, significant intramedullary reaming is often required.

ANKLE INJURY

Congruity and stability are both required for normal function of this weight-bearing joint. Injuries are common and may be open or closed. Fractures and ligament ruptures are often combined. Additionally, important tendons, nerves, and blood vessels cross the ankle, and all are at risk of injury and should be specifically examined. AP, lateral, and mortise roentgenograms are essential for evaluation of ankle injuries.

Fractures of the distal tibia may involve only the malleoli or may disrupt the horizontal tibial plafond. Malleolar fractures may be undisplaced and stable, minimally displaced, and acceptably aligned or significantly displaced. Whether or not the talus is normally located under the plafond is the major issue, for the contact area between the two is seriously reduced by only a slight sideways shift of the talus. Fractures disrupting the weight-bearing surface of the plafond are usually obvious and may be severe. When the condition of patient and soft tissues permits, anatomic reconstruction of the articular surface and precise realignment of the talus with the mating tibia are key steps toward recovery of normal ankle function. This can require extensive exposure with risk of skin slough and infection. An alternative is traction via the calcaneous or fixed distraction with an external fixator or pins-and-plaster from tibia to calcaneus. If at all possible, after repair, early motion (but delayed weight-bearing) seems to improve the prognosis of severe injuries. I think that movement should be delayed until the patient is able to do it comfortably, and the ankle must be splinted in a neutral position initially to avoid development of an equinus contracture.

Ligament injuries most commonly involve the lateral collateral. Initial treatment is with a well-padded splint that holds the ankle in neutral. Severe sprains should be protected in a short leg cast for 6 weeks. The medial collateral (deltoid) ligament is rarely injured in isolation, but may be one component of a significantly unstable "bimalleolar" injury when the fibular fracture is much more obvious on the x-ray film. In addition to the status of the malleoli and collateral ligaments, it is essential to assess the syndesmotic ligaments that bind together the distal tibia and fibula. Mortise widening due to syndesmosis disruption requires temporary internal fixation of the distal fibula to the tibia.

Undisplaced malleolar ankle fractures often are treated satisfactorily in plaster, but some of these are unstable and lose alignment. Careful roentgenographic monitoring through the cast demonstrates this and permits timely repair. Most *displaced bimalleolar injuries* can be well reduced closed. Subsequent loss of reduction in plaster is so common that I generally prefer ORIF for these patients. An additional benefit is the ability to avoid a long leg cast and, often, to permit earlier weight-bearing.

When soft tissue condition, multiple injuries, or other factors contraindicate ORIF of unstable malleolar fractures, a helpful maneuver is transfixion of the joint with a stout Steinmann pin, inserted from the sole of the foot through calcaneus, talus, and well into the tibia. The foot and ankle should be held reduced and in neutral position during insertion of this pin.

Dislocations of the talus require prompt reduction, usually open, as do its displaced fractures.

FOOT INJURY

The ability to walk normally can be significantly compromised by residua of foot injuries. Their early recognition prevents complications. Prompt treatment is often more effective than that postponed "until he's over the other injuries." Foot trauma may appear relatively insignificant, but it must not be ignored.

Subtalar dislocations require prompt reduction to avoid skin slough. Closed reduction is usually possible, but a general anesthetic is often needed. Manual traction with correction of deformity, inversion or eversion, is the technique for reduction.

Calcaneal fractures are often severe bursting injuries that signify major damage to the heel. Associated vertebral fractures are not unusual. Swelling may be marked, occasionally to the point of delayed skin slough. Bed rest, leg elevation, and a well-padded splint to hold the foot in neutral position are advisable. ORIF may be used in the management of selected calcaneal fractures, but in general its results seem little better than those of closed treatment. Treatment might include manipulation to correct gross deformity, perhaps with the use of a Steinmann pin in the tuberosity for reduction and fixation of the posterior subtalar facet. I think it is most important to maintain a plantigrade foot and to mobilize the ankle.

Midtarsal and tarsometatarsal joint disruptions may be obvious roentgenographically or may be minimally displaced, with small avulsion fractures and slight deformity being the only indication of the gross instability obvious on physical examination. These severe injuries may include damage to skin and neurovascular structures and place the patient's foot at risk of amputation. Open reduction may be required, but closed manipulation usually suffices. Because of marked swelling, position is hard to maintain in plaster. Therefore percutaneous pinning is helpful if closed reduction is acceptable. A normally shaped foot with its sole perpendicular to the leg is the primary goal, and open reduction should be done if needed to achieve this.

Metatarsal and phalangeal fractures may be displaced enough to inferfere with normal weight-bearing. If they are, reduction, usually closed, is required. Small Kirschner wires usually hold an unstable reduction. A well-padded splint is advisable to hold foot and ankle in neutral position during the early phases of recovery. As soon as foot and other injuries permit, weight-bearing begins in a well-molded cast.

REHABILITATION AFTER MUSCULOSKELETAL TRAUMA

Unlike most trauma to other organ systems, the ultimate result of musculoskeletal injuries does not depend exclusively on the effectiveness of the initial therapy. In fact, several months of well-directed rehabilitation often contribute more to the outcome than whatever "definitive fracture treatment" is chosen. Although early aggressive fracture stabilization greatly facilitates the initial management of a multiply injured patient, it does not guarantee a satisfactory recovery. Injured bones usually heal, and deformity is generally preventable, but joint injuries always present the challenges of impaired mobility, instability, and pain. Muscles, weakened by injury and inactivity, require sustained use to regain their strength. The injured patient's cardiorespiratory reserve diminishes rapidly while his activity is limited, and is restored only by prolonged aerobic reconditioning.

Whenever possible, motion (passive, active, or both) should begin promptly for all injured joints. This is especially crucial for the shoulder, hand, and knee. If early movement is not possible, immobilization must be in a functional position. Mobilization is vital for mild injuries as well. For example, in an older patient with a flail chest, a contused shoulder may stiffen irreversibly unless assisted range-of-motion exercises are begun promptly, even while the patient is on a respirator in the intensive care unit.

The planning of rehabilitation begins simultaneously with diagnosis and early treatment of injuries. It must continue until maximal recovery is achieved. Follow-up orthopaedic supervision is thus required until the patient has clearly reached an acceptable plateau.

BURNS

JURIS BUNKIS, M.D.
ROBERT L. WALTON, M.D.

Given the ubiquitous nature of thermal injuries, it behooves all physicians to understand the basic physiologic alterations occurring as a result of thermal injuries and to at least possess the ability to provide first aid to the burn victim. At least two million people in the United States annually sustain burns serious enough to warrant medical attention, but most require little more than first aid treatment for relief of pain. A quarter of a million patients with minor burns can be adequately managed on an outpatient basis. Approximately 100,000 patients annually will sustain burns severe enough to warrant hospitalization, and of these approximately 12,000 will die as a result of their injuries. Such statistics exemplify the importance of thermal injury as a disease entity. The economic effects are magnified when one considers the number of working years lost due to the fact that the majority of burn patients are males under the age of 40. Half of all burns serious enough to require hospitalization occur in the home, and of these at least two-thirds are considered preventable. The cause of burns varies from one part of the world to another. Numerically, flame and scald victims constitute the largest percentage of patients sustaining thermal injuries. In the United States, approximately 75 percent of burns are due to flame injuries, 13 percent to scalds, 5 percent to contact burns, 3 percent to electrical burns, 1 percent to chemical burns, and less than 1 percent to radiation injuries. Whether produced by flame, scald, chemical, contact, or electricity, many of the pathophysiologic mechanisms of hyperthermic injuries are similar—extensive tissue destruction is accompanied by an increased capillary permeability and massive extravascular fluid loss.

PATHOPHYSIOLOGY

Cutaneous Response

An understanding of the basic physiologic responses to burn injury is essential in caring for the burn patient. Thermal injury results in injury to the skin. One must remember, however, that a severe burn causes alteration of virtually every organ system in the body.

The skin is one of the largest organs of the body and constitutes 15 percent of total body weight. The average adult has a skin surface area of 4.7 square meters. The skin is a vital organ and loss of substantial areas of it impairs the homeostatic mechanism and expose the body to the damaging elements of the environment. If the lost skin is not replaced by the patient's own skin, death may result. Destruction of the protective layers of the skin eliminates the normal vapor barrier and allows body water to evaporate through areas of injury at the same rate as it would from an open pan. The average insensible water loss through intact skin is approximately 15 ml per square meter per hour (700 to 1,000 ml per day), but water loss through areas of full-thickness burn may reach 200 ml per square meter per hour. Slightly less water loss is experienced with partial-thickness burns. The evaporative water loss is accompanied by a 560 Kcal heat loss with the evaporation of each liter of water. With major burns, total energy expenditures associated with the increased evaporative water loss may result in a 7,000 Kcal day deficit. This energy expenditure is accompanied by a significant rise in oxygen consumption and basal metabolic rate.

The second major protective function of skin is the prevention of invasive infection. Subsequent to thermal injury, surface microorganisms persisting in the skin appendages begin to multiply, reaching quantitative bacteriologic counts as high as 10^8 organisms per gram of tissue by the second or third post-burn day. The predominant bacteria constituting this initial proliferation are gram-positive staphylococci, but by the fifth to seventh post-burn day, gram-negative bacilli, particularly *Pseudomonas aeruginosa* are dominant. With partial-thickness injuries, some protection against invasive sepsis persists. All burns are contaminated, but every effort must be made to prevent burn wound sepsis (defined quantitatively as a burn wound containing more than 10^5 microorganisms per gram of tissue). Following partial-thickness injuries, infection may cause a conversion of the wound to a full-thickness injury. Wound cultures obtained by swabbing the surface and visual inspection of the wound provide little information about the degree of infection; every unit providing care of the seriously burned patient should have the capability to monitor wound bacteriologic status with frequent quantitative cultures.

With full-thickness injuries, cell death occurs as a result of coagulation necrosis. Thermal injury may result in interference with cell metabolism, denaturation of cell protein, and secondary interference with vascular supply. A decrease in the severity of injury is noted vertically from the surface to the depth of the wound and peripherally in all directions from the central point of injury. Three concentric zones of injury directly related to the intensity of the thermal stimulus have been described. The central "zone of coagulation" contains permanently irreversible coagulation and lacks capillary blood flow. Tissue in this area is irreversibly damaged from the outset. Surrounding the necrotic tissue is a "zone of stasis" characterized by a sluggish capillary blood flow. Any further injury (e.g, secondary to desiccation or infection) may result in total cessation of blood flow and necrosis with enlargement of the "zone of coagulation." A peripheral "zone of hyperemia" constitutes the third concentric zone of thermal injury. The hyperemia results from the usual inflammatory response of healthy tissue to nonlethal injury and, unless complicating factors develop, this injury is usually healed by the seventh day.

Cardiovascular and Metabolic Response

Immediately following a burn, the most striking physiologic alteration is related to the circulatory system. Increased capillary permeability allows water, electrolytes, and protein to escape from vascular compartments into the burn wound. Following minor burns, this immediate and reversible vascular response to burning is confined to the burned area, but with involvement of more than 30 percent of the body surface area, increased capillary permeability is systemic. The most significant loss from the vascular compartment is the loss of serum (i.e., the saline component). Increased capillary permeability is accompanied by a sudden marked decrease in cardiac output concomitant with increased pulse rate, decreased stroke volume, and a marked rise in peripheral vascular resistance. Within 3 hours following major thermal injury, 50 percent of the total plasma volume can be lost through the open wound. Appropriate fluid resuscitation must be undertaken to prevent hypovolemic shock, progression of burn injury, and acute renal tubular necrosis secondary to hypovolemia.

The initial loss of large volumes of protein-rich fluid presents the same physiologic threat to life as acute external hemorrhage. Marked loss of plasma results in hemoconcentration with subsequent sludging, the possibility of a further decrease in peripheral tissue perfusion and oxygenation, and then cell death, particularly in the "zone of stasis."

Plasma volume reduction is accompanied by hemoconcentration, blood cell agglutination, and sludging of the microcirculation. A variable amount of red blood cell destruction takes place in the burn area, but due to the relatively more significant loss of plasma with resultant hemoconcentration, transfusion of whole blood is rarely necessary during the first 72 hours.

Serum protein levels may drop precipitously in the first 4 days following burn injury, with protein losses equalling twice the total plasma pool. Approximately half of this protein is lost through the wound, but the remainder may lie sequestered in the extravascular space for as long as 3 weeks before being returned to the vascular compartment. In addition, catabolism of all proteins proceeds at twice the normal rate.

The increased capillary permeability in response to burning is greatest within the first 12 hours post-burn, although additional loss at a much slower rate may continue for another 6 to 24 hours. Capillary permeability returns to normal 48 hours after injury and the resorption of edema fluid begins. This process is expressed clinically as a diuresis. The subacute phase following the shock phase is manifested clinically by diuresis and mobilization of sodium. Anemia generally becomes manifest as the clinical edema subsides, and blood transfusions may be necessary.

Immediately following a burn, the metabolically active zones of the wound are flooded with fluid, plasma proteins, and polymorphonuclear leukocytes. As with any major injury, the patient experiences an increased basal metabolic rate, increased secretion of multiple hormones (e.g., catecholamines, cortisol, renin-angiotensin, antidiuretic hormone, aldosterone), negative potassium and phosphorous balance, disturbed carbohydrate utilization, fat mobilization, salt and water retention, alteration in the metabolism of certain vitamins, and a negative nitrogen balance with resultant weight loss. The severity of these alterations generally parallels the extent of injury. Fluid loss, hypermetabolism, and caloric requirements may be decreased by the application of biological dressings and by placing the burned victim in a warm humidified environment. It is difficult, however, to obtain a positive nitrogen balance prior to closure of the wound. Following wound closure, the anabolic phase of injury is entered.

Pulmonary Response

Pulmonary changes are noted even in the absence of "inhalation injury." Initial depression of arterial oxygen tension is noted, but normal levels return by the end of the first week unless complications supervene. With burns involving more than 40 percent of the body surface area, increased minute ventilation occurs by the third post-burn day, peaks by the fifth day, and gradually declines. However, airway resistance does not appear to be significantly increased except in the presence of inhalation injury. Interestingly, increased pulmonary capillary permeability is not believed to occur, even with extensive burns, in the absence of inhalation injury. Pulmonary edema, when it occurs, is thought to be the result of overaggressive resuscitation and not of increased capillary permeability.

It is impossible to produce a thermal injury below the larynx by inhalation of hot air. Steam, however, has a heat-carrying capacity four thousand times that of air, and can cause an actual burn of the pulmonary tree. Most patients with inhalation injuries damage the tracheobronchial mucosa as a result of the inhalation of the noxious products of combustion. Severe inflammation, congestion of the submucosal blood vessels, and marked edema of the mucosa occur. These changes classically occur 24 hours post-burn. With severe injuries, sloughing of the entire trachobronchial mucosa can occur. Most deaths following burn injuries today are due to accompanying inhalation injuries or the result of complicating pulmonary infections.

Gastrointestinal Response

An adynamic intestinal ileus develops in all patients with burns involving more than 30 percent body surface area. This generally subsides in 48 to 72 hours, following which the gastrointestinal tract may be employed for nutritional purposes.

In the past, 25 percent of hospitalized burn patients developed massive melena or hematemesis due to "Curling's ulcers." Now that all major burn victims are treated with antacids or histamine blockers, clinically significant gastrointestinal bleeding is rarely encountered. Colonic mucosal ulcerations may also cause lower gastrointestinal bleeding, but these are rarely encountered.

Immunologic Response

The immune system is depressed by thermal injury. Impaired cellular immunity is demonstrated by lymphocytopenia, delayed rejection of allografts, and anergy to common antigens.

Humoral defects are characterized by a depression of immunoglobulins, specifically IgG, IgA, and IgM. Serum immunoglobulin levels are maximally depressed 2 to 5 days after injury. Complement titers also decrease following burn injury, but this may be due to protein leakage from permeable capillaries.

Burn patients are more susceptible to infection. These infections are frequently refractory to treatment with antibiotics. It has been shown experimentally that neutrophil phagocytosis progresses normally, but the efficiency of intracellular killing is diminished. Impaired chemotaxis delays neutrophil migration. An overall deficit in host-defense mechanisms results.

PATIENT EVALUATION

The severity of burn injury is related to the depth of the burn, the total body surface area involved, the patient's age, the severity of associated injuries, and the pre-injury state of health of the victim. Information regarding each of these categories must be sought in order to establish therapeutic priorities, devise a treatment plan, and determine the eventual prognosis.

History

A thorough history provides the surgeon with clues as to the magnitude of the burn, as well as information regarding associated injuries and preexisting medical conditions. When, where, and how the injury occurred must be established. The patient—as well as other family members, firemen, policemen, emergency medical technicians, and other eye witnesses—may provide illuminating details of the accident. Most patients, even those with extensive burns, are alert immediately following the accident, thus allowing a full history to be obtained while the examination is being performed and treatment initiated.

Burns result from the application of an energy source to the skin, with energy transfer occurring directly by contact or indirectly by radiance. The depth of the burn varies with the intensity and duration of the applied heat as well as the conductivity of the involved tissues. The speed with which the transfer takes place is much more important than the total amount of heat transferred. As the rate of heat transfer exceeds the body's ability to dissipate the energy, heat damage occurs. Tissue conductivity is influenced by water content, surface oils and secretions, insulating material such as the cornified keratin layer of the skin, and the density of local pigmentation. A 0.54-second exposure of human skin to 3.9 cal per square centimeter per second of radiant heat results in a second-degree burn; increasing the heat delivered to 4.8 cal per square centimeter per second would lead to a third-degree injury. Cell damage rarely occurs with a heat source below 45 °C, but with temperatures greater than 50 °C, denaturation of various protein elements begins, although the damage may be reversible. Above 65 °C, protein denaturation is usually complete, and cell death results from protein coagulation. Knowledge of these facts, combined with an appreciation of the mechanism of thermal injury, may have a predictive value clinically in determining the depth of injury. Therefore, one can predict that a brief flash burn or spill scald will result in partial-thickness burns, whereas flame burns and immersion scalds, owing to prolonged contact with the heat source, are more likely to produce a full-thickness burn injury. Immersion injuries expose the tissue to uniform intensity of heat for a prolonged duration and result in homogeneous tissue destruction. Flame burns, on the other hand, are more likely to expose the skin to varying intensities of exposure and frequently produce a patchy distribution of full thickness and partial-thickness destruction. Flash and scald burns are unlikely to produce inhalation injury, but flame burns sustained within an enclosed space or steam burns may be associated with an inhalation injury.

The patient's age is closely linked to the predicted mortality for the burn injury. For any given extent of burn, patients under the age of 2 and those over the age of 65 have a higher predicted mortality. The very young and the very old may have a greater susceptibility to infection owing to incompletely developed or depressed immune systems. The very young (immature dermal papillae) and the very old (atrophic dermal papillae) also have thinner skin than do people between these extremes of age and thus develop deeper burns from the same heat intensity. In addition, cardiac disease, diabetes, or chronic obstructive pulmonary disease may significantly worsen the prognosis in the elderly. Information regarding antecedent illnesses, allergies, and medications is useful in the planning of management of the burn patient. Chronically administered cardiac, hormonal, and anticonvulsant medications must be continued during the hospitalization.

A thorough history—including the setting and events leading to the burn, the alleged mechanism of injury, and the appropriateness of parental response—must all be evaluated to rule out the possibility of child abuse or neglect. Evidence of a suicide attempt is a signal for early psychiatric intervention to prevent a repeat performance and to minimize problems in social adjustment to the injury.

Physical Examination

A rapid preliminary evaluation to assess the magnitude of injury and to establish the priorities for treatment must precede the recording of a detailed history and physical examination. Most pertinent aspects of the history can usually be obtained and the initial evaluation performed while the patient is being undressed and placed on the examining table. Following severe burns, it is necessary to establish an airway and to initiate the resuscitation concurrently during the initial evaluation.

As with any major trauma patient, a thorough physical examination must be performed. This requires removal of all clothing, dressings, make-up, jewelry, and dentures. The presence of associated injuries must be determined. Hyperemic oral or nasal mucosal surfaces, singed nasal hairs, or the presence of intranasal or intraoral soot may herald a significant inhalation injury. The patient's age, extent and depth of burn, as well as the presence of pre-existing or associated injuries will influence prognosis and immediate therapeutic decisions.

Extent of Burn. The age of the patient and the extent of the burn are the two most important factors in predicting the prognosis of the burn victim (Table 1). Extent of a burn is expressed as a percentage of the total body surface area (percent BSA) injured. A careful calculation of the percent BSA of involvement forms the basis for predicting the amount of fluid required for resuscitation, forms the basis of the American Burn Association severity index, and allows the surgeon to prognosticate with regard to final outcome. Knowledge of the extent, depth, and location of the burn, the presence of associated injuries, and pre-existing medical conditions allows the surgeon to classify the burn as mild, moderate, or severe, thus forming the basis of initial triage decisions and allowing determination of the initial treatment protocol (Table 2).

TABLE 1   Predicted Mortality Following Burn Injury

Age (Years)	% BSA Burned									
	10	20	30	40	50	60	70	80	90	100
10	0	4	14	37	60	78	91	97	99	100
20	0	3	13	35	59	77	90	97	99	100
30	0	4	16	39	62	79	92	97	99	100
40	1	7	22	47	69	84	94	98	100	
50	3	13	35	59	77	90	96	99	100	
60	9	27	53	72	87	96	99	100		
70	24	49	70	85	95	99	100			
80	51	71	86	95	99	100				
90	75	89	97	99	100					

TABLE 2 American Burn Association Burn Severity Categorization

Burn Classification	Characteristics	Implications for Treatment
Minor burn injury	1° burns 2° burn <15% BSA in adults 2° burn < 5% in children/aged 3° burn < 2% BSA	These patients may qualify for outpatient therapy.
Moderate burn injury	2° 15–25% BSA in adults 2° burn 10–20% BSA in children/aged 3° burn <10% BSA	Hospitalization is required. Given adequate staff and facilities, a community hospital may suffice.
Major burn injury	2° burn >25% BSA in adults 2° burn >20% BSA in children/aged 3° burn >10% BSA Burns involving hands, face, eyes, ears, feet, or perineum Most patients with inhalation injury, electrical injury, concomitant major trauma, or significant pre-existing diseases	Care in a specialized burn center is indicated.

The palmar surface of each hand equals approximately 1.25 percent BSA. The extent of small burns can be calculated rapidly by comparing the size of the burned area to multiples of the area of the hand; thus, a burn the size of two hands would be equivalent to 2.5 percent BSA. For larger burns, the percent BSA involved can be calucated rapidly and accurately by application of the "Rule of Nines." This rule divides the body surface into areas representing multiples of 9 percent. In the adult, approximately 9 percent is allowed for each upper extremity, 18 percent for the anterior thorax and abdomen, 18 percent for the back and buttocks, 18 percent for each lower extremity, and the remaining 1 percent for the neck. In the child, the relatively larger BSA of the head and proportionally smaller BSA of each lower extremity must be taken into consideration. The age-related charts modified by Lund and Brower provide a more accurate determination of the extent of burn. Each emergency room and burn unit should have these charts available and one should be filled out initially for every burn victim.

Depth of Burn. Frequently, the most difficult aspect of burn wound evaluation involves determining the depth of the burn. Several classifications have been employed to differentiate various depths of injury. The simplest and most useful divides burn wounds into two basic categories: partial-thickness injuries (those which under ideal circumstances will epithelialize spontaneously from retained skin appendages) versus full-thickness injuries (those in which the entire thickness of skin has been destroyed, thus requiring wound contraction, migration of epithelial cells from the periphery, or surgical intervention to produce healing).

Traditionally, burn wounds have been divided into three categories by degree. The first-degree wound is characterized by erythema, which blanches on pressure, and tenderness and edema of the skin (probably related to the release of various amines from reversibly injured cells). The damage is confined to the epidermal layer, although dermal blood vessels are dilated and congested. Most first-degree burns are the result of prolonged exposure to the sun or of minor scalding injuries. Pain normally subsides after 48 to 72 hours and healing takes place uneventfully. As the involved epithelium peels off within 5 to 10 days, it is replaced by new cells from the basal layer of the epidermis. The burned area usually heals without residual scarring. Owing to the superficial nature of the injury, the protective barrier of the skin is retained, thus minimizing fluid loss and any danger of infection.

Second-degree injuries involve the epidermis and varying depths of the dermis, while leaving viable dermis containing skin appendages (hair follicles, sweat or sebaceous glands) from which epidermal repopulation can occur. Such burns are characterized by vesicle formation due to detachment of the epidermis from the underlying dermis. The presence of intact bullae is usually a good sign that circulation in the deeper areas of the dermis has been preserved, and that spontaneous healing can be expected. More superficial wounds are erythematous, progressing to a waxy, white coloration with increasing depth. With deeper injuries, waxy, insensate skin may be difficult to differentiate from full-thickness injury. The burn surface appears moist, owing to the loss of the protective barrier function of the epidermis and subsequent serous fluid loss. Varying degrees of thrombosis of the dermal vessels and wound edema are seen. Such burns are likely to be painful. The rate of healing of a second-degree burn is directly proportional to the depth of injury. Superficial second-degree wounds can be expected to heal uneventfully within 7 to 10 days unless infection supervenes. Deep partial-thickness injuries may require a month for epithelial regeneration from the remaining glands and hair follicles. Minimal scarring results from healing of a superficial second-degree burn, but prominent scarring with unstable overlying epithelium can be expected following healing of deep partial-thickness injuries. Fluid loss and metabolic derangements likewise are progressively more severe as the depth and extent of burn injury increases. Any partial-thickness wound can be converted to a full-thickness injury by infection, desiccation, or maceration.

Third-degree burn wounds are characterized by destruction of the entire thickness of dermis along with all the contained skin appendages, and by thrombosis of the subdermal vascular plexus. Following third-degree flame, electrical, or chemical burns, the skin appears dry, hard, insensate, inelastic, waxy, and white. With full-thickness scald burns, the epidermal layer frequently sloughs immediately following the injury, and the patient presents with a lobster-red, insensate coagulated dermis. Such burn wounds are insensate owing to the destruction of terminal, sensory nerve endings in the dermis. In addition, one may suspect third-degree injury if hair shafts can be pulled from their follicles easily and painlessly. Increased capillary permeability and wound edema are more severe than in second-degree injuries. In the untreated burn wound, the coagulated collagenous eschar can be expected to begin separating in 10 to 14 days, partially as a result of autolysis and leukocyte digestion accompanied by suppuration, revealing a granulating tissue bed. Since such wounds lack epidermal appendages, healing can only occur by wound contraction (frequently complicated by severe contractures), by migration of epithelial cells from the periphery, or by surgical intervention. Chronic open wounds, or those with unstable epithelium, are at an increased risk of undergoing malignant degeneration many years later.

Tissue fluorometry can distinguish between deep-partial and full-thickness burns for diagnostic purposes. Practically speaking, however, better results, both functionally and aesthetically, are obtained by treating deep dermal and full-thickness wounds in a similar fashion by early excision and grafting, thus obviating the necessity to distinguish clinically between the two levels of injury prior to the initiation of therapy.

TREATMENT

First Aid

At the scene of the accident, the first priority is to remove the victim from the heat source. Burn victims should be moved to well-ventilated areas away from flaming material to minimize the possibility of continued inhalation injury. A burning patient should be placed in a horizontal position and the flames smothered by rolling the patient in a blanket, rug, or large garment, or the flames can be extinguished by water. Frequently, a patient whose clothes are on fire may instinctively begin to run, but this should be avoided as running only fans the flames. Similarly, maintaining the erect position allows clothing and hair to burn more vigorously in a wick-like fashion, thus once again stressing the importance of assuming the horizontal position in order to allow the flames to be extinguished rapidly.

Following electrical injury, power should be shut off if possible and the patient removed from the source of electricity. The rescuer must not touch a patient who is still in contact with a live electric wire lest he be electrocuted or sustain a similar electrical burn injury. Following contact with a noxious chemical, the burned area should be washed with copious quantities of water. Following inadvertent contact with hot tar or molten metals, the involved part should be cooled with water, but efforts to remove the tar or metal should not be started at the scene of the accident.

All burned parts should be cooled with water as soon as possible following a burn. Although the beneficial effects of cooling remain controversial, we believe that application of cold water (4 °C) minimizes progression of the burn injury in the zone-of-stasis. Experimentally, retention of intact blisters has been shown to prevent dehydration necrosis in the zone of stasis much more effectively than does cooling. However, cooling does appear to have a beneficial effect on the dermal microvascular circulation at the burn site. In addition, the use of ice compresses brings almost immediate relief from burn pain. Cold compresses are applied to the burned areas for 30 minutes following the injury.

Clean, moist dressings should be applied to the burn wound to minimize wound contamination and to maximize patient comfort. Any clean sheet, towel, or cloth may be used as an emergency dressing. Frequently, the lay person applies topical first-aid medications or home remedies such as butter, petroleum jelly, or antibiotic creams before seeking professional assistance. Public education efforts should discourage use of such medications, as there is no evidence of a beneficial effect from such remedies and they may be difficult to remove later. Following application of the clean dressings, the patient should be positioned for comfort and, if appropriate, the burned areas elevated to minimize subsequent edema.

Burn patients may develop an ileus with the subsequent risk of aspiration. Oral fluids should be avoided initially; alcoholic beverages should definitely be prohibited.

All burn victims with full-thickness burns, partial-thickness burns involving more than 5 percent BSA, burns involving vital body parts (such as the hand, face or perineum), significant associated injuries, or pre-existing diseases should be evaluated by a physician. Arrangements must be made to transport the patient to a medical facility as soon as possible following the burn injury. Most communites are served by well-trained emergency medical technicians and suitable transportation verhicles that are available for transport of the seriously injured burn patient to the emergency room. Following minor burns, the patient may be brought to the emergency room by any appropriate available means.

Outpatient Burn Therapy

"Minor burns," as defined by the American Burn Association severity categorization index, may be treated on an outpatient basis provided the patient and/or his parents are considered reliable and other complicating factors are absent (see Table 2). The majority of burn patients presenting to an emergency room can be treated in this way.

Following any burn injury, the initial evaluation must include a determination of the extent, depth, and location of the burn as well as the patient's age, the presence of pre-existing illness, and associated injuries. The extent of the burn must be diagrammed in the medical record, and if there is any question of subsequent legal action, photographs should be obtained for further documentation. Vital signs must be determined and a complete physical examination performed. Social factors must be considered. Only then can the decision be made to treat the patient on an outpatient basis. Occasionally, hospitalization of a patient with a minor burn may be indicated for the first day or two while the patient or his family are educated in dressing changes and wound care. Criteria for admission to the hospital are frequently liberalized when dealing with the pediatric and geriatric populations.

Severe anxiety and pain frequently accompany a burn injury. A calm and reassuring approach by the physician is of prime importance in minimizing the patient's anxiety and apprehension. Relatively minor injuries treated on an outpatient basis can be extremely painful. The requirement for sedation is usually inversely proportional to the depth of the initial thermal injury. Narcotics and other vasodilating agents must not be administered to the hypotensive or hypovolemic patient. Once the vital signs have stabilized, a full therapeutic dose of parenteral narcotic (up to 1.5 mg per kilogram body weight of meperidine or 0.2 mg per kilogram of morphine sulfate) may be necessary to provide initial pain control. The narcotic must be given in small increments, however, to minimize complications that could result from vasodilation or respiratory depression. Most minor burns do not require continued narcotic support following initial debridement and application of dressings. Topical analgesics, while quite effective, should be avoided in all but small burns to avoid absorption of the potentially semitoxic medications.

Partial-thickness wounds should be washed gently but thoroughly with balanced salt solutions to remove all surface contaminants. Irritating soaps and antiseptics should be avoided, as these produce further tissue injury. Ruptured blisters should be debrided, but the temptation to aspirate or debride intact blisters definitely should be avoided. Blister fluid provides the most physiologic microenvironment for rapid wound healing.

In general, dressings are recommended for all burns treated on an outpatient basis, except for second-degree burns of the face. A well-applied occlusive dressing minimizes pain and contamination and frequently allows the patient to continue usual activities. A layer of nonadherent petrolatum gauze can be placed against the superficial partial-thickness burn and incorporated in a bulky, comfortable dressing. Furacin mesh gauze may be employed as an alternative to the petrolatum gauze. Topical antimicrobial agents generally are not necessary for the treatment of small superficial burns. Such agents diminish the rate of epithelialization and, thus, wound healing. In areas subject to excessive contamination (e.g., perineum, groin) and in the treatment of deep partial-thickness burns, however, topical antimicrobial agents (e.g., silver sulfadiazine) minimize the possibility of infection. Allografts, xenografts, and synthetic biological dressings are occasionally advocated, but are prohibitively expensive and usually unnecessary for small wounds typically handled on an outpatient basis. It is difficult to keep a tidy facial dressing in place, and for this reason, partial-thickness facial injuries are best managed by frequent application of moist compresses followed by application of neosporin or bacitracin antibiotic ointment to avoid desiccation.

Prophylactic antibiotics are not indicated in the treatment of uncomplicated burns. Should peripheral erythema, tenderness, or fever suggest streptococcal infection, however, cultures must be obtained and appropriate antibiotic therapy instituted. In addition, tetanus prophylaxis must be considered in all patients with burn injuries.

Limited deep dermal or full-thickness burns involving nonvital areas can be excised and closed primarily by approximation of the wound edges or covered by a split-thickness skin graft in an outpatient surgical facility. This is usually performed within the first 48 hours following the burn injury to minimize the possibility of wound infection and graft loss. Patients suitable for outpatient burn surgery must be selected carefully to avoid complications involving donor sites or the grafted wounds.

At least initially, the patient should be seen in the outpatient burn clinic or physician's office on a daily basis for wound re-evaluation and redressing. Burn wound classification is not static and, particularly if a partial-thickness wound becomes infected, conversion to a full-thickness injury may result, with the accompanying need for hospitalization. As the wound begins to show signs of epithelialization, outpatient visits may become less frequent, until total wound healing has been achieved. All patients with partial-thickness burn injuries should be followed closely until the wounds are completely epithelialized. Subsequently, the patient should be re-examined every 1 to 3 months for evidence of scar hypertrophy. Pressure garments, special exercises, and splints may be indicated to avoid or minimize hypertrophic scarring. The patient must be instructed to avoid excessive exposure to sunlight for at least a one-year period to minimize scar or graft hyperpigmentation.

Burns usually result in damage to the normal lubricating mechanism of the skin. Following epithelialization or grafting, healing areas may benefit from a mild lanolin lotion to decrease dryness. Pruritus in particular is a common complaint following burn injury. An antihistamine, such as diphenhydramine hydrochloride (i.e., Bendaryl), may provide symptomatic relief.

Appropriate rehabilitation—physical, psychological and social—must be directed by the physician. Optimal patient care is provided by specialized personnel trained in the management of the burn patient; outpatients with burns should be seen in the same area as those who have been discharged from a burn unit and are returning for follow-up care. The superior results can be attributed to the specialized training and facilities and the personal interest expressed by the burn clinic personnel.

Hospital Burn Care

Criteria for inpatient care of the burn patient must be individualized to take into consideration general medical and social factors. Generally, adult patients sustaining partial-thickness burns exceeding 15 percent BSA (10% in children) or full-thickness burns exceeding 2 percent BSA require hospitalization. In addition, patients with burns involving the hands, face, eyes, ears, feet, or perineum; inhalation or electrical injury; major associated injuries; or serious pre-existing illnesses should be admitted for treatment of their injuries.

Care of a patient with a major burn proceeds more smoothly if a pre-established protocol is followed. Such a protocol is particularly helpful to physicians who do not deal with acutely burned patients on a daily basis. Such a protocol should include information regarding the following categories:

1. Patient evaluation including required laboratory data.
2. Establishment of airway and maintenance of breathing.
3. Insertion of indwelling intravenous lines and initiation of resuscitation.
4. Insertion of indwelling bladder catheter +/− CVP line for patient monitoring.
5. Confirmation of peripheral circulation, escharotomies PRN.
6. Initiation of nasogastric suctioning.
7. Sedation.
8. Initiation of tetanus and antibiotic prophylaxis.
9. Burn wound care.
10. General supportive measures.

Patient Evaluation.   Rapid preliminary evaluation will allow determination of the magnitude of injury and the establishment of treatment priorities. A quick history, determination of the extent and depth of burn, drawing of blood samples for baseline laboratory tests and crossmatching, a portable chest roentgenogram, and an electrocardiogram can be obtained while resuscitation is being initiated. Charting of the depth and extent of the burn wound should also be delayed until resuscitation is underway and the patient is in stable condition, but should definitely be performed before dressings are applied to the burned areas.

Establishment of Airway and Maintenance of Breathing.   The patient's history and physical examination are helpful in raising the suspicion of an inhalation injury. The most sensitive indicators of the degree of pulmonary injury are provided by arterial blood gas and carboxyhemoglobin determination. A patient with a suspected inhalation injury should be initially treated with a mask providing humidified air with high oxygen content and meticulous tracheobronchial toilet. If bronchospasm and wheezing are present, bronchodilators and mucolytic agents may be helpful. Flexible bronchoscopy may be employed to assess the degree of damage and to remove carbonaceous sputum plugs, but routine repeated bronchoscopy has not been shown to be significantly helpful. Indications for intubation and respiratory support are the same as those for any patient following major trauma. If hypoxemia (PaO_2 < 60 mm Hg) or hypercarbia ($PaCO_2$ > 55 mm Hg) persists following the application of an oxygen mask, the patient should be intubated to ensure an adequate airway and respiration. Any patient who demonstrates marginal respiratory status during the initial evaluation should be intubated immediately. Gas exchange predictably deteriorates during the first few days following an inhalation injury. In addition, massive edema during the resuscitative phase can be expected to further compromise the airway and make intubation difficult later. Generally, patients requiring prolonged ventilatory support tolerate nasotracheal intubation better than orotracheal tubes. In burned victims, a formal tracheostomy is accompanied by a markedly increased complication rate and thus tracheostomy should be avoided unless absolutely necessary. Antibiotics should be reserved for treatment of documented infections. Prophylactic steroid therapy likewise has not been shown to be beneficial in the treatment of inhalation injury.

Circumferential burns involving the chest or neck may interfere with ventilation. A thick, unyielding circumferential eschar may prevent normal chest excursion during respiration. A leathery, circumferential eschar around the neck may prevent external swelling during the resuscitative phase; internal fluid shifts can result in a sufficient pressure elevation to occlude the neck veins or to compromise the airway. If the patient presents with circumferential chest or neck eschar, prophylactic escharotomies are indicated. The longitudinal decompression incisions must be extended beyond the constricting eschar proximally and distally. As many incisions as necessary to relieve the compression should be made under sterile conditions, but anesthesia is not required as the full-thickness burn wound is insensate.

Fluid Resuscitation. Resuscitation of burn shock by aggressive intravenous fluid administration is of paramount importance during the initial phase following injury. The goals of fluid resuscitation are to replace and maintain effective plasma volume during the period of increased capillary permeability and evaporated surface losses, as well as to provide maintenance fluid during the immediate post-burn period associated with intestinal ileus. Intravenous fluid resuscitation is generally required if burns exceed 20 percent BSA in adults and 10 to 15 percent BSA in children or the elderly.

A large-bore intravenous cannula must be inserted to allow administration of the large quantities of fluid required for resuscitation. Suppurative thrombophlebitis remains a possibility during the entire treatment period. Antibiotic ointment and a sterile dressing are applied around the catheter entry site to minimize the incidence of phlebitis. Frequently, finding adequate intravenous access is difficult, especially following burns involving all four extremities. If at all possible, intravenous lines, whether inserted by percutaneous puncture or cutdown, should not be placed through burned tissue to avoid the almost certain occurrence of subsequent phlebitis. During the resuscitative phase, however, reliability of venous access is more important than violation of the burn wound. Similarly, use of the upper extremities for vascular access is preferable to use of lower extremities because of the lesser incidence of phlebitis. Central venous lines occasionally provide the only reasonable route for fluid administration, but owing to potentially lethal infectious complications, the placement of central lines solely for the purpose of fluid administration should be avoided if peripheral alternatives are available.

Most burn formulas are based on the patient's body weight and the percent BSA burned. Always remember to calculate fluid requirements from the time of burn injury, not from the time the patient is first seen in the emergency room. However, all burn formulas should be treated as mere guidelines for the calculation of fluid deficits during the initiation of resuscitation. Each patient must be monitored continuously and therapy modified according to the individual patient's responses.

A number of formulas have been proposed to help the surgeon determine the amount of electrolyte solution, colloid solution, and free water necessary to effect the resuscitation. The most commonly recommended formulas guiding resuscitation are the Brooke, Evans, and Baxter formulas (Table 3). Analysis of these formulas reveals that the total volume and the total sodium load recommended for the initial 48-hour period vary little, the major differences being in the timing of the colloid administration. Colloid administration within the first 24 hours post-burn is of little benefit as osmotic pressure cannot be maintained over freely permeable capillary membranes. During the initial 24 hours following the burn, the colloid leaks into the extravascular space and actually augments extravascular fluid retention. Therefore, most major burn centers no longer provide a colloid component during the initial 24 hours of fluid resuscitation and rely instead on a sodium-containing electrolyte solution. Measurements of cardiac output, plasma volume, and extracellular fluid have demonstrated that plasma volume replacement during the first 24 hours post-burn is dependent only upon the rate, not the type, of fluid administered. The sodium load administered during the resuscitation is a prime determinant of the return of cardiac function. For these reasons, the Baxter formula is the most frequently employed in the United States today. Electrolyte solutions during the first 24 hours restore plasma volume. During the second 24 hours, maintenance fluid is given as free water to maintain serum sodium near 140 mEq per liter, and sufficient colloid solutions are administered to maintain normal plasma volume. One must appreciate, however, that very little difference exists between the different formulas. For this reason, physicians should select a single resuscitation method and learn to use it well instead of attempting to mix the several approaches found in the current literature.

Certain investigators have advocated hypertonic salt solutions for burn shock resuscitation in order to inhibit weight gain and wound edema. Hypertonic solution resuscitation allows adequate vascular volume restoration by inducing extracellular movement of intracellular water. The argument of isotonic versus hypertonic fluids for resuscitation becomes one of whether it is more physiologic to have a normal serum sodium concentration with extensive edema or an elevated sodium serum concentration with cellular dehydration. Each theory has its proponents, but definitive studies demonstrating the superiority of one method over the other are lacking.

TABLE 3 Fluid Replacement Formulas for Initial 48 Hours

| Burn Formula | 1st 24 Hours | | | | 2nd 24 Hours | | |
	Colloid	Electrolyte	Water	Rate of Administration	Colloid	Electrolyte	Water
Evans	1 ml/kg/% BSA burn	1 ml/kg/% BSA burn (up to 50% max.)	2,000 ml	½ first 8 hr ¼ second 8 hr ¼ third 8 hr	0.5 ml/kg/% BSA burn	0.5 ml/kg/% BSA burn	2,000 ml
Brooke	0.5 ml/kg/% BSA burn	1.5 ml/kg/% BSA burn (up to 50% max.)	2,000 ml	½ first 8 hr ¼ second 8 hr ¼ third 8 hr	0.5 ml/kg/% BSA burn	0.75 ml/kg/% BSA burn	2,000 ml
Brooke (revised 1979)	--	2–3 ml/kg/% BSA burn (no upper limit)	--		Sufficient to replace vascular volume and maintain normal urine output	--	Sufficient to maintain normal serum sodium concentration
Baxter	--	4 ml/kg/% BSA burn (no upper limit)	--	½ first 8 hr ¼ second 8 hr ¼ third 8 hr	Sufficient to replace vascular volume and to maintain urine output		

Patient Monitoring. Response to resuscitation can be measured by several criteria including clinical observation (e.g., vital signs, mental status, central venous pressure, urine output) and laboratory data (e.g., hematocrit, electrolytes, osmolalities). During the early post-burn period, however, the blood pressure and pulse are unreliable guides to the adequacy of resuscitation. Hematocrit, electrolyte, and protein levels should be determined initially and followed throughout the hospitalization. These laboratory values likewise do not provide a reliable guide to the adequacy of initial fluid resuscitation.

An adequate urine output (1.0 ml per kilogram per hour) is the best single guide to the adequacy of fluid replacement. An indwelling bladder catheter should be inserted immediately upon the patient's admission to the emergency room and urine output monitored closely. If urine output drops below 30 ml per hour in the average adult patient, the rate of fluid administration should be increased. Similarly, if the urine output exceeds 100 ml per hour the patient should be re-evaluated to ascertain that fluid requirements have not been overestimated. A low urine output unresponsive to a fluid challenge may herald acute renal insufficiency.

The adequacy of resuscitation can be determined by following the urinary output in most burned patients. Patients failing to respond to an apparently adequate fluid challenge and those with pre-existing pulmonary or cardiac abnormalities may benefit from monitoring of central pressures. The best indicator of adequate fluid replacement is left ventricular end diastolic filling pressure, but in most patients determination of right-sided central venous pressure will suffice. CVP less than 7 cm of water indicates a need for more vigorous fluid resuscitation. Caution should be exercised if the CVP rises above 15 cm of water and the need for prophylactic digitalization considered.

Circulation. With burns involving the extremities, peripheral circulation may be compromised by the circumferential, thick leathery eschar. Internal fluid shifts occur beneath the unyielding eschar, and tissue pressures may rise sufficiently to threaten limb viability. The inelastic eschar acts as a limb tourniquet; as tissue pressure increases, lymphatic, venous, and arterial flow are interrupted in a sequential manner. The extremity may appear pale, cool, and pulseless. If the circumferential burn is isolated to a proximal segment of the extremity, the spared area distal to the eschar may develop severe edema and may similarly become pulseless.

Escharotomies must be performed early to prevent irreversible ischemic insult. Following obvious full-thickness circumferential extremity burns, prophylactic escharotomies are performed in the emergency room. With circumferential extremity burns of indeterminate depth, clinical reevaluation must be performed frequently to determine the necessity for escharotomies. The onset of neurologic signs such as paresthesia, anesthesia, or deep tissue pain mandates immediate decompressing escharotomies. Absent, severely delayed, or extremely rapid nail bed capillary filling may provide a useful clinical sign indicating compromised peripheral circulation due to the constricting eschar. One must remember that arterial occlusion occurs later than venous obstruction.

Longitudinal escharotomies, which extend beyond the limits of the burn, are performed under sterile conditions. The decompression must extend down into the subcutaneous tissue, but care must be taken to avoid injury to the underlying veins, lymphatics, and cutaneous nerves. The incisions must be carried just deep enough to allow the wound edges to separate. Except during treatment of electrical injury, fasciotomies usually are not required. Following severe hand burns, the escharotomies must be carried along the midaxial lines of the digits to the fingertips, care being taken to avoid injury to the underlying neurovascular structures. All involved digits must be released bilaterally with the incisions joining within the web spaces. In addition, multiple dorsal incisions may be necessary to fully decompress the hand. Due to the thicker nature of the palmar skin, full-thickness burns of the volar surface of the hand are most unusual, and palmar escharotomies are rarely indicated.

Enzymatic debridement can provide a nonsurgical decompression of burned extremities. When decompressing circumferential eschar, we limit the use of Sutilains ointment (Travase), which contains a proteolytic enzyme derived from *Bacillus subtilis*, to extremities that are well-perfused at the time of admission. If the extremity is cold and pulseless initially, or if it becomes so subsequently, immediate surgical escharotomies must be performed.

Burned extremities should be elevated to minimize edema. With lower extremity burns, the foot of the bed should be elevated. Elevation of the upper extremities is facilitated by the use of stockinettes. The hand is maintained in the protective position by applying splints and comfortable bulky dressings. The wrist should be extended 15 or 20 degrees, the thumb maintained in abduction, the metacarpal phalangeal joints flexed maximally, and the interphalangeal joints fully extended.

Although patients with severe burns spend considerable amounts of time in bed and are hypercoagulable, clinical deep vein thrombophlebitis or pulmonary emboli are rarely seen. Prophylactic anticoagulation is not indicated.

Nasogastric Suctioning. Adynamic ileus frequently accompanies extensive burns. Initial therapy of major burns should include nasogastric intubation for at least the first 24 to 72 hours. Burn patients frequently experience an intense thirst, but oral solutions should be avoided. Given unlimited access to oral fluids, such patients may develop acute gastric dilatation and the subsequent risk of aspiration. Oral and nasogastric feedings should be avoided until peristalsis returns. Although of little consequence in itself, the effect of ileus may be detrimental to the patient in that it prevents enteral alimentation during a time that large amounts of fluid and calories are required. If the ileus persists beyond the resuscitative phase, consideration should be given to total parenteral nutrition. Ileus that persists or develops following the resuscitative phase is generally indicative of a complication such as burn wound sepsis or gastrointestinal tract perforation.

The nasogastric tube also allows sampling of gastric secretions to permit accurate titration of the gastric pH with antacids. However, administration of cimetidine (Tagament, 400 mg IV every 4 hours) is technically simpler and better tolerated by the patient than is frequent administration of large quantities of antacids. The nasogastric tube is particularly useful in patients with altered levels of consciousness to prevent regurgitation and vomiting with possible aspiration. A nasogastric tube must be inserted in all patients during the initial evaluation prior to transfer to a major burn center to prevent a catastrophe en route.

Sedation. All conscious burn patients exhibit severe anxiety and experience pain requiring sedation and analgesia. However, the patient must not be reflexly given a large dose of narcotics by a sympathetic physician or nurse. Cold compresses may be applied to the wounds initially to provide relief while the patient is being evaluated. Narcotics should be withheld while the patient is in profound shock. One must also remember that agitation may not be a sign of discomfort, but of cerebral hypoxia, a state that might be aggravated by the administration of narcotics. All sedatives and analgesics administered during the acute period should be given intravenously and in small doses to provide prompt pain relief. Intramuscular or subcutaneous administration during this period of hemodynamic instability results in variable absorption and may allow drug accumulation with later sudden absorption leading to fatal apnea. In the adult patient, a small dose of morphine sulfate, 1 to 3 mg intravenously, usually provides satisfactory sedation and analgesia. This dose may be repeated every 1 to 3 hours as needed, but the patient must be carefully observed for signs of respiratory depression. Inadvertent narcotic overdosage is treated by intravenous administration of the specific antagonist, naloxone. A small dose of diazepam (Valium), 2 to 5 mg intravenously, provides satisfactory sedation in the extremely anxious patient. In addition, diazepam provides an extremely beneficial amnesic effect, which is particularly helpful during subsequent dressing changes.

Subsequent dressing changes are usually anticipated by the burn patient with great anxiety. Judicious doses of appropriately timed analgesics usually are sufficient, but occasionally, particularly in children, additional sedation is required. In such cases, intravenous diazepam (0.1 mg per kilogram), followed by a subanesthetic dose of intravenous ketamine (Ketalar, 0.5 mg per kilogram), allow the dressings to be changed without inflicting further psychologic trauma. If such a regimen is to be used, an anesthesiologist should be available, resuscitative equipment present, and the patient must have an empty stomach to prevent aspiration. Long-term analgesia for a patient with extensive burns presents a difficult clinical problem. Every effort must be made to provide the patient satisfactory pain relief while avoiding drug addiction. Hypnosis has been of value in the long-term management of patients with chronic pain.

Tetanus and Antibiotic Therapy. Intensive use of prophylactic antibiotics is ineffective in decreasing the incidence of infectious complications following burn injury. Traditionally, prophylactic penicillin therapy has been recommended during the early post-burn period to prevent group A beta-hemolytic streptococcal cellulitis. Burn wound sepsis and other infectious complications occasionally seen in the burn victim are not prevented by prophylactic antibiotic therapy.

Should streptococcal cellulitis occur in a patient who had not been treated prophylactically with antibiotics, the infection will be very sensitive to intravenous penicillin therapy. Prophylactic penicillin therapy, however, hastens the emergence of antibiotic-resistant gram-negative organisms. The risks of prophylactic antibiotic therapy are outweighed by any possible benefits, and therefore we agree with the general principle that systemic antibiotics are not indicated on a prophylactic basis for the burn victim.

The majority of pathogenic bacteria gain entrance to the burn surface from foci within the nasopharynx and hands of burn unit personnel, from other patients, from various pieces of hospital equipment, and from the patient's own respiratory and alimentary tracts. Gross contamination of the wounds should be minimized by isolation techniques and meticulous handwashing. Surface cultures of the wounds, nares, throat, urine, and sputum should be obtained at the time of admission and at regular intervals thereafter. Bacteriologic data dictate the need for specific antibiotic coverage of infectious complications.

Intact burn eschar provides initial protection from burn wound sepsis. Following successful resuscitation, however, consideration should be given to excising the eschar and grafting the wounds before the onset of clinical infection. All open wounds quickly become contaminated and yield a variety of organisms by qualitative surface swab cultures. Surface swab cultures demonstrate the presence of bacteria, but yield little information regarding the magnitude of risk of burn wound sepsis. The presence of burn wound sepsis can be definitively confirmed by quantitative wound biopsy assays; burn wounds containing more than 10^5 organisms per gram of tissue, by definition, represent burn wound sepsis. Histologic examination of a portion of the biopsy specimen demonstrates the depth of bacterial invasion.

Recent comparative studies of bacterial quantification in burn wounds have shown a high correlation coefficient between samples obtained by standard biopsy techniques and the new, absorbent paper disc techniques. The absorbent disc technique is simple, convenient, noninvasive, and appears to yield reproducible results, thus increasing its appeal and justifying further investigation of its efficacy. *Pseudomonas aeruginosa* and *Staphylococcus aureus* are the organisms most commonly implicated in burn wound sepsis. Quantitative cultures demonstrating burn wound sepsis or consistently positive blood cultures require wound debridement, systemic antibiotic therapy, and a probable change of topical antimicrobial agents. Subeschar antibiotic injections may serve as a temporizing maneuver, but total wound excision and appropriate antibiotic coverage—systemic and topical—are more efficacious.

The avascular nature of the burn eschar and the sluggish blood flow in the surrounding zone of stasis contribute to the inability of parenterally administered antibiotics to reach the burn wound, to modify the bacterial flora, or to influence the mortality rate in the burn population. Topical chemotherapeutic agents, however, have been efficacious in the prevention of burn wound sepsis with resultant improvement in mortality rates. Ideally, the topical antimicrobial agent should

TABLE 4 Topical Antimicrobial Agents

Agent	Composition	Application	Bacterial Spectrum	Resistance	Advantages	Disadvantages
Silver nitrate	0.5% solution of the inorganic silver salt $AgNO_3$, in distilled water	Moist compresses changed b.i.d. and saturated q4h Painless	Bacteriostatic to entire spectrum	None	No sensitivities Not inactivated by specific antagonists	Does not penetrate eschar well Dilutional hyponatremia and hypokalemia due to leaching of electrolytes into wound Discolors wound, unburned skin, and environment Hypochloremia due to AgCl precipitation
Mafenide acetate	Methylated sulfonamide, 11.1% suspension in a water dispersible cream base	Applied topically b.i.d. as a cream; medication washed off daily Painful for 20–30 minutes following application to 2° burn	Bacteriostatic to entire spectrum, but minimally effective against staphylococci and fungi	Occasionally to staphylococci	Penetrates eschar well	Potent carbonic anhydrase inhibitor Tends to produce acidosis Sensitivity in 5 percent, manifested by a maculopopular rash
Silver sulfadiazine	1% suspension in a hydrophilic cream base	Applied topically b.i.d. as a cream; medication washed off daily	Bacteriostatic to entire spectrum	Occasionally to *Pseudomonas* and Enterobacter	No significant effect on fluids or electrolytes	Penetrates eschar poorly Can cause granulocytosis

be effective against the organisms proliferating in the burn wound, lack local and systemic toxicity, be readily available and easily applied, rapidly excreted or easily metabolized, and should not interfere with wound healing. No single agent satisfies all these requirements, but several excellent topical preparations have met most of these requirements. These include 0.5 percent silver nitrate solution, mafenide acetate (Sulfamylon), and silver sulfadiazine (Silvadene) creams. Advantages and disadvantages of these agents are summarized in Table 4. Topical antimicrobial agents, applied in solution or as water-soluble creams, markedly reduce evaporative water loss, and thus caloric demands. Reduced wound bacterial levels also result in lessened caloric requirements.

Tetanus prophylaxis is indicated for all patients with injuries resulting in a break in epithelial integrity. All second- and third-degree burns result in necrotic tissue, thus providing an ideal milieu for tetanus infection. Although this disease is rare, tetanus in the burn victim is almost always fatal. The prior immunization status of the patient determines the need for tetanus prophylaxis (see Table 3 in chapter on *Wound Management*).

Wound Care. The principal aims of wound care are to allow survival of any remaining viable tissue, to prevent infection, and to provide suitable circumstances to allow the best possible functional and aesthetic results to occur as the wounds heal. The use of topical antimicrobial agents has resulted in a dramatic improvement in survival from major burns, but 70 percent of all burn deaths are still the result of burn wound sepsis. Sterile techniques must be employed when burn wounds are handled. This includes wearing a cap, mask, sterile gown, and gloves whenever handling the burn victim or his wounds.

The burn victim must first be undressed and the wounds inspected while the history is being obtained, physical examination performed, and resuscitation initiated. Immediate cooling by immersion in ice water or by application of ice compresses for 20 minutes diminishes pain, subsequent edema, and progression of the burn injury. Cooling should be limited to patients with burns involving less than 30 percent BSA to avoid complications stemming from hypothermia.

The surface of all burn wounds should be cleansed with a mild antiseptic solution. Intact blisters protect the wound and therefore should be left undisturbed. Loose necrotic tissue may be debrided after the patient has been placed in the hydrotherapy tank. Vigorous mechanical debridement may further damage the injured tissue and should be avoided initially. Since discomfort is aggravated by air currents over the burn wound, the wounds are covered with a topical antimicrobial agent and dressed. Silver sulfadiazine and mafenide acetate creams are the most commmonly employed topical antimicrobial agents. Subsequently, the burn wound should be bathed daily to remove necrotic debris and the topical antimicrobial agent; the burn wound should be inspected, the cream reapplied, and the wound redressed. Silver sulfadiazine is employed most frequently because it causes little pain, is easy to apply, and has an effective antibacterial spectrum. Mafenide acetate has better eschar penetrating ability and therefore is the agent of choice for burns with thick eschar or those infected with anaerobic or gram-negative organisms. The topical antimicrobial agents may be applied to areas of partial-thickness and full-thickness burns. Superficial partial-thickness burns should heal in 7 to 14 days. Deeper burns generally require removal of the eschar and skin grafting to obtain wound coverage. One must remember that topical antimicrobial agents do not sterilize the burn wound, but only reduce the number of bacteria present, thus minimizing the incidence of invasive infection.

Following application of the topical antimicrobial agent, a single layer of fine mesh gauze is placed next to the wound. Several layers of multiple-ply, coarse-mesh gauze without cotton filling are next applied. The outer layer consists of bias stockinette. Splints are incorporated into the dressing between the coarse mesh gauze and the outer wrap in extremity burns to immobilize joints in the positions of function. Extremities should be elevated to minimize edema. At each dressing change, joints should be put through active and passive range of motion exercises. The splints may be discarded after the wounds have healed. During the resuscitative phase, occlusive extremity dressings must be modified to allow monitoring of blood supply in order to determine the need for escharotomies.

Partial-thickness burns of the face and neck are more easily treated by the open technique. The wound is rinsed gently twice a day with a sterile physiologic saline solution. This is followed by application of an antibiotic ointment (e.g., Bacitracin, Neomycin) or standard topical antimicrobial agents.

The full-thickness burn wound must be free of eschar before skin grafts can be applied. Different options for obtaining a satisfactory bed for grafting include waiting for spontaneous separation of eschar, enzymatic debridement, total burn wound excision to fascia, or tangential debridement.

Spontaneous separation of eschar begins between the tenth and fourteenth post-burn days in the untreated wound. This separation of the eschar from the underlying burn wound results from bacterial growth and autolysis of necrotic tissue. Treatment with topical antimicrobial agents will delay eschar separation. Following eschar separation, a granulating bed is usually present which may require minor debridement in preparation for grafting. Unfortunately, however, the burn wound remains susceptible to invasive sepsis during this entire phase. For this reason, enzymatic or surgical debridement of the eschar and early skin grafting are now practiced in most major burn centers.

Enzymatic debridement has proved to be particularly effective for debridement of burned hands. Sutilains ointment (Travase), applied 3 times daily, effectively dissolves an eschar in 24 to 36 hours. Twenty-four hours following initiation of enzymatic therapy, the wound can be debrided with the edge of a scalpel handle, scraping rather than cutting, to expose underlying viable tissue which will accept a skin graft. The operative time is short and simple. Blood loss is negligible and long-term function results are excellent. Proteolytic enzymes, however, allow bacterial proliferation; when they are used alone, cellulitis and even invasive burn wound sepsis can occur. To lessen the possibility of infection during this phase, the Sutilains ointment is combined with silver sulfadiazine cream prior to application to the burn wound. This method is effective when applied to small, localized wounds such as those occurring on the dorsum of the hand.

More extensive deep-dermal and full-thickness burn wounds require surgical debridement. This may take the form of early, total excision of the burn wound down to the underlying fascia or tangential debridement to bleeding tissue. Excision of the entire burn wound down to underlying fascia can be performed rapidly by means of the cutting current of the electrocautery unit, produces minimal blood loss, and results in a satisfactory bed for immediate skin grafting. Burn wound excision to fascia, however, removes subcutaneous tissue and can result in a significant contour deformity. Tangential escharectomy is more tedious, is accompanied by significant blood loss, and with full-thickness burns, results in a poorly vascularized adipose tissue bed for subsequent skin grafting. Hemostasis is simpler to obtain following fascial than tangential escharectomy. Following tangential escharectomy, delayed skin grafting (24 hours later, prior to the onset of significant bacterial proliferation) may be necessary if perfect hemostasis cannot be achieved initially. The method employed to rid the patient of the necrotic eschar in preparation for skin grafting is not as important as the timing of the debridement. Debridement must be individualized according to patients' needs. Every effort should be made, however, to remove all necrotic tissue and to close the wound with skin grafts before significant bacterial proliferation occurs. Except in unusual circumstances (e.g., a concomitant brain injury or myocardial infarction), escharectomies are performed within 48 hours of the burn injury and wound closure begun. Should a delay be necessary, quantitative bacterial assays must be employed to insure that wound bacterial counts are less than 10^5 bacteria per gram of tissue before grafts are applied.

A free hand knife or any of the standard dermatomes can be employed to obtain the skin grafts. The thighs and buttocks are the most common donor sites for split-thickness skin grafts. Following injury to these sites or in the presence of an extensive burn, skin grafts may be obtained from any unburned site. It is rarely possible to skin graft areas larger than 30 percent BSA at any one time. Following extensive burns, sufficient donor sites may not be available initially to provide total wound coverage. In these instances, the entire eschar is initially removed, the available autografts are applied, and biological dressings employed to cover the remaining open wounds. In such instances, the initial autografts are usually applied to the hands or other joint areas (in order to allow early restoration of function), or to aesthetically important sites such as the face. Temporary biological dressings reduce fluid and protein exudation from the wound, promote patient comfort, and preserve bacteriologic control of the wound until donor sites have had the opportunity to re-epithelialize prior to reharvesting. A variety of biological dressings have been proposed, including cadaver allografts, amniotic membranes, xenografts, and synthetic biocomposite wound dressings (e.g., Biobrane). The synthetic biomembranes are as effective as the other biological dressings, but the ease of handling and storage and the universal availability of the biocomposite dressings have made them the material of choice, in our experience, when we are faced with a shortage of autografts.

Donor sites are often dressed with an impregnated fine mesh gauze dressing. Op-Site, a hypoallergenic, moisture vapor permeable synthetic membrane that allows rapid epithelialization of the donor site is easy to use, promotes patient comfort, and is our material of choice for a donor site dressing. If thin grafts are harvested, donor site re-epithelialization can be expected in 10 to 14 days and the donor sites may be reused every 2 to 3 weeks. Donor site infection delays re-epithelialization and may even result in loss of remaining dermal and epidermal elements with conversion to a full-thickness wound.

Sheet grafts are employed to cover small wounds and aesthetically important areas such as the face. Grafts can be meshed (allowing expansion from 1.5 to 9 times the original size). Although theoretically sheet and mesh grafts should display a similar incidence of take, clinically, mesh grafts appear to do better over extremity and trunk wounds. The mesh grafts allow egress of serum and better contouring of the graft to an irregular bed, and they increase the area covered per graft. The remaining raw interstices epithelialize rapidly and the final aesthetic result is usually acceptable.

Complete immobilization of the graft on its bed is essential to allow the graft to take. Grafts may be immobilized by any combination including sutures, surgical staples, adhesive tapes, or conforming dressings. Staples provide the most rapid method of graft fixation. Staples are removed on the fifth day following grafting. Grafted extremities are dressed with immobilizing, conforming, circumferential dressings. A single layer of Furacin-impregnated fine mesh gauze is applied directly to the skin grafts. Coarse mesh gauze, prefabricated orthoplast splints, and bias stockinette complete the extremity dressing. Furacin solution is employed to keep the dressings moist until the first dressing change 48 to 36 hours following grafting. It is much more difficult to apply an effective dressing over trunk or facial skin grafts. Respiratory or normal facial movements beneath a dressing may cause shearing between the skin graft and its bed. Following grafting of trunk or facial wounds, a sheet graft may be left exposed to allow constant observation, but a single layer of Xeroform gauze should be applied to meshed grafts to prevent desiccation. These patients frequently require sedation, and occasionally even restraints, to minimize patient motion in order to enhance graft take during the initial postoperative period. Rarely, in the well-selected patient, it may be necessary to paralyze and mechanically ventilate the patient for a few days following application of crucial split-thickness skin grafts.

External splints and percutaneous pins serve two main functions. First, splints and pins can be employed to immobilized extremities during the post-grafting phase to allow successful vascularization of the skin grafts. Second, pins and splints can be employed to maintain joints in the position of function to minimize joint contractures and to facilitate subsequent rehabilitation. This is particularly important following burns to the hand, but other joints should not be forgotten.

Interphalangeal joints should be held in extension, metacarpal phalangeal joints maximally flexed, the thumb abducted, the wrist slightly extended, the elbow almost completely extended, the shoulder abducted, the knee almost completely extended, and the ankle in neutral position. External splints may also be designed to keep the neck extended. This aspect of burn wound care is frequently performed by physical therapists, occupational therapists, or burn unit nurses. The patient's physician, however, must have a thorough understanding of basic principles of physical medicine and maintain a leadership role in the patient's rehabilitation.

Burn wounds that have been skin grafted or have healed secondarily are frequently unsightly, particularly during the early hypertrophic phase. The patient must take special care of the skin during this period. The patient should be fitted with custom-made pressure garments (e.g., Jobst garments) prior to discharge from the hospital in order to minimize scar hypertrophy and keloid formation. Topical or intralesional steroids may be employed to reduce hypertrophic scars but their use is confined to small areas. Patients with healing wounds frequently complain of pruritus and dryness, which can be helped by lanolin creams. Lanolin ointment and gentle massage facilitate scar maturation and improve patient comfort. Exposure of the burned areas to sunlight must be avoided. Ultraviolet radiation may further damage the scarred skin and produce permanent hyperpigmentation. The patients must be educated in the use of sun-screening agents—these should be applied to all exposed areas whenever the patient anticipates outdoor activity.

In spite of optimal wound care, severe scarring may dictate the need for subsequent reconstructive surgery in order to return the burn victim to a reasonable social situation. The most common procedures include release of burn scar contractures and resurfacing of unacceptable areas, preferably in aesthetic units.

Supportive Measures

One of the most significant advances in the management of burn patients during the past few decades has been the increasing realization of the need for adequate nutrition and the development of means to provide it. Negative nitrogen balance and increased metabolic needs begin abruptly at the time of injury and continue until the wound is closed. Protein loss into the wound, loss of muscle from disuse, and increased metabolic rate from evaporative water loss all contribute to the negative nitrogen balance. An increased secretion of catabolic hormones such as glucocorticoids, catecholamines, and glucagon occurs concomitantly with an impaired secretion of the anabolic hormone insulin, contributing to the hypermetabolic, negative nitrogen balance state. The duration and magnitude of the negative nitrogen balance are influenced by the severity of the burn and the nutritional regimen employed. The basal metabolic rate and oxygen consumption increase in a linear fashion parallel with the extent of the burn injury up to a maximum level corresponding with a 40 to 50 percent BSA maximum. Energy expenditures seem to peak toward the end of the first week, but nitrogen balance does not return to normal (3 to 4 g of nitrogen per square meter per day) until wound closure has been achieved. Malnutrition increases the incidence of infection and reduces the efficiency of wound healing in the nutritionally depleted burn patient. Therefore, every effort must be made to maintain nutritional status during this period of hypermetabolism.

Oral feeding is preferred whenever possible. By the second day following extensive burns, the obligatory intestinal hypoperistalsis has usually resolved and oral feedings may be started. It is preferable to start oral intake with limited amounts of fluids at frequent intervals, but the diet may progress as tolerated by the patient. A lack of appetite frequently occurs in the post-burn patient. Attention should be directed toward attractively presented and tastefully prepared meals. Total caloric needs may be calculated employing the ''Curreri formula'' (caloric requirement = 25 Kcal per kilogram + 40 Kcal per percent burn). Nitrogen requirements can be met by supplying 1 g protein per 50 Kcal. Most patients find it difficult to consume sufficient quantities of protein and calories during regular mealtimes. A high-protein, high-caloric liquid supplement can be given between meals via a nasogastric feeding tube. Such supplements usually consist of a concentrated protein and milk formula and are well tolerated by the majority of burn patients, but occasionally, particularly in black adults, a galactase deficiency may produce intolerance to milk feedings. Provision of adequate protein and calories does not return metabolism to preinjury levels, but does reduce nitrogen loss, promote healing, and hasten the patient's recovery.

In addition to protein and calories, routine vitamin supplements are recommended as follows: ascorbic acid, 1,500 mg; thiamine, 50 mg; riboflavin, 50 mg; and nicotinamide, 500 mg daily. The vitamin supplements and increased caloric diet should be continued until burn wounds are healed.

It is imperative not to fall behind caloric requirements in the burn patient. Should the gastrointestinal tract be unavailable for feedings, total parenteral nutrition must be instituted promptly, employing the same guidelines used for any other seriously injured patient.

Periodic transfusions and therapeutic administration of albumin or gamma globulin may be necessary in patients with extreme emaciation and hypoproteinemia following delayed referral to a burn center.

Finally, total rehabilitation of the burn patient necessitates a return to adequate social function. This requires the cooperation of a large number of individuals including not only physicians, nurses, nutritionists, and physical therapists, but also psychologic and social support teams. All burn unit personnel must contribute to a supportive environment during the patient's recovery. Skin is man's outer cover. Burn injury induces severe anxiety, an altered body image, a physical, and possibly a social handicap. A burn injury may produce devastating emotional and social consequences. Initially, the patient is apprehensive for his life, but later is plagued by fear of permanent disability and disfigurement. Patients frequently develop a mild depression when preparing to leave the hospital and to face the potentially hostile community environment. Specific psychologic support eases the transition to the outside world. Although all burn patients may benefit from psychologic intervention, studies have indicated that the success of therapy depends more on the patient's pre-burn personality than on any single factor.

Burned children are particularly apt to have difficulties with psychosocial adjustment following hospitalization for their injuries. Parents of burned children frequently require psychiatric counseling to alleviate feelings of guilt regarding their responsibility for the child's accident. Psychologic counseling may also be required for spouses and other relatives of burn victims. Despite relative marital satisfaction, studies have demonstrated dissatisfaction in sexual relations involving rehabilitated burn injured patients. A number of regional and national support groups consisting of rehabilitated burn victims have been organized. Such peer groups can provide the burn victim much needed support. In the presence of an effective rehabilitative team, better than 95 percent of burn victims are able to return to their pre-burn socioeconomic status.

ELECTRICAL INJURIES

Damage due to electrical injury is frequently referred to as an electrical burn. The intensity of current, the duration of contact, the resistance at points of contact, the efficiency of grounding, and the pathway of the current through the body determine the extent of injury. Higher voltage and prolonged contact increase the severity of injury. Thin skin and surface moisture decrease resistance to the electrical current, whereas thick skin and surface oil increase it. A larger area of grounding will encourage greater current flow and consequently increase the degree of injury. The current flows in a direct line between the points of grounding. Cardiac or respiratory arrest may occur if the pathway of the current includes the heart or brain. The current rarely causes irreversible damage to the heart or lungs; prompt cardiopulmonary resuscitation should allow return of vital functions to an unimpaired level and residual cardiopulmonary disease is rarely encountered in these patients. Direct current produces muscular spasms only at the start and stop of current flow, whereas alternating current produces muscular contraction and relaxation with each cycle. Thus, low-voltage direct current is less dangerous than the alternating variety.

The electric current produces tissue disruption by thermal necrosis. Treatment of electrical injury should be modified considerably from that of thermal injury because tissue damage is much deeper. The amount of heat generated is directly proportional to the resistance to current flow. The lowest resistances are offered by nerves, followed by blood vessels, muscle, skin, tendons, fat, and bone. Thus, tissues located near the center of the limb may be injured while more superficial tissues may be spared. In many aspects, an electrical injury more nearly simulates crush injury than it does a thermal burn. More tissue is always destroyed by an electrical injury than is apparent at first inspection.

Three types of skin damage are associated with electrical injures: (1) contact burns (entry and exit sites), (2) arc burns, and (3) flame burns resulting from the ignition of clothing by electrical sparks. Initial treatment of electrical and thermal burns is similar, but a high-voltage electrical injury must be treated more like a crush injury. The current may cause thrombosis, even at some distance from the original injury. Peripheral perfusion must be monitored and a fasciotomy performed at the first sign of vascular compromise. Viability of tissues in patients with high-voltage electrical injuries can be determined only by direct visualization, and early exploration of such tissues is mandatory. Obvious necrotic tissue must be excised and daily debridement performed to extirpate remaining nonviable tissue to prevent sepsis and minimize the need for amputations. An excessive release of myoglobin into the circulation may produce renal damage, and therefore massive replacement fluid therapy is essential. Frequently, an osmotic diuretic also is indicated.

Failure to remove extensively damaged muscle may lead to anaerobic clostridial infections and death. Anticlostridial prophylaxis with large doses of penicillin and tetanus prophylaxis are necessary. Mafenide acetate cream is preferred to other topical antimicrobials for its ability to penetrate into the deeper tissues.

Fractures due to severe muscular contractions must be suspected in patients following electrical injury. Such patients must also be observed for spontaneous vascular rupture (false aneurysms), visceral injury, and vascular thrombosis.

Physical therapy is of paramount importance in the rehabilitation of the patient following electrical injury. Prosthetic training is frequently required due to the high incidence of amputations.

Unattended children frequently bite electrical cords and sustain low intensity electrical burns of the oral commissures. Such injuries are caused by the heat of the arc and are true thermal injuries without distal sequelae. Classically, children with electrical burns of the lips were admitted to the hospital for wound care and observation during the 7 to 21 days required for secondary healing. Potential hemorrhage from the labial arteries following separation of eschar provided the rationale for hospitalization. Outpatient management of children with electrical burns of the lip in conjunction with parental education, however, is in most cases safe and cost effective. Parents can be taught to control hemorrhage by direct pressure and to immediately bring the child to an emergency facility should bleeding occur. Such wounds are kept clean by frequent cleansing with physiologic saline, and antibiotic ointments are applied until secondary healing is obtained. Splinting of the oral commissures following electrical injury of the lips to prevent contracture has become increasingly accepted in the past several years. Good results have been reported utilizing intraoral splints constructed from acrylic and fixed to the teeth by the pediorthodontist. Secondary surgery may be required for microstomia.

CHEMICAL INJURY

Chemical burns tend to be progressive as long as the active agent remains in contact with the skin. Tissue destruction ceases only when the offending agent has been removed or neutralized. Initial therapy, irrespective of the causative agent, should consist of copious irrigation of the affected part with physiologic saline or water, removal of clothing, and repeated irrigation. Attempting to identify the offending agent and to locate the proper neutralizing agent will only result in delay of treatment and a progression of tissue destruction. Most chemical burns result from contact with acid or alkali. A careful search should be made for retained foreign material, particularly following contact with white phosphorus since in situ re-ignition may occur if particles are allowed to remain. Burns known to be due to white phosphorus may be washed with a 1 percent copper sulfate solution (0.5 ml per square centimeter of burn), which coats the particles with black cupric phosphide, thus impeding oxidation and allowing easy identification. Ten percent calcium gluconate solution may be injected into wounds caused by hydrofluoric acid to limit progression of tissue destruction. All wounds caused by chemical burns should be observed frequently and, if progressive tissue destruction occurs despite copious irrigation, surgical excision of the involved areas considered.

Following initial management, the basic principles described for thermal injury are applicable. Tangential escharectomy may be employed to debride wounds of uncertain depth. All deep dermal and full-thickness burns should be debrided and wounds closed with skin grafts as soon as feasible.

SPECIAL PROBLEMS

FRANK R. LEWIS Jr., M.D.

ACCIDENTAL HYPOTHERMIA

Accidental hypothermia has been reported with a number of preexistent medical conditions, but for practical purposes is seen in the urban setting principally in three conditions: outdoor exposure while intoxicated, prolonged unconsciousness due to drug overdosage, and cold water immersion or near drowning. Under normal circumstances, exposure in cold climates results in profound cutaneous vasoconstriction, so that little heat is lost through the skin to the air. Although it is possible, in cold climates, for hypothermia to develop in a normal person who is inadequately clothed and insulated (backpackers, mountain climbers), such an occurrence is uncommon. Hypothermia is seen most commonly in urban areas with relatively moderate or cool temperatures (30 to 60 °F) in patients who are acutely intoxicated and unable to vasoconstrict effectively, and who are inadequately clothed. In such patients hypothermia typically develops over several hours. Ingestion of drugs that produce sedation or unconsciousness, such as barbiturates and other tranquilizer/hypnotics, may also result in hypothermia. These drugs generally have mild vasodilatory properties, so that heat is lost more freely, but the sedated patient fails to awaken in response to cooling.

Much less commonly, hypothermia is seen after cold water immersion following boating accidents. Because water has a greater heat capacity and penetrates most clothing, cooling occurs far more rapidly in water. Thus exposure for more than one hour to water that is cooler than 50 °F is usually fatal, and even at 50 to 60 °F, exposure for more than 2 hours is commonly fatal. In addition to cutaneous exposure, immersion may result in aspiration of cold water, and this produces the most rapid cooling of all, with core temperature reduced into the 80 to 90 °F range within a few minutes. It has recently been shown that this is the result of cooling via the lung, with its extensive surface area for heat exchange. It has also become clear that successful resuscitation of drowning victims in cardiac arrest, even after documented periods of arrest of 15 to 25 minutes are due to this "instant hypothermia." It produces a rapid decrease in oxygen consumption and metabolic requirements, so that the arrested hypothermia victim can be successfully resuscitated well beyond the limits that are normally thought to be irreversible.

For purposes of prognosis, hypothermia to levels no lower than 90 to 92 °F is rarely fatal and is usually easily treated. Most cases of severe complications, often fatal, are caused by temperatures below 90 °F, but usually above 75 °F. Survival when cooling below 75 °F has occurred is rare, although one patient has been reported to survive with a body temperature of 67 °F. It seems likely that both the degree of hypothermia and the length of time the patient remains at low temperature levels govern the magnitude and severity of complications seen, but these relationships have not been clearly documented in the literature. In general, mortality of 50 percent is seen with hypothermia in the 75 to 90 °F range.

The clinical signs of hypothermia are not specific, but one is usually led to think of it as soon as he lays hand on the patient to examine him. Normal clinical thermometers are inadequate to measure temperatures below 94 °F, and either laboratory thermometers or electric thermometers, which are commonly available, must be used. The core temperature should be monitored continuously during treatment until normothermia is attained. The cerebral signs of hypothermia are those of decreased cortical function, but they are not localized. They are progressive with decreasing temperature below approximately 94 °F, to the point where coma usually is present at temperatures below 80 °F. With milder degrees of cooling the patient may be apathetic, confused, or noncommunicative. As the level of cooling progresses, mental processes become more deranged, and the patient may be disoriented, somnolent, uncooperative, or totally withdrawn. Muscular rigidity and difficulty with movement and coordination are progressive with cooling below 90 °F.

The acute metabolic effects that accompany hypothermia are multiple and produce complex changes in the cardiopulmonary system. Oxygen consumption decreases rapidly with cooling, and cardiac output falls in proportion to oxygen consumption. Patients who are cooled below 90 °F typically have cardiac outputs of less than 2 liters per minute; with more profound cooling, cardiac output decreases below 1 liter per minute. Blood viscosity is increased and, in conjunction with peripheral vasoconstriction, produces marked increases in systemic vascular resistance. This tends to prevent the decreased cardiac output from causing profound hypotension, and the hypothermic patient usually has a blood pressure in the low normal to moderately hypotensive range. Diuresis accompanies severe hypothermia, but the cause has not been clearly defined. Renal tubular damage is a common sequela of moderate-to-severe hypothermia, and acute renal failure, either oliguric or nonoliguric, is common. Whether the early diuresis is a manifestation of tubular damage or a response to humoral mechanisms is unknown. It is important to recognize, however, that the hypothermic patient may be severely hypovolemic if the condition has been present for 12 hours or more, and he or she needs vigorous resuscitation and intensive cardiac monitoring. It is probable that many of the reported adverse results of rewarming from hypothermia are simply a result of failure to recognize and aggressively treat the hypovolemia that is present.

At the cellular level, the oxyhemoglobin dissociation curve is shifted to the left with hypothermia, which means that oxygen unloading peripherally is impaired. This is partially compensated by the increased amount of dissolved oxygen that is carried in the cooled plasma as well as by the decreased oxygen requirements. Thus, although peripheral hypoxia is a theoretic problem, the protective effects appear to outweigh the detrimental ones, so that overall the tissues are protected, not damaged, by cooling, at least as far as oxygenation is concerned.

Treatment of the hypothermic victim entails either passive or active rewarming, correction of metabolic and intravascular volume abnormalities, intensive cardiac and respiratory monitoring with ventilator support as needed, and close evaluation for the development of predictable complications. The method of rewarming has evoked considerable controversy in the literature, and on one extreme there are advocates of immediate rewarming using extracorporeal bypass via the femoral vessels, while on the other extreme there are those who advocate only passive rewarming. Logically, it would seem that a rapid return of body temperature to normal is desirable, for it is clear that the hypothermic state produces significant tissue damage when present over a prolonged period. However, rapid rewarming by immersion of the victim in a warm tub of water or by placing heating blankets over and below him in bed has been associated, in some studies, with a greater incidence of cardiac arrhythmias or refractory hypotension. The concept has developed that rapid rewarming produces peripheral warming prior to "core" warming and, by so doing, creates vasodilation and lowered systemic resistance in excess of the ability of the heart to increase cardiac output. The actual evidence that this occurs is lacking in the literature, and it seems more likely that most of the effects attributed to it are a result of inadequate intravascular volume replacement, as was mentioned earlier. Given the rate of blood circulation between the extremities and the core, even in a profound hypothermic state, it is not possible that a significant temperature difference between them can be maintained. Despite this, the concept is often repeated in the literature and frequently governs management. It is my practice to actively rewarm all patients who have temperatures below 92 °F by means of heating blankets surrounding the patient. Continuous monitoring of core temperature by esophageal or rectal probe is essential to attain a rewarming rate of at least 1 °C, and preferably 2 °C, per hour. I have had no experience with the use of extracorporeal bypass for rewarming, but the reports have been favorable, and in patients with life-threatening complications such as refractory cardiac arrhythmias due to the lowered temperature, it seems indicated. In the average patient, active rewarming as described is adequate, and more aggressive means generally are not necessary.

Cardiac arrhythmias are the greatest acute threat to patients, and continuous ECG monitoring is essential. Atrial fibrillation is common, but usually resolves as normal temperature is attained and does not require treatment. If rapid ventricular response occurs and produces hypotension, conventional treatment with intravenous rapid-acting digitalis preparations is indicated. The less common but more life-threatening arrhythmias are ventricular tachycardia and fibrillation. These are treated in the conventional way with lidocaine, Pronestyl, or defibrillation, but may be difficult to convert. Least common are varying degrees of atrioventricular conduction block ranging from bundle branch blocks to complete A-V block. Only if this is severe enough to produce hypotension is treatment usually necessary.

Adequate cardiac and pulmonary monitoring of the hypothermic patient necessitates an indwelling arterial line and a central venous line for pressure measurement. Some have advocated routine placement of pulmonary artery catheters for improved definition of cardiac function, but the greater hazard of ventricular arrhythmias in this group of patients has led us to defer it until the patient's temperature is brought up to normal. A Foley catheter is placed to allow hourly monitoring of urine output, and replacement intravenous fluids are gauged by the urine output and central venous pressure. Normally we would administer balanced salt solutions rapidly until urine output is restored to 0.5 to 1 ml per kilogram per hour, or until the central venous pressure rises to 12 to 14 cm H_2O. Hypokalemia is a uniform occurrence in these patients, and aggressive potassium replacement is also required. I have found it most effective and safest to administer potassium via intravenous drip, at the rate of 5 to 10 mEq per hour over 1 to 3 days, with close monitoring of serum potassium levels.

Acute respiratory failure and the development of interstitial infiltrates are common complications of moderate or severe hypothermia; they typically appear after rewarming is complete, usually 2 to 5 days after admission. The edema is noncardiogenic, due to permeability increases, and the cause has not been determined. In severe cases in which the patient has been comatose, aspiration pneumonia may be a cause of respiratory failure, but in many patients this seems improbable. Disseminated intravascular coagulation (DIC) is frequently present on the second to fifth day and is associated with acute respiratory failure. It is usually diagnosed by thrombocytopenia and by the presence of fibrin degradation products and soluble fibrin monomer in the blood. Whether DIC is the cause of the respiratory failure has not been determined, but it seems likely.

The frequency of respiratory problems dictates that arterial blood gas be monitored closely. If the patient develops significant hypoxemia and/or clinical respiratory failure with tachypnea and increased work of breathing, endotracheal intubation and mechanical ventilation may be needed. We have found this to be necessary in more than 50 percent of hypothermia patients. Irreversible respiratory failure, frequently complicated by sepsis, is the most common cause of death in these patients. As a result, it should be aggressively sought and treated.

Other common complications are acute renal failure, as has been noted, and pancreatitis. If the renal failure remains nonoliguric, management is simplified, as potassium management is not usually a problem, and dialysis often can be avoided. Other than early and aggressive fluid resuscitation, I know of no specific way to avoid renal failure. Its frequent occurrence should lead one to suspect it and to carry out daily creatinine clearances during the first 3 or 4 hospital days to detect it as early as possible.

Pancreatitis is often a rather subtle diagnosis, manifested by epigastric pain and tenderness with some abdominal distention, but minimal peritoneal signs of rebound tenderness. Serum amylases are frequently elevated and may confirm the clinical impression. Etiology is obscure, and treatment is supportive. In rare instances, the pancreatitis is hemorrhagic in type and produces extreme morbidity and mortality.

The final typical finding after profound hypothermia is peripheral edema that is unusually persistent and seemingly indicative of a prolonged permeability defect in the peripheral circulation. As far as I am aware, this has not been discussed in the literature, but it has been a frequent finding in my experience.

It is interesting to conjecture that most of the complications of hypothermia result from a shedding of capillary endothelial cells throughout the vascular system, and that this produces increased permeability which leads to the failure of the lung, kidney, and pancreas, as well as the peripheral edema. It also provides an explanation for the persistent DIC that is often seen, as exposure of basement membrane collagen would provide an ongoing stimulus for platelet aggregation and initiation of coagulation.

FROSTBITE

Frostbite is a cold injury of peripheral tissues in which freezing of the tissues, with ice crystal formation, occurs. It most commonly involves the feet, but also affects the hands and, on occasion, the nose and ears. The injury occurs because of direct exposure of the tissues with inadequate protection or insulation.

Tissue temperature is normally a balance between heat loss through the skin and heat inflow via the circulation. When peripheral tissues begin to cool, vasoconstriction decreases the inflow and makes the part more susceptible to the effects of environmental cooling. If external compression is present, as a result of overly tight clothing, this may further reduce inflow and predispose to freezing. Obviously, cooling is enhanced by immersion in cold water or by moisture-saturated clothing.

For frostbite to occur, the temperature of the part must decrease below 32 °F, and theoretically any external temperatures below this might produce it. Practically, however, it usually does not occur unless ambient temperatures of 10 to 15 °F or lower are encountered, or unless other adverse circumstances are present. The depth to which freezing in tissue occurs appears to determine the extent of the cold injury, and it may be superficial or deep. The subsequent extent of tissue loss is also principally dependent on the level to which freezing occurs, and it is usually graded as first-, second-, third-, or fourth-degree—depending, respectively, on whether the involvement is superficial, partial-thickness, full-thickness of skin, or extending into deeper structures.

The initial symptom experienced by all patients is intense coldness followed by numbness. This numbness persists as long as the part remains frozen, but after thawing occurs a number of other sensory changes are noted. The most common complaint is pain, but it is usually accompanied by paresthesias, burning, tingling, or a "pins and needles" sensation. Although these sensory disturbances are most severe in the early phases of rewarming, they tend to persist for long periods of time, and some may be permanent. Even after many years, patients may complain of pain brought on by cold and of excessive sweating. In the late phases, the extremities appear to have increased sympathetic tone, and this no doubt accounts for some of the symptoms.

If the patient is seen early, the frozen part is obviously cold, hard, and numb. More commonly, however, partial or complete thawing has occurred before the patient is seen by medical personnel, and the extent of damage may be initially underestimated. It has been well documented in the literature that prediction of extent of damage and ultimate viability is difficult during the early period, and only when there has been a chance for gangrene to develop into a line of demarcation can one be sure of the extent of tissue loss. Retrospectively, the classification into first-, second-, third-, and fourth-degree tissue loss is possible, but prospectively this judgment cannot be made. Even severely injured tissue is reperfused after thawing and may be flushed and hyperemic transiently. Ultimate tissue damage and loss are due to vascular spasm and occlusion, red cell and protein extravasation with edema formation, and membrane damage.

Acute treatment, if the part has not been completely rewarmed, is to immerse it in warm water for approximately 30 minutes, until the extremity has been rewarmed to normal temperature. One method for accomplishing this has been to immerse the frozen part in progressively warmer water, starting at 20 °C and increasing by 5 °C at 5-minute intervals until 40 °C is reached. Alternatively, water at 38 to 42 °C may be used initially and maintained at that temperature throughout.

Other methods of treatment have been advocated, but relatively few have achieved any objective evidence of benefit. The one modality that seems to have value at present is intra-arterial injection of reserpine or other alpha-blocking agents early after thawing, with a repeat injection at 2 to 3 days. Available evidence, both clinical and arteriographic, indicates that this may improve and maintain perfusion. Other modalities, including heparin, dextran, and indomethacin, have not been shown to have prolonged benefit. Sympathectomy has not been shown to have any value in early treatment, but in the patient who has pain and excessive sympathetic tone late after the frostbite injury, the procedure appears to produce subjective improvement with increased skin perfusion.

When tissue loss occurs, the extent of gangrene usually becomes apparent within a week or 10 days. When this is extensive, for example, extending to the ankle level, there seems little reason to temporize, and it is our practice to proceed immediately to definitive amputation. In situations in which the gangrene involves only part of a digit, it is probably better to wait and allow the part of autoamputate, so that the greatest tissue length is preserved.

SNAKEBITE

Four species of poisonous snakes are present in the United States—

rattlesnakes, copperheads, water moccasins, and coral snakes. The first three are pit vipers in the genus Crotalidae, whereas coral snakes belong to the family Elapidea. As a practical problem, pit vipers account for virtually all the snake bites seen, and coral snakes are reported to cause less than 1 percent of the total. In addition, coral snakes envenomation is less frequent when a bite occurs and appears to produce fewer toxic effects, so that it is rarely a threat to life. The following discussion will therefore focus entirely on the effects of pit vipers.

Although pit vipers are present in all parts of the United States, the incidence of snake bite is most common in the southern and southwestern states. Bites usually occur in rural settings as a result of accidental encounters with the snake, though a suprising number of people in urban areas also keep poisonous snakes for pets and are bitten when handling them. It is stated that snakes do not actively pursue humans, but when surprised or confronted they do not necessarily retreat. Snakes have poor eyesight and hearing, but a unique ability to detect prey by means of two pits on each side of the head, which are exquisitely heat-sensitive. Heat detection is thought to be the principal means by which the snake gauges the direction of strike, and even perhaps the amount of envenomation, dependent on what size the prey is thought to be. The damage inflicted by pit vipers is not strictly a bite, but rather a penetration of the skin by two fangs in the upper jaw, which are as long as 15 to 18 mm. Venom is injected through the fangs into subcutaneous tissue, where it diffuses rapidly, causing local damage. If moderate-to-large envenomations occur, systemic absorption of venom produces severe systemic effects. The quantity of venom injected is variable, dependent on the size and age of the snake as well as the size of the prey, as noted. Nearly all snakebites are on the extremities, and envenomation can occur through clothing unless it is thick, but rarely through leather boots or other protective wear.

Pit viper venom is a potent cocktail of proteolytic enzymes and other proteins that produce multiple toxic effects. The ones that are recognized to cause greatest damage are (1) hyaluronidase, which softens connective tissue and enhances spreading of venom to adjacent tissues, (2) multiple proteolytic enzymes, which digest most proteins including collagen, reticulin, and elastin, (3) procoagulants, which activate fibrinogen and result in fibrin clot formation, and (4) phospholipase A, which cleaves lecithin, releasing lysolecithin, a particularly damaging substance that destroys cell walls and membranes.

When a snake bite occurs, one should try to identify the type of snake, since the majority are nonpoisonous. The victim can sometimes identify or describe it, but if possible, the snake should be killed and examined by a knowledgeable expert. If this is not possible, the patient must be observed medically or be hospitalized until the extent of local and systemic reaction becomes evident and the need for treatment is determined.

Most of the traditionally recommended methods of snakebite treatment are without benefit and should not be practiced. Chief among these is the application of ice to the injury since this will not inactivate the venom nor prevent its spread, but may do additional tissue damage. Incising the punctured area and sucking out the venom appears to have value only if done within the first 5 minutes of envenomation. If the victim is seen later than this, it should not be attempted. Tourniquets inflated to 50 mm Hg, to impede venous and lymphatic return without producing arterial ischemia, have been recommended, but in my opinion, this measure increases local pain and accentuates swelling in the affected limb, and its overall efficacy is questionable. Perhaps the best compromise is wrapping the entire extremity in an elastic bandage, which impedes systemic spread of the venom without increasing local edema. It is worthwhile to keep the patient as quiet as possible and keep him from using the bitten extremity if possible. Rapid transport to a medical facility is imperative so that the patient can be observed and treated as needed.

The effects of envenomation are both local and systemic. Locally, pain develops, and swelling begins within minutes to an hour or two, progressing to severe edema over several hours. The patient may report local paresthesias, and after several hours vesicles may form. Cyanosis is uncommon, but has been reported. After a day or more, ecchymoses may develop. The systemic symptoms are generalized weakness, nausea, and vomiting, and hypotension may occur. Later the signs of failure of specific organ systems are seen.

The degree of envenomation should be graded as mild if there are only local symptoms with minimal regional and no systemic involvement; moderate if local symptoms are severe and regional involvement of the entire extremity is present; and severe and life-threatening if, in addition to the aforementioned symptoms, systemic manifestations are present. The systemic organ systems that are primarily affected are cardiovascular, pulmonary, hematologic, and renal. The cardiac effects are due to fluid loss from increased capillary permeability and third space leakage of plasma, as well as vasodilatation and perhaps cardiac depression. Hypotension is common when systemic effects are present, and it requires standard methods of cardiovascular support. Pulmonary effects appear to be related primarily to interstitial edema, which in turn creates hypoxemia and decreased pulmonary compliance. Arterial blood gas monitoring is essential, and institution of ventilatory support may be necessary. The hematologic effects are similar to generalized intravascular clotting, with defibrination in severe cases. Prothrombin time and partial thromboplastin time are prolonged, and thrombocytopenia is present. Renal failure may occur if significant red cell lysis is present with hemoglobinuria, or if the patient has prolonged hypotension.

The principal care that can be given to snakebite victims is supportive when systemic manifestations are present. The usual indications and methods of cardiovascular and pulmonary support are utilized. The only specific therapy that can be administered is antivenin, which is polyvalent and effective against all pit vipers seen in the United States. When envenomation is mild, it is recommended that 50 ml (5 vials) of antivenin be used; when moderate, 100 ml, and when severe, 150 ml or more. The danger of using antivenin is that the patient may be sensitive to horse serum, from which it is made, and so sensitivity testing should precede intravenous administration. Serum sickness afterward may be anticipated in a high percentage of patients.

For severe local effects, continuous elevation and immobilization of the affected part are mandatory during the first few days, followed later by aggressive physical therapy to re-establish normal range of motion in affected parts. The edema seen is persistent, and if it is severe, a compartment syndrome can develop. If this occurs, fasciotomy is necessary, but this is uncommon as the edema is usually maximal in subcutaneous tissues rather than in muscle compartments.

Overall mortality from snakebite is low, with less than 1 percent of poisonous snake bites resulting in death. The local effects, and disability from them, are far more common.

SPIDER BITES

Two spiders account for most of the severe bites seen in the United States—the black widow and the brown recluse. The black widow is usually 1 to 2 cm in size and is shiny black with a characteristic red hourglass mark on the underside of the body. This species is widely distributed in all of the continental United States as well as in South America. They tend to be found outdoors, under objects such as rocks or logs or in piles of rubbish or wood.

When a bite occurs, venom is injected and then absorbed into the circulation, as the principal effects are systemic. Local effects are minimal, consisting only of slight pain and swelling. The systemic effects appear to be due to a cholinergic reaction and consist of diffuse muscle cramps and spasm, abdominal rigidity being common. Nonspecific CNS signs, such as nausea, vomiting, headache, and swelling, may be present as well. Cardiovascular or pulmonary effects appear to be minimal, although hypertension has sometimes been reported. Most patients recover after a few days. If symptoms are severe, intravenous calcium gluconate (10 ml of 10% solution) is used to relieve muscle cramps and spasm, and other symptoms may be treated with sedatives or analgesics as needed.

The brown recluse spider is somewhat larger than the black widow, reaching 3 to 4 cm in overall diameter. It is reddish brown with a characteristic violin-shaped mark at the anterior end of the dorsal side of the body. The venom injected by the brown recluse is a mixture of nucleases and proteases, which produce severe local tissue damage and necrosis. The initial bite may not be noticed, but after a few hours a reddish painful lesion, 1 to 3 mm in size, is noted. With time this enlarges and is surrounded by an area of vasoconstriction. After several hours, extravasation of red cells may develop in a circular pattern around the central lesion. During the next few days the lesion proceeds indolently, with progressive tissue destruction and ulceration. There is local swelling, red cell extravasation, and erythema, and cellulitis may develop. The skin and subcutaneous tissue progressively necrose in the area, and debridement may be necessary. Systemic symptoms can occur in addition to the local lesions, but are not common and have been seen mainly in the pediatric population. When present, they take the form of acute hemolytic reactions with fever, chills, hemoglobinuria, and later, jaundice and renal failure. If a brown recluse bite can definitely be identified, early excision of the lesion and adjacent involved tissue appears to offer the most rapid resolution. The lesion otherwise tends to be indolent and ultimately requires sharp debridement in most cases. It is not certain that the amount of tissue loss is lessened by early debridement, but the course of the illness probably is shortened, allowing for earlier skin grafting of the area, as is usually required. Although deaths from brown recluse bites have been reported in South America, they appear to be rare in the United States, being reported only in children.

INDEX

The letter *f* following a page number indicates a figure; the letter *t* following a page number indicates a table.

MEFOXIN®

(STERILE CEFOXITIN SODIUM, MSD)

DESCRIPTION

MEFOXIN* (Sterile Cefoxitin Sodium, MSD) is a semi-synthetic, broad-spectrum cepha antibiotic for parenteral administration. It is derived from cephamycin C, which is produced by *Streptomyces lactamdurans.* It is the sodium salt of 3-(hydroxymethyl)-7α-methoxy-8-oxo-7-[2-(2-thienyl)acetamido]-5-thia-1-azabicyclo [4.2.0] oct-2-ene-2-carboxylate carbamate (ester). The empirical formula is $C_{16}H_{16}N_3NaO_7S_2$, and the structural formula is:

MEFOXIN contains approximately 53.8 mg (2.3 milliequivalents) of sodium per gram of cefoxitin activity. Solutions of MEFOXIN range from clear to light amber in color. The pH of freshly constituted solutions usually ranges from 4.2 to 7.0.

CLINICAL PHARMACOLOGY

Clinical Pharmacology

After intramuscular administration of a 1 gram dose of MEFOXIN to normal volunteers, the mean peak serum concentration was 24 mcg/mL. The peak occurred at 20 to 30 minutes. Following an intravenous dose of 1 gram, serum concentrations were 110 mcg/mL at 5 minutes, declining to less than 1 mcg/mL at 4 hours. The half-life after an intravenous dose is 41 to 59 minutes; after intramuscular administration, the half-life is 64.8 minutes. Approximately 85 percent of cefoxitin is excreted unchanged by the kidneys over a 6-hour period, resulting in high urinary concentrations. Following an intramuscular dose of 1 gram, urinary concentrations greater than 3000 mcg/mL were observed. Probenecid slows tubular excretion and produces higher serum levels and increases the duration of measurable serum concentrations.

Cefoxitin passes into pleural and joint fluids and is detectable in antibacterial concentrations in bile.

*Registered trademark of MERCK & CO., INC.
COPYRIGHT © MERCK & CO., INC., 1984
All rights reserved

MEFOXIN®
(Sterile Cefoxitin Sodium, MSD)

Clinical experience has demonstrated that MEFOXIN can be administered to patients who are also receiving carbenicillin, kanamycin, gentamicin, tobramycin, or amikacin (see PRECAUTIONS and ADMINISTRATION).

Microbiology

The bactericidal action of cefoxitin results from inhibition of cell wall synthesis. Cefoxitin has *in vitro* activity against a wide range of gram-positive and gram-negative organisms. The methoxy group in the 7α position provides MEFOXIN with a high degree of stability in the presence of beta-lactamases, both penicillinases and cephalosporinases, of gram-negative bacteria. Cefoxitin is usually active against the following organisms *in vitro* and in clinical infections:

Gram-positive

Staphylococcus aureus, including penicillinase and non-penicillinase producing strains

Staphylococcus epidermidis

Beta-hemolytic and other streptococci (most strains of enterococci, e.g., *Streptococcus faecalis,* are resistant)

Streptococcus pneumoniae (formerly *Diplococcus pneumoniae*)

Gram-negative

Escherichia coli

Klebsiella species (including *K. pneumoniae*)

Hemophilus influenzae

Neisseria gonorrhoeae, including penicillinase and non-penicillinase producing strains

Proteus mirabilis

Morganella morganii (formerly *Proteus morganii*)

Proteus vulgaris

Providencia species, including *Providencia rettgeri* (formerly *Proteus rettgeri*)

Anaerobic organisms

Peptococcus species

Peptostreptococcus species

Clostridium species

Bacteroides species, including the *B. fragilis* group (includes *B. fragilis, B. distasonis, B. ovatus, B. thetaiotaomicron, B. vulgatus*)

MEFOXIN is inactive *in vitro* against most strains of *Pseudomonas aeruginosa* and enterococci and many strains of *Enterobacter cloacae.*

Methicillin-resistant staphylococci are almost uniformly resistant to MEFOXIN.

Susceptibility Tests

For fast-growing aerobic organisms, quantitative methods that require measurements of zone diameters give the most precise estimates of antibiotic susceptibility. One such procedure* has been recommended for use with discs to test susceptibility to cefoxitin. Interpretation involves correlation of the diameters obtained in the disc test with minimal inhibitory concentration (MIC) values for cefoxitin.

Reports from the laboratory giving results of the standardized single disc susceptibility test* using a 30 mcg cefoxitin disc should be interpreted according to the following criteria:

Organisms producing zones of 18 mm or greater are considered susceptible, indicating that the tested organism is likely to respond to therapy.

Organisms of intermediate susceptibility produce zones of 15 to 17 mm, indicating that the tested organism would be susceptible if high dosage is used or if the infection is confined to tissues and fluids (e.g., urine) in which high antibiotic levels are attained.

Resistant organisms produce zones of 14 mm or less, indicating that other therapy should be selected.

The cefoxitin disc should be used for testing cefoxitin susceptibility.

Cefoxitin has been shown by in vitro tests to have activity against certain strains of *Enterobacteriaceae* found resistant when tested with the cephalosporin class disc. For this reason, the cefoxitin disc should not be used for testing susceptibility to cephalosporins, and cephalosporin discs should not be used for testing susceptibility to cefoxitin.

Dilution methods, preferably the agar plate dilution procedure, are most accurate for susceptibility testing of obligate anaerobes.

A bacterial isolate may be considered susceptible if the MIC value for cefoxitin** is not more than 16 mcg/mL. Organisms are considered resistant if the MIC is greater than 32 mcg/mL.

---

*Bauer, A. W.; Kirby, W.M.M.; Sherris, J.C.; Turck, M.: Antibiotic susceptibility testing by a standardized single disc method. Amer. J. Clin. Path. *45*:493-496, Apr. 1966. Standardized disc susceptibility test. Federal Register 37:20527-20529, 1972. National Committee for Clinical Laboratory Standards: Approved Standard: ASM-2, Performance Standards for Antimicrobial Disc Susceptibility Tests, July 1975.
**Determined by the ICS agar dilution method (Ericsson and Sherris, Acta Path. Microbiol. Scand. [B] Suppl. No. 217, 1971) or any other method that has been shown to give equivalent results.

INDICATIONS AND USAGE

Treatment

MEFOXIN is indicated for the treatment of serious infections caused by susceptible strains of the designated microorganisms in the diseases listed below.

(1) **Lower respiratory tract infections,** including pneumonia and lung abscess, caused by *Streptococcus pneumoniae* (formerly *Diplococcus pneumoniae*), other streptococci (excluding enterococci, e.g., *Streptococcus faecalis*), *Staphylococcus aureus* (penicillinase and non-penicillinase producing), *Escherichia coli, Klebsiella* species, *Hemophilus influenzae,* and *Bacteroides* species.

(2) **Genitourinary infections.** Urinary tract infections caused by *Escherichia coli, Klebsiella* species, *Proteus mirabilis,* indole-positive Proteus (i.e., *Proteus morganii, rettgeri,* and *vulgaris*), and *Providencia* species. Uncomplicated gonorrhea due to *Neisseria gonorrhoeae* (penicillinase and non-penicillinase producing).

(3) **Intra-abdominal infections,** including peritonitis and intra-abdominal abscess, caused by *Escherichia coli, Klebsiella* species, *Bacteroides* species including the *Bacteroides fragilis* group*, and *Clostridium* species.

(4) **Gynecological infections,** including endometritis, pelvic cellulitis, and pelvic inflammatory disease caused by *Escherichia coli, Neisseria gonorrhoeae* (penicillinase and non-penicillinase producing), *Bacteroides* species including the *Bacteroides fragilis* group*, *Clostridium* species, *Peptococcus* species, *Peptostreptococcus* species, and Group B streptococci.

(5) **Septicemia** caused by *Streptococcus pneumoniae* (formerly *Diplococcus pneumoniae*), *Staphylococcus aureus* (penicillinase and non-penicillinase producing), *Escherichia coli, Klebsiella* species, and *Bacteroides* species including the *Bacteroides fragilis* group.*

(6) **Bone and joint infections** caused by *Staphylococcus aureus* (penicillinase and non-penicillinase producing).

(7) **Skin and skin structure infections** caused by *Staphylococcus aureus* (penicillinase and non-penicillinase producing), *Staphylococcus epidermidis,* streptococci (excluding enterococci, e.g., *Streptococcus faecalis*), *Escherichia coli, Proteus mirabilis,*

---

*B. fragilis, B. distasonis, B. ovatus, B. thetaiotaomicron, B. vulgatus.

Klebsiella species, *Bacteroides* species including the *Bacteroides fragilis* group*, *Clostridium* species, *Peptococcus* species, and *Peptostreptococcus* species.

Appropriate culture and susceptibility studies should be performed to determine the susceptibility of the causative organisms to MEFOXIN. Therapy may be started while awaiting the results of these studies.

In randomized comparative studies, MEFOXIN and cephalothin were comparably safe and effective in the management of infections caused by gram-positive cocci and gram-negative rods susceptible to the cephalosporins. MEFOXIN has a high degree of stability in the presence of bacterial beta-lactamases, both penicillinases and cephalosporinases.

Many infections caused by aerobic and anaerobic gram-negative bacteria resistant to some cephalosporins respond to MEFOXIN. Similarly, many infections caused by aerobic and anaerobic bacteria resistant to some penicillin antibiotics (ampicillin, carbenicillin, penicillin G) respond to treatment with MEFOXIN. Many infections caused by mixtures of susceptible aerobic and anaerobic bacteria respond to treatment with MEFOXIN.

Prevention

When compared to placebo in randomized controlled studies in patients undergoing gastrointestinal surgery, vaginal hysterectomy, abdominal hysterectomy and cesarean section, the prophylactic use of MEFOXIN resulted in a significant reduction in the number of postoperative infections.

The prophylactic administration of MEFOXIN perioperatively (preoperatively, intraoperatively, and postoperatively) may reduce the incidence of certain postoperative infections in patients undergoing surgical procedures (e.g., hysterectomy, gastrointestinal surgery and transurethral prostatectomy) that are classified as contaminated or potentially contaminated.

The perioperative use of MEFOXIN may be effective in surgical patients in whom infection at the operative site would present a serious risk, e.g., prosthetic arthroplasty.

In patients undergoing cesarean section, intraoperative (after clamping the umbilical cord) and postoperative use of MEFOXIN may reduce the incidence of certain postoperative infections.

Effective prophylactic use depends on the

*B. fragilis, B. distasonis, B. ovatus, B. thetaiotaomicron, B. vulgatus.

time of administration. MEFOXIN usually should be given one-half to one hour before the operation, which is sufficient time to achieve effective levels in the wound during the procedure. Prophylactic administration should usually be stopped within 24 hours since continuing administration of any antibiotic increases the possibility of adverse reactions but, in the majority of surgical procedures, does not reduce the incidence of subsequent infection. However, in patients undergoing prosthetic arthroplasty, it is recommended that MEFOXIN be continued for 72 hours after the surgical procedure.

If there are signs of infection, specimens for culture should be obtained for identification of the causative organism so that appropriate therapy may be instituted.

CONTRAINDICATIONS

MEFOXIN is contraindicated in patients who have shown hypersensitivity to cefoxitin and the cephalosporin group of antibiotics.

WARNINGS

BEFORE THERAPY WITH MEFOXIN IS INSTITUTED, CAREFUL INQUIRY SHOULD BE MADE TO DETERMINE WHETHER THE PATIENT HAS HAD PREVIOUS HYPERSENSITIVITY REACTIONS TO CEFOXITIN, CEPHALOSPORINS, PENICILLINS, OR OTHER DRUGS. THIS PRODUCT SHOULD BE GIVEN WITH CAUTION TO PENICILLIN-SENSITIVE PATIENTS. ANTIBIOTICS SHOULD BE ADMINISTERED WITH CAUTION TO ANY PATIENT WHO HAS DEMONSTRATED SOME FORM OF ALLERGY, PARTICULARLY TO DRUGS. IF AN ALLERGIC REACTION TO MEFOXIN OCCURS, DISCONTINUE THE DRUG. SERIOUS HYPERSENSITIVITY REACTIONS MAY REQUIRE EPINEPHRINE AND OTHER EMERGENCY MEASURES.

Pseudomembranous colitis has been reported with virtually all antibiotics (including cephalosporins); therefore, it is important to consider its diagnosis in patients who develop diarrhea in association with antibiotic use. This colitis may range from mild to life threatening in severity.

Treatment with broad-spectrum antibiotics alters normal flora of the colon and may permit overgrowth of clostridia. Studies indicate a toxin produced by *Clostridium difficile* is one primary cause of antibiotic-associated colitis.

Mild cases of pseudomembranous colitis may

MEFOXIN®
(Sterile Cefoxitin Sodium, MSD)

respond to drug discontinuance alone. In more severe cases, management may include sigmoidoscopy, appropriate bacteriological studies, fluid, electrolyte and protein supplementation, and the use of a drug such as oral vancomycin as indicated. Isolation of the patient may be advisable. Other causes of colitis should also be considered.

PRECAUTIONS

General

The total daily dose should be reduced when MEFOXIN is administered to patients with transient or persistent reduction of urinary output due to renal insufficiency (see DOSAGE), because high and prolonged serum antibiotic concentrations can occur in such individuals from usual doses.

Antibiotics (including cephalosporins) should be prescribed with caution in individuals with a history of gastrointestinal disease, particularly colitis.

As with other antibiotics, prolonged use of MEFOXIN may result in overgrowth of nonsusceptible organisms. Repeated evaluation of the patient's condition is essential. If superinfection occurs during therapy, appropriate measures should be taken.

Drug Interactions

Increased nephrotoxicity has been reported following concomitant administration of cephalosporins and aminoglycoside antibiotics.

Drug/Laboratory Test Interactions

As with cephalothin, high concentrations of cefoxitin (>100 micrograms/mL) may interfere with measurement of serum and urine creatinine levels by the Jaffé reaction, and produce false increases of modest degree in the levels of creatinine reported. Serum samples from patients treated with cefoxitin should not be analyzed for creatinine if withdrawn within 2 hours of drug administration.

High concentrations of cefoxitin in the urine may interfere with measurement of urinary 17-hydroxy-corticosteroids by the Porter-Silber reaction, and produce false increases of modest degree in the levels reported.

A false-positive reaction for glucose in the urine may occur. This has been observed with CLINITEST* reagent tablets.

Carcinogenesis, Mutagenesis, Impairment of Fertility

Long-term studies in animals have not been

*Registered trademark of Ames Company, Division of Miles Laboratories, Inc.

MEFOXIN®
(Sterile Cefoxitin Sodium, MSD)

performed with cefoxitin to evaluate carcinogenic or mutagenic potential. Studies in rats treated intravenously with 400 mg/kg of cefoxitin (approximately three times the maximum recommended human dose) revealed no effects on fertility or mating ability.

Pregnancy

Pregnancy Category B. Reproduction studies performed in rats and mice at parenteral doses of approximately one to seven and one-half times the maximum recommended human dose did not reveal teratogenic or fetal toxic effects, although a slight decrease in fetal weight was observed.

There are, however, no adequate and well-controlled studies in pregnant women. Because animal reproduction studies are not always predictive of human response, this drug should be used during pregnancy only if clearly needed.

In the rabbit, cefoxitin was associated with a high incidence of abortion and maternal death. This was not considered to be a teratogenic effect but an expected consequence of the rabbit's unusual sensitivity to antibiotic-induced changes in the population of the microflora of the intestine.

Nursing Mothers

MEFOXIN is excreted in human milk in low concentrations. Caution should be exercised when MEFOXIN is administered to a nursing woman.

Pediatric Use

Safety and efficacy in infants from birth to three months of age have not yet been established. In children three months of age and older, higher doses of MEFOXIN have been associated with an increased incidence of eosinophilia and elevated SGOT.

ADVERSE REACTIONS

MEFOXIN is generally well tolerated. The most common adverse reactions have been local reactions following intravenous or intramuscular injection. Other adverse reactions have been encountered infrequently.

Local Reactions

Thrombophlebitis has occurred with intravenous administration. Pain, induration, and tenderness after intramuscular injections have been reported.

Allergic Reactions

Rash (including exfoliative dermatitis), pruritus, eosinophilia, fever, and other allergic reactions including anaphylaxis have been noted.

Cardiovascular

Hypotension

Gastrointestinal

Diarrhea, including documented pseudo-membranous colitis which can appear during or after antibiotic treatment. Nausea and vomiting have been reported rarely.

Blood

Eosinophilia, leukopenia, including granulo-cytopenia, neutropenia, anemia, including he-molytic anemia, thrombocytopenia, and bone marrow depression. A positive direct Coombs test may develop in some individuals, especially those with azotemia.

Liver Function

Transient elevations in SGOT, SGPT, serum LDH, and serum alkaline phosphatase have been reported.

Renal Function

Elevations in serum creatinine and/or blood urea nitrogen levels have been observed. As with the cephalosporins, acute renal failure has been reported rarely. The role of MEFOXIN in changes in renal function tests is difficult to assess, since factors predisposing to prerenal azotemia or to impaired renal function usually have been present.

OVERDOSAGE

The acute intravenous LD_{50} in the adult female mouse and rabbit was about 8.0 g/kg and greater than 1.0 g/kg respectively. The acute intraperitoneal LD_{50} in the adult rat was greater than 10.0 g/kg.

DOSAGE

TREATMENT

Adults

The usual adult dosage range is 1 gram to 2 grams every six to eight hours. Dosage and route of administration should be determined by susceptibility of the causative organisms, sever-ity of infection, and the condition of the patient (see Table 1 for dosage guidelines).

In adults with renal insufficiency, an initial loading dose of 1 gram to 2 grams may be giv-en. After a loading dose, the recommendations for *maintenance dosage* (Table 2) may be used as a guide.

When only the serum creatinine level is available, the following formula (based on sex, weight, and age of the patient) may be used to convert this value into creatinine clearance. The serum creatinine should represent a steady state of renal function.

Table 1—Guidelines for Dosage of MEFOXIN		
Type of Infection	Daily Dosage	Frequency and Route
Uncomplicated forms* of infections such as pneumonia, urinary tract infection, cutaneous infection	3-4 grams	1 gram every 6-8 hours IV or IM
Moderately severe or severe infections	6-8 grams	1 gram every 4 hours *or* 2 grams every 6-8 hours IV
Infections commonly needing antibiotics in higher dosage (e.g., gas gangrene)	12 grams	2 grams every 4 hours *or* 3 grams every 6 hours IV

*Including patients in whom bacteremia is ab-sent or unlikely.

$$\text{Males:} \quad \frac{\text{Weight (kg)} \times (140 - \text{age})}{72 \times \text{serum creatinine (mg/100 mL)}}$$

Females: $0.85 \times$ above value

MEFOXIN may be used in patients with re-duced renal function with the following dosage adjustments:

Table 2—Maintenance Dosage of MEFOXIN in Adults with Reduced Renal Function			
Renal Function	Creatinine Clearance (mL/min)	Dose (grams)	Frequency
Mild impairment	50-30	1-2	every 8-12 hours
Moderate impairment	29-10	1-2	every 12-24 hours
Severe impairment	9-5	0.5-1	every 12-24 hours
Essentially no function	<5	0.5-1	every 24-48 hours

In patients undergoing hemodialysis, the loading dose of 1 to 2 grams should be given after each hemodialysis, and the maintenance dose should be given as indicated in Table 2.

Antibiotic therapy for group A beta-hemolytic streptococcal infections should be maintained for at least 10 days to guard against the risk of rheumatic fever or glomerulonephritis. In staph-ylococcal and other infections involving a collec-tion of pus, surgical drainage should be carried out where indicated.

The recommended dosage of MEFOXIN **for uncomplicated gonorrhea** is 2 grams intra-muscularly, with 1 gram of BENEMID* (Pro-

*Registered trademark of MERCK & CO., INC.

benecid, MSD) given by mouth at the same time or up to ½ hour before MEFOXIN.

Infants and Children

The recommended dosage in children three months of age and older is 80 to 160 mg/kg of body weight per day divided into four to six equal doses. The higher dosages should be used for more severe or serious infections. The total daily dosage should not exceed 12 grams.

At this time no recommendation is made for children from birth to three months of age (See PRECAUTIONS).

In children with renal insufficiency the dosage and frequency of dosage should be modified consistent with the recommendations for adults (see Table 2).

PREVENTION

For prophylactic use, the following doses are recommended:

Adults:

(1) 2 grams administered intravenously or intramuscularly just prior to surgery (approximately one-half to one hour before the initial incision).

(2) 2 grams every 6 hours after the first dose for no more than 24 hours (continued for 72 hours after prosthetic arthroplasty).

Children (3 months and older):

30 to 40 mg/kg doses may be given at the times designated above.

Cesarean section patients:

The first dose of 2.0 grams is administered intravenously as soon as the umbilical cord is clamped. The second and third doses should be given as 2.0 grams intravenously or intramuscularly 4 hours and 8 hours after the first dose. Subsequent doses may be given every 6 hours for no more than 24 hours.

Transurethral prostatectomy patients:

One gram administered just prior to surgery; 1 gram every 8 hours for up to five days.

PREPARATION OF SOLUTION

Table 3 is provided for convenience in constituting MEFOXIN for both intravenous and intramuscular administration.

For intravenous use, 1 gram should be constituted with at least 10 mL of Sterile Water for Injection, and 2 grams, with 10 or 20 mL. The 10 gram bulk package should be constituted with 50 or 100 mL of Sterile Water for Injection or any of the solutions listed under the *Intravenous* portion of the COMPATIBILITY AND STABILITY section. CAUTION: NOT FOR DIRECT INFU-

Table 3—Preparation of Solution			
Strength	Amount of Diluent to be Added (mL)*	Approximate Withdrawable Volume (mL)	Approximate Average Concentration (mg/mL)
1 gram Vial	2 (Intramuscular)	2.5	400
2 gram Vial	4 (Intramuscular)	5	400
1 gram Vial	10 (IV)	10.5	95
2 gram Vial	10 or 20 (IV)	11.1 or 21.0	180 or 95
1 gram Infusion Bottle	50 or 100 (IV)	50 or 100	20 or 10
2 gram Infusion Bottle	50 or 100 (IV)	50 or 100	40 or 20
10 gram Bulk	50 or 100 (IV)	55 or 105	180 or 95

*Shake to dissolve and let stand until clear.

SION. One or 2 grams of MEFOXIN for infusion may be constituted with 50 or 100 mL of 0.9 percent Sodium Chloride Injection, 5 percent or 10 percent Dextrose Injection, or any of the solutions listed under the *Intravenous* portion of the COMPATIBILITY AND STABILITY section.

Benzyl alcohol as a preservative has been associated with toxicity in neonates. While toxicity has not been demonstrated in infants greater than three months of age, in whom use of MEFOXIN may be indicated, small infants in this age range may also be at risk for benzyl alcohol toxicity. Therefore, diluent containing benzyl alcohol should not be used when MEFOXIN is constituted for administration to infants.

For intramuscular use, each gram of MEFOXIN may be constituted with 2 mL of Sterile Water for Injection, *or—*

For intramuscular use ONLY: each gram of MEFOXIN may be constituted with 2 mL of 0.5 percent lidocaine hydrochloride solution* (without epinephrine) to minimize the discomfort of intramuscular injection.

ADMINISTRATION

MEFOXIN may be administered intravenously or intramuscularly after constitution.

Parenteral drug products should be inspected

*See package circular of manufacturer for detailed information concerning contraindications, warnings, precautions, and adverse reactions.

visually for particulate matter and discoloration prior to administration whenever solution and container permit.

Intravenous Administration

The intravenous route is preferable for patients with bacteremia, bacterial septicemia, or other severe or life-threatening infections, or for patients who may be poor risks because of lowered resistance resulting from such debilitating conditions as malnutrition, trauma, surgery, diabetes, heart failure, or malignancy, particularly if shock is present or impending.

For intermittent intravenous administration, a solution containing 1 gram or 2 grams in 10 mL of Sterile Water for Injection can be injected over a period of three to five minutes. Using an infusion system, it may also be given over a longer period of time through the tubing system by which the patient may be receiving other intravenous solutions. However, during infusion of the solution containing MEFOXIN, it is advisable to temporarily discontinue administration of any other solutions at the same site.

For the administration of higher doses by continuous intravenous infusion, a solution of MEFOXIN may be added to an intravenous bottle containing 5 percent Dextrose Injection, 0.9 percent Sodium Chloride Injection, 5 percent Dextrose and 0.9 percent Sodium Chloride Injection, or 5 percent Dextrose Injection with 0.02 percent sodium bicarbonate solution. BUTTERFLY* or scalp vein-type needles are preferred for this type of infusion.

Solutions of MEFOXIN, like those of most beta-lactam antibiotics, should not be added to aminoglycoside solutions (e.g., gentamicin sulfate, tobramycin sulfate, amikacin sulfate) because of potential interaction. However, MEFOXIN and aminoglycosides may be administered separately to the same patient.

Intramuscular Administration

As with all intramuscular preparations, MEFOXIN should be injected well within the body of a relatively large muscle such as the upper outer quadrant of the buttock (i.e., gluteus maximus); aspiration is necessary to avoid inadvertent injection into a blood vessel.

COMPATIBILITY AND STABILITY

Intravenous

MEFOXIN, as supplied in vials or the bulk package and constituted to 1 gram/10 mL with

---

*Registered trademark of Abbott Laboratories.

Sterile Water for Injection, Bacteriostatic Water for Injection, (see PREPARATION OF SOLUTION), 0.9 percent Sodium Chloride Injection, or 5 percent Dextrose Injection, maintains satisfactory potency for 24 hours at room temperature, for one week under refrigeration (below 5°C), and for at least 30 weeks in the frozen state.

These primary solutions may be futher diluted in 50 to 1000 mL of the following solutions and maintain potency for 24 hours at room temperature and at least 48 hours under refrigeration:

Sterile Water for Injection[†]
0.9 percent Sodium Chloride Injection
5 percent or 10 percent Dextrose Injection[†]
5 percent Dextrose and 0.9 percent Sodium Chloride Injection
5 percent Dextrose Injection with 0.02 percent sodium bicarbonate solution
5 percent Dextrose Injection with 0.2 percent or 0.45 percent saline solution
Ringer's Injection
Lactated Ringer's Injection[†]
5 percent Dextrose in Lactated Ringer's Injection[†]
5 percent or 10 percent invert sugar in water
10 percent invert sugar in saline solution
5 percent Sodium Bicarbonate Injection
Neut (sodium bicarbonate)*[†]
M/6 sodium lactate solution
AMINOSOL* 5 percent Solution
NORMOSOL-M in D5-W*[†]
IONOSOL B w/Dextrose 5 percent*[†]
POLYONIC M 56 in 5 percent Dextrose**
Mannitol 5% and 2.5%
Mannitol 10%[†]
ISOLYTE*** E
ISOLYTE*** E with 5% Dextrose

MEFOXIN, as supplied in infusion bottles and constituted with 50 to 100 mL of 0.9 percent Sodium Chloride Injection, or 5 percent or 10 percent Dextrose Injection, maintains satisfactory potency for 24 hours at room temperature or for 1 week under refrigeration (below 5°C).

Limited studies with solutions of MEFOXIN in 0.9 percent Sodium Chloride Injection, Lactated Ringer's Injection, and 5 percent Dextrose Injec-

---

*Registered trademark of Abbott Laboratories.
**Registered trademark of Cutter Laboratories, Inc.
***Registered trademark of American Hospital Supply Corporation.
[†]In these solutions, MEFOXIN has been found to be stable for a period of one week under refrigeration.

MEFOXIN®
(Sterile Cefoxitin Sodium, MSD)

tion in VIAFLEX* intravenous bags show stability for 24 hours at room temperature, 48 hours under refrigeration, 26 weeks in the frozen state, and 24 hours at room temperature thereafter. Also, solutions of MEFOXIN in 0.9 percent Sodium Chloride Injection show similar stability in plastic tubing, drip chambers, and volume control devices of common intravenous infusion sets.

After constitution with Sterile Water for Injection and subsequent storage in disposable plastic syringes, MEFOXIN is stable for 24 hours at room temperature and 48 hours under refrigeration.

After the periods mentioned above, any unused solutions or frozen material should be discarded. Do not refreeze.

Intramuscular

MEFOXIN, as constituted with Sterile Water for Injection, Bacteriostatic Water for Injection, or 0.5 percent or 1 percent lidocaine hydrochloride solution (without epinephrine), maintains satisfactory potency for 24 hours at room temperature, for one week under refrigeration (below 5°C), and for at least 30 weeks in the frozen state.

After the periods mentioned above, any unused solutions or frozen material should be discarded. Do not refreeze.

MEFOXIN has also been found compatible when admixed in intravenous infusions with the following:

Heparin 0.1 units/mL at room temperature—8 hours

Heparin 100 units/mL at room temperature—24 hours.

M.V.I.** concentrate at room temperature 24 hours; under refrigeration 48 hours

BEROCCA*** C-500 at room temperature 24 hours; under refrigeration 48 hours

Insulin in Normal Saline at room temperature 24 hours; under refrigeration 48 hours

Insulin in 10% invert sugar at room temperature 24 hours; under refrigeration 48 hours

HOW SUPPLIED

Sterile MEFOXIN is a dry white to off-white powder supplied in vials and infusion bottles containing cefoxitin sodium as follows:
No. 3356—1 gram cefoxitin equivalent
   NDC 0006-3356-71 in trays of 10 vials.

*Registered trademark of Travenol Laboratories, Inc.
**Registered trademark of USV Pharmaceutical Corp.
***Registered trademark of Roche Laboratories.

MEFOXIN®
(Sterile Cefoxitin Sodium, MSD)

NDC 0006-3356-45 in trays of 25 vials.
No. 3368—1 gram cefoxitin equivalent
   NDC 0006-3368-71 in trays of 10 infusion bottles.
No. 3357—2 gram cefoxitin equivalent
   NDC 0006-3357-73 in trays of 10 vials.
   NDC 0006-3357-53 in trays of 25 vials.
No. 3369—2 gram cefoxitin equivalent
   NDC 0006-3369-73 in trays of 10 infusion bottles.
No. 3388—10 gram cefoxitin equivalent
   NDC 0006-3388-10 in bulk bottles.

Special storage instructions

MEFOXIN in the dry state should be stored below 30°C. Avoid exposure to temperatures above 50°C. The dry material as well as solutions tend to darken, depending on storage conditions; product potency, however, is not adversely affected.

A.H.F.S. Category: 8:12.28

Issued July 1985   DC 7057120

INJECTION

PRIMAXIN®

(IMIPENEM-CILASTATIN SODIUM, MSD)

DESCRIPTION

PRIMAXIN† (Imipenem-Cilastatin Sodium, MSD) is a formulation of imipenem, a thienamycin antibiotic, and cilastatin sodium, the inhibitor of the renal dipeptidase, dehydropeptidase I, with sodium bicarbonate added as a buffer. PRIMAXIN is a potent broad spectrum antibacterial agent for intravenous administration.

Imipenem (N-formimidoylthienamycin monohydrate) is a crystalline derivative of thienamycin, which is produced by *Streptomyces cattleya*. Its chemical name is [5R-[5α, 6α (R*)]]-6-(1-hydroxyethyl)-3-[[2-[(iminomethyl)amino] ethyl]thio]-7-oxo-1-azabicyclo [3.2.0] hept-2-ene-2-carboxylic

†Registered Trademark of Merck & CO., INC.
COPYRIGHT © MERCK & CO., INC., 1985
All rights reserved

PRIMAXIN®
(Imipenem-Cilastatin Sodium, MSD)

acid monohydrate. It is an off-white, non-hygroscopic crystalline compound with a molecular weight of 317.37. It is sparingly soluble in water, and slightly soluble in methanol. Its empirical formula is $C_{12}H_{17}N_3O_4S \cdot H_2O$, and its structural formula is:

Cilastatin sodium is the sodium salt of a derivatized heptenoic acid. Its chemical name is [Z, 7(R),2(S)]-7-[(2-amino-2-carboxyethyl)thio]-2-[[(2,2-dimethyl-cyclopropyl)carbonyl]amino]-2-heptenoic acid mono-sodium salt. It is an off-white to yellowish-white, hygroscopic, amorphous compound with a molecular weight of 380.43. It is very soluble in water and in methanol. Its empirical formula is $C_{16}H_{25}N_2O_5S$ Na, and its structural formula is:

PRIMAXIN is buffered to provide solutions in the pH range of 6.5 to 7.5. There is no significant change in pH when solutions are prepared and used as directed. (See COMPATIBILITY AND STABILITY.) PRIMAXIN 250 contains 18.8 mg of sodium (0.8 mEq) and PRIMAXIN 500 contains 37.5 mg of sodium (1.6 mEq). Solutions of PRIMAXIN range from colorless to yellow. Variations of color within this range do not affect the potency of the product.

CLINICAL PHARMACOLOGY

Intravenous Administration

Intravenous infusion of PRIMAXIN over 20 minutes results in peak plasma levels of imipenem antimicrobial activity that range from 14 to 24 mcg/mL for the 250 mg dose, from 21 to 58 mcg/mL for the 500 mg dose and from 41 to 83 mcg/mL for the 1000 mg dose. At these doses, plasma levels of imipenem antimicrobial activity decline to below 1 mcg/mL

or less in 4 to 6 hours. Peak plasma levels of cilastatin following a 20-minute intravenous infusion of PRIMAXIN, range from 15 to 25 mcg/mL for the 250 mg dose, from 31 to 49 mcg/mL for the 500 mg dose and from 56 to 88 mcg/mL for the 1000 mg dose.

General

The plasma half-life of each component is approximately 1 hour. The binding of imipenem to human serum proteins is approximately 20% and that of cilastatin is approximately 40%. Approximately 70% of the administered imipenem is recovered in the urine within 10 hours after which no further urinary excretion is detectable. Urine concentrations of imipenem in excess of 10 mcg/mL can be maintained for up to 8 hours with PRIMAXIN at the 500 mg dose. Approximately 70% of the cilastatin sodium dose is recovered in the urine within 10 hours of administration of PRIMAXIN.

No accumulation of PRIMAXIN in plasma or urine is observed with regimens administered as frequently as every 6 hours in patients with normal renal function.

Imipenem, when administered alone, is metabolized in the kidneys by dehydropeptidase I resulting in relatively low levels in urine. Cilastatin sodium, an inhibitor of this enzyme, effectively prevents renal metabolism of imipenem so that when imipenem and cilastatin sodium are given concomitantly fully adequate antibacterial levels of imipenem are achieved in the urine.

After a 1 gram dose, the following average levels of imipenem were measured (usually at 1 hour post-dose) in the tissues and fluids listed:

sputum	2.1 mcg/mL
pleural	22.0 mcg/mL
peritoneal	3.9 mcg/mL
bile	2.5 mcg/mL
aqueous humor	1.8 mcg/mL
interstitial fluid	16.0 mcg/mL
CSF (uninflamed meninges)	0.8 mcg/mL
reproductive organs	4.3 mcg/g (2½ hours post-dose)
bone	2.4 mcg/g

Microbiology

The bactericidal activity of imipenem results from the inhibition of cell wall synthesis. Its greatest affinity is for penicillin binding proteins (PBP) 1A, 1B, 2, 4, 5, and 6 of *Escherichia coli*, and 1A, 1B, 2, 4 and 5 of *Pseudomonas aeruginosa*. The lethal effect is related to binding to PBP 2 and PBP 1B. Imipenem has *in vitro* activity against a wide range of gram-positive and gram-negative organisms.

Imipenem has a high degree of stability in the presence of beta-lactamases, both penicillinases and cephalosporinases produced by gram-negative and gram-positive bacteria. It is a potent inhibitor of beta-lactamases from certain gram-negative bacteria which are inherently resistant to most beta-lactam antibiotics, e.g., *Pseudomonas aeruginosa*, *Serratia* spp., and *Enterobacter* spp.

In vitro, imipenem is active against most strains of clinical isolates of the following microorganisms:

Gram-positive:
Group D streptococci (including enterococci e.g., *Streptococcus faecalis*)
NOTE: Imipenem is inactive against *Streptococcus faecium*.
Streptococcus pyogenes (Group A streptococci)
Streptococcus agalactiae (Group B streptococci)
Group C streptococci
Group G streptococci
Viridans streptococci
Streptococcus pneumoniae (formerly *Diplococcus pneumoniae*)
Staphylococcus aureus including penicillinase producing strains
Staphylococcus epidermidis including penicillinase producing strains
NOTE: Many strains of methicillin-resistant staphylococci are resistant to imipenem.

Gram-negative:
Escherichia coli
Proteus mirabilis
Proteus vulgaris
Morganella morganii
Providencia rettgeri
Providencia stuartii
Citrobacter spp.
Klebsiella spp. including *K. pneumoniae* and *K. oxytoca*
Enterobacter spp.
Hafnia spp. including *H. alvei*
Serratia marcescens
Serratia spp. including *S. liquefaciens*
Haemophilus parainfluenzae
H. influenzae
Gardnerella vaginalis
Acinetobacter spp.
Pseudomonas aeruginosa
NOTE: Imipenem is inactive against *P. maltophilia* and some strains of *P. cepacia*

Anaerobes:
Bacteroides spp. including *Bacteroides bivius*, *Bacteroides fragilis*, *Bacteroides melaninogenicus*
Clostridium spp. including *C. perfringens*
Eubacterium spp.
Fusobacterium spp.
Peptococcus spp.
Peptostreptococcus spp.
Propionibacterium spp. including *P. acnes*
Actinomyces spp.
Veillonella spp.

Imipenem has been shown to be active *in vitro* against the following microorganisms; however, clinical efficacy has not yet been established.

Gram-positive:
Listeria monocytogenes
Nocardia spp.

Gram-negative:
Salmonella spp.
Shigella spp.
Yersinia spp. including *Yersinia enterocolitica*, *Yersinia pseudotuberculosis*
Bordetella bronchiseptica
Campylobacter spp.
Achromobacter spp.
Alcaligenes spp.
Moraxella spp.
Pasteurella multocida
Aeromonas hydrophila
Plesiomonas shigelloides
Neisseria gonorrhoeae (including penicillinase-producing strains)

Anaerobes:
Bacteroides asaccharolyticus
Bacteroides disiens
Bacteroides distasonis
Bacteroides ovatus
Bacteroides thetaiotaomicron
Bacteroides vulgatus

In vitro tests show imipenem to act synergistically with aminoglycoside antibiotics against some isolates of *Pseudomonas aeruginosa*.

PRIMAXIN®
(Imipenem-Cilastatin Sodium, MSD)

Susceptibility Testing

Quantitative methods that require measurement of zone diameters give the most precise estimate of antibiotic susceptibility. One such procedure has been recommended for use with discs to test susceptibility to imipenem.

Reports from the laboratory giving results of the standard single-disc susceptibility test with a 10 mcg imipenem disc should be interpreted according to the following criteria.

Susceptible organisms produce zones of 16 mm or greater, indicating that the test organism is likely to respond to therapy.

Organisms that produce zones of 14 to 15 mm are expected to be susceptible if high dosage is used or if the infection is confined to tissues and fluids in which high antibiotic levels are attained.

Resistant organisms produce zones of 13 mm or less, indicating that other therapy should be selected.

A bacterial isolate may be considered susceptible if the MIC value for imipenem is equal to or less than 8 mcg/mL. Organisms are considered resistant if the MIC is equal to or greater than 16 mcg/mL.

The standardized quality control procedure requires use of control organisms. The 10 mcg imipenem disc should give the zone diameters listed below for the quality control strains.

Organism	ATCC	Zone Size Range
E. coli	25922	27-31 mm
Ps. aeruginosa	27853	20-28 mm

Dilution susceptibility tests should give MICs between the ranges listed below for the quality control strains.

Organism	ATCC	MIC (mcg/mL)
E. coli	25922	0.06-0.25
S. aureus	29213	0.008-0.03
S. faecalis	29212	0.25-1.0
Ps. aeruginosa	27853	1.0-4.0

Based on blood levels of imipenem achieved in man, breakpoint criteria have been established for imipenem.

Category	Zone Diameter (mm)	Recommended MIC Breakpoint (mcg/mL)
Susceptible	≥16	≤8
Moderately Susceptible	14-15	
Resistant	≤13	≥16

INDICATIONS AND USAGE

PRIMAXIN is indicated for the treatment of serious infections caused by susceptible strains of the designated microorganisms in the diseases listed below:

(1) **Lower respiratory tract infections.** *Staphylococcus aureus* (penicillinase producing strains)*, *Escherichia coli, Klebsiella* species, *Enterobacter* species, *Haemophilus influenzae, Haemophilus parainfluenzae**, *Acinetobacter* species*, *Serratia marcescens**.

(2) **Urinary tract infections** (Complicated and uncomplicated). *Staphylococcus aureus* (penicillinase producing strains)*, Group D streptococci (enterococci), *Escherichia coli, Klebsiella* species, *Enterobacter* species, *Proteus vulgaris**, *Providencia rettgeri**, *Morganella morganii**, *Pseudomonas aeruginosa*.

(3) **Intra-abdominal infections.** *Staphylococcus aureus* (penicillinase producing strains)*, *Staphylococcus epidermidis**, Group D streptococci (enterococci), *Escherichia coli, Klebsiella* species, *Enterobacter* species, *Proteus* species (indole positive and indole negative), *Morganella morganii**, *Pseudomonas aeruginosa, Citrobacter* species*, *Clostridium* species, Gram-positive anaerobes, including *Peptococcus* species*, *Peptostreptococcus* species*, *Eubacterium* species, *Propionibacterium* species*, *Bifidobacterium* species, *Bacteroides* species, including *B. fragilis, Fusobacterium* species*.

(4) **Gynecologic infections.** *Staphylococcus aureus* (penicillinase producing strains)*, *Staphylococcus epidermidis,* Group B streptococci, Group D streptococci (enterococci), *Escherichia coli, Klebsiella* species*, *Proteus* species (indole positive and indole negative)*, *Enterobacter* species*, Gram-positive anaerobes, including *Peptococcus* species*, *Peptostreptococcus* species*, *Propionibacterium* species*, *Bifidobacterium* species*, *Bacteroides* species, *B. fragilis**, *Gardnerella vaginalis**.

(5) **Bacterial septicemia.** *Staphylococcus aureus* (penicillinase producing strains), Group D streptococci (enterococci)*, *Escherichia coli, Klebsiella* species*, *Pseudomonas aeruginosa**, *Serratia* species*, *Enterobacter* species*, *Bacteroides* species, *B. fragilis**.

*Efficacy for this organism in this organ system was demonstrated in less than 10 infections.

(6) **Bone and joint infections.** *Staphylococcus aureus* (penicillinase producing strains), *Staphylococcus epidermidis**, Group D streptococci (enterococci)*, *Enterobacter* species*, *Pseudomonas aeruginosa*.

(7) **Skin and skin structure infections.** *Staphylococcus aureus* (penicillinase producing strains), *Staphylococcus epidermidis*, Group D streptococci (enterococci), *Escherichia coli*, *Klebsiella* species, *Enterobacter* species, *Proteus vulgaris**, *Providencia rettgeri**, *Morganella morganii*, *Pseudomonas aeruginosa*, *Serratia* species, *Citrobacter* species*, *Acinetobacter* species*, Gram-positive anaerobes, including *Peptococcus* species and *Peptostreptococcus* species, *Bacteroides* species, including *B. fragilis*, *Fusobacterium* species*.

(8) **Endocarditis.** *Staphylococcus aureus* (penicillinase producing strains).

(9) **Polymicrobic infections.** PRIMAXIN is indicated for polymicrobic infections including those in which *S. pneumoniae* (pneumonia, septicemia), Group A beta-hemolytic streptococcus (skin and skin structure), or nonpenicillinase-producing *S. aureus* is one of the causative organisms. However monobacterial infections due to these organisms are usually treated with narrower spectrum antibiotics, such as penicillin G.

Although clinical improvement has been observed in patients with cystic fibrosis, chronic pulmonary disease, and lower respiratory tract infections caused by *Pseudomonas aeruginosa*, bacterial eradication may not necessarily be achieved.

As with other beta-lactam antibiotics, some strains of *Pseudomonas aeruginosa* may develop resistance fairly rapidly on treatment with PRIMAXIN. When clinically appropriate during therapy of *Pseudomonas aeruginosa* infections, periodic susceptibility testing should be done.

Infections resistant to other antibiotics, for example, cephalosporins, penicillin, and aminoglycosides, have been shown to respond to treatment with PRIMAXIN.

CONTRAINDICATIONS

PRIMAXIN is contraindicated in patients who have shown hypersensitivity to any component of this product.

*Efficacy for this organism in this organ system was demonstrated in less than 10 infections.

PRIMAXIN®
(Imipenem-Cilastatin Sodium, MSD)

WARNINGS

SERIOUS AND OCCASIONALLY FATAL HYPERSENSITIVITY (anaphylactic) REACTIONS HAVE BEEN REPORTED IN PATIENTS RECEIVING THERAPY WITH BETA-LACTAMS. THESE REACTIONS ARE MORE APT TO OCCUR IN PERSONS WITH A HISTORY OF SENSITIVITY TO MULTIPLE ALLERGENS.

THERE HAVE BEEN REPORTS OF PATIENTS WITH A HISTORY OF PENICILLIN HYPERSENSITIVITY WHO HAVE EXPERIENCED SEVERE HYPERSENSITIVITY REACTIONS WHEN TREATED WITH ANOTHER BETA-LACTAM. BEFORE INITIATING THERAPY WITH PRIMAXIN, CAREFUL INQUIRY SHOULD BE MADE CONCERNING PREVIOUS HYPERSENSITIVITY REACTIONS TO PENICILLINS, CEPHALOSPORINS, OTHER BETA-LACTAMS, AND OTHER ALLERGENS. IF AN ALLERGIC REACTION TO PRIMAXIN OCCURS, DISCONTINUE THE DRUG. SERIOUS HYPERSENSITIVITY REACTIONS MAY REQUIRE EPINEPHRINE AND OTHER EMERGENCY MEASURES.

Pseudomembranous colitis has been reported with virtually all antibiotics, including PRIMAXIN; therefore it is important to consider its diagnosis in patients who develop diarrhea in association with antibiotic use. This colitis may range in severity from mild to life threatening.

Mild cases of pseudomembranous colitis may respond to drug discontinuance alone. In more severe cases, management may include sigmoidoscopy, appropriate bacteriological studies, fluid, electrolyte and protein supplementation, and the use of a drug such as oral vancomycin, as indicated. Isolation of the patient may be advisable. Other causes of colitis should also be considered.

PRECAUTIONS

General

CNS adverse experiences such as myoclonic activity, confusional states, or seizures have been reported with PRIMAXIN. These experiences have occurred most commonly in patients with CNS disorders (e.g., brain lesions or history of seizures) who also have compromised renal function. However, there were rare reports in which there was no recognized or documented underlying CNS disorder. Close adherence to recommended dosage schedules is urged especially in patients with known factors that predispose to seizures (see DOSAGE AND ADMINISTRATION). Anticonvulsant therapy should be continued in patients with a known seizure disorder. If focal tremors, myoclonus, or seizures occur, patients should be placed on anticonvulsant therapy. If CNS symptoms continue, the dosage of PRIMAXIN should be decreased or discontinued.

As with other antibiotics, prolonged use of PRIMAXIN may result in overgrowth of non-susceptible organisms. Repeated evaluation of the patient's condition is essential. If super-infection occurs during therapy, appropriate measures should be taken.

While PRIMAXIN possesses the characteristic low toxicity of the beta-lactam group of antibiotics, periodic assessment of organ system function during prolonged therapy is advisable.

Drug Interactions

Since concomitant administration of PRIMAXIN and probenecid results in only minimal increases in plasma levels of imipenem and plasma half-life, it is not recommended that probenecid be given with PRIMAXIN.

PRIMAXIN should not be mixed with or physically added to other antibiotics. However, PRIMAXIN may be administered concomitantly with other antibiotics, such as aminoglycosides.

Carcinogenesis, Mutagenesis, Impairment of Fertility

Gene toxicity studies were performed in a variety of bacterial and mammalian tests *in vivo* and *in vitro*. The tests were: V79 mammalian cell mutation assay (PRIMAXIN alone and imipenem alone), Ames test (cilastatin sodium alone), unscheduled DNA synthesis assay (PRIMAXIN) and *in vivo* mouse cytogenicity test (PRIMAXIN). None of these tests showed any evidence of genetic damage.

Reproduction tests in male and female rats were performed with PRIMAXIN at dosage levels up to 8 times the usual human dose. Slight decreases in live fetal body weight were restricted to the highest dosage level. No other adverse effects were observed on fertility, reproductive performance, fetal

viability, growth or postnatal development of pups. Similarly, no adverse effects on the fetus or on lactation were observed when PRIMAXIN was administered to rats late in gestation.

Pregnancy

Pregnancy Category C. Teratogenicity studies with cilastatin sodium in rabbits and rats at 10 and 33 times the usual human dose, respectively, showed no evidence of adverse effect on the fetus. No evidence of teratogenicity or adverse effect on postnatal growth or behavior was observed in rats given imipenem at dosage levels up to 30 times the usual human dose. Similarly, no evidence of adverse effect on the fetus was observed in teratology studies in rabbits with imipenem at dosage levels at the usual human dose.

Teratology studies with PRIMAXIN at doses up to 11 times the usual human dose in pregnant mice and rats during the period of major organogenesis revealed no evidence of teratogenicity.

Data from preliminary studies suggests an apparent intolerance to PRIMAXIN (including emesis, inappetence, body weight loss, diarrhea and death) at doses equivalent to the average human dose in pregnant rabbits and cynomolgus monkeys that is not seen in non-pregnant animals in these or other species. In other studies, PRIMAXIN was well tolerated in equivalent or higher doses (up to 11 times the average human dose) in pregnant rats and mice. Further studies are underway to evaluate these findings.

There are, however, no adequate and well-controlled studies in pregnant women. PRIMAXIN should be used during pregnancy only if the potential benefit justifies the potential risk to the fetus.

Nursing Mothers

It is not known whether this drug is excreted in human milk. Because many drugs are excreted in human milk, caution should be exercised when PRIMAXIN is administered to a nursing woman.

Pediatric Use

Safety and effectiveness in infants and children below 12 years of age have not yet been established.

ADVERSE REACTIONS

PRIMAXIN is generally well tolerated.

Many of the 1,723 patients treated in clinical trials were severely ill and had multiple background diseases and physiological impairments, making it difficult to determine causal relationship of adverse experiences to therapy with PRIMAXIN.

Local Adverse Reactions

Adverse local clinical reactions that were reported as possibly, probably or definitely related to therapy with PRIMAXIN were:

Phlebitis/thrombophlebitis—3.1%
Pain at the injection site—0.7%
Erythema at the injection site—0.4%
Vein induration—0.2%
Infused vein infection—0.1%

Systemic Adverse Reactions

The most frequently reported systemic adverse clinical reactions that were reported as possibly, probably, or definitely related to PRIMAXIN were nausea (2.0%), diarrhea (1.8%), vomiting (1.5%), rash (0.9%), fever (0.5%), hypotension (0.4%), seizures (0.4%) (see *PRECAUTIONS*), dizziness (0.3%), pruritus (0.3%), urticaria (0.2%), somnolence (0.2%).

Additional adverse systemic clinical reactions reported as possibly, probably or definitely drug related occurring in less than 0.2% of the patients are listed within each body system in order of decreasing severity: *Gastrointestinal*—pseudomembranous colitis (see WARNINGS), hemorrhagic colitis, gastroenteritis, abdominal pain, glossitis, tongue papillar hypertrophy, heartburn, pharyngeal pain, increased salivation; *CNS*—encephalopathy, confusion, myoclonus, paresthesia, vertigo, headache; *Special Senses*—transient hearing loss in patients with impaired hearing, tinnitus; *Respiratory*—chest discomfort, dyspnea, hyperventilation, thoracic spine pain; *Cardiovascular*—palpitations, tachycardia; *Renal*—oliguria/anuria, polyuria; *Skin*—erythema multiforme, facial edema, flushing, cyanosis, hyperhidrosis, skin texture changes, candidiasis, pruritis vulvae; *Body as a whole*—polyarthralgia, asthenia/weakness.

Adverse Laboratory Changes

Adverse laboratory changes without regard to drug relationship that were reported during clinical trials were:

Hepatic: Increased SGPT, SGOT, alkaline phosphatase, bilirubin and LDH.

Hemic: Increased eosinophils, positive Coombs test, decreased WBC and neutrophils, increased WBC, increased platelets, decreased platelets, decreased hemoglobin and hematocrit, increased monocytes, abnormal prothrombin time, increased lymphocytes, increased basophils.

Electrolytes: Decreased serum sodium, increased potassium, increased chloride.

Renal: Increased BUN, creatinine.

Urinalysis: Presence of urine protein, urine red blood cells, urine white blood cells, urine casts, urine bilirubin, and urine urobilinogen.

OVERDOSAGE

The intravenous LD_{50} of imipenem is greater than 2000 mg/kg in the rat and approximately 1500 mg/kg in the mouse.

The intravenous LD_{50} of cilastatin sodium is approximately 5000 mg/kg in the rat and approximately 8700 mg/kg in the mouse.

The intravenous LD_{50} of PRIMAXIN is approximately 1000 mg/kg/day in the rat and approximately 1100 mg/kg/day in the mouse.

Information on overdosage in humans is not available.

DOSAGE AND ADMINISTRATION

The dosage recommendations for PRIMAXIN represent the quantity of imipenem to be administered. An equivalent amount of cilastatin is also present in the solution.

Initially, the total daily dosage for PRIMAXIN should be based on the type or severity of infection and given in equally divided doses. Subsequent dosing must be based on consideration of severity of illness, degree of susceptibility of the pathogen(s), age, weight, and creatinine clearance.

Serum creatinine alone may not be a sufficiently accurate measure of renal function. Creatinine clearance (T_{cc}) may be estimated from the following equation:

$$T_{cc} \text{ (Males)} = \frac{\text{(wt. in kg) (140 - age)}}{\text{(72) (creatinine in mg/dL)}}$$

T_{cc} (Female) = 0.85 x above value

Each 250 mg or 500 mg dose should be given by intravenous infusion over twenty to thirty minutes. Each 1000 mg dose should be infused over forty to sixty minutes. In patients who develop nausea during the infusion, the rate of infusion may be slowed.

PRIMAXIN®
(Imipenem-Cilastatin Sodium, MSD)

INTRAVENOUS DOSING SCHEDULE
FOR ADULTS WITH
NORMAL RENAL FUNCTION

Type or severity of infection	Gram-positive organisms Anaerobes Highly susceptible gram-negative organisms	Other gram-negative organisms
Mild	250 mg q6h	500 mg q6h
Moderate	500 mg q8h- 500 mg q6h	500 mg q6h- 1 g q8h
Severe, life threatening	500 mg q6h	1 g q8h- 1 g q6h
Uncomplicated urinary tract infection	250 mg q6h	250 mg q6h
Complicated urinary tract infection	500 mg q6h	500 mg q6h

Due to the high antimicrobial activity of PRIMAXIN, it is recommended that the maximum total daily dosage not exceed 50 mg/kg/day or 4.0g/day, whichever is lower. There is no evidence that higher doses provide greater efficacy.

INTRAVENOUS DOSING SCHEDULE
FOR ADULTS WITH
IMPAIRED RENAL FUNCTION

Patients with creatinine clearance of ≤ 70 mL/min/1.73 m^2 require adjustment of the dosage of PRIMAXIN as indicated in the table below. Doses cited are in every case the imipenem component of a 1:1 ratio of imipenem:cilastatin Na and are based on a body weight of 70 kg. Proportionate reduction in dose administered should be made for patients with reduced body weight.

Intravenous Dosage of PRIMAXIN in Adults
With Impaired Renal Function

Creatinine Clearance (mL/min/ 1.73 m2)	Renal Function	Less Severe Infections or Presence of Highly Susceptible Organisms	Life Threatening Infections— Maximum Dosage
30-70	Mild Impairment	500 mg q8h	500 mg q6h
20-30	Moderate Impairment	500 mg q12h	500 mg q8h
5-20	Severe to Marked Impairment	250 mg q12h	500 mg q12h
0-5	None, but on hemodialysis	250 mg q12h	500 mg q12h

PRIMAXIN is cleared by hemodialysis. In patients undergoing hemodialysis, a supple-

PRIMAXIN®
(Imipenem-Cilastatin Sodium, MSD)

mental dose of PRIMAXIN should be given after hemodialysis unless the next dose is scheduled within four hours. The benefits versus the risks should be considered in patients on hemodialysis. Dialysis patients, especially those with CNS background diseases, should be carefully monitored (see PRECAUTIONS).

PREPARATION OF SOLUTION
120 mL Infusion Bottles

Contents of the 120 mL infusion bottles of PRIMAXIN Powder should be restored with 100 mL of diluent (see list of diluents under COMPATIBILITY AND STABILITY) and shaken until a clear solution is obtained.
13 mL Vials

Contents of the 13 mL vials must be suspended and transferred to 100 mL of an appropriate infusion solution.

A suggested procedure is to add approximately 10 mL from the appropriate infusion solution (see list of diluents under COMPATIBILITY AND STABILITY) to the vial. Shake well and transfer the resulting suspension to the infusion solution container.

CAUTION: THE SUSPENSION IS NOT FOR DIRECT INFUSION.

Repeat with an additional 10 mL of infusion solution to ensure complete transfer of vial contents to the infusion solution. **The resulting mixture should be agitated until clear.**

COMPATIBILITY AND STABILITY
Before reconstitution:

The dry powder should be stored at a temperature below 30°C.
Reconstituted solutions:

Solutions of PRIMAXIN range from colorless to yellow. Variations of color within this range do not affect the potency of the product.

PRIMAXIN, as supplied in infusion bottles and vials and reconstituted as above with the following diluents, maintains satisfactory potency for four hours at room temperature and for 24 hours under refrigeration (4°C) (note exception below). Solutions of PRIMAXIN should not be frozen.

0.9% Sodium Chloride Injection*
5% or 10% Dextrose Injection

---

*PRIMAXIN has been found to be stable in 0.9% Sodium Chloride Injection for 10 hours at room temperature and 48 hours under refrigeration.

PRIMAXIN®
(Imipenem-Cilastatin Sodium, MSD)

5% Dextrose Injection with 0.02% sodium bicarbonate solution

5% Dextrose and 0.9% Sodium Chloride Injection

5% Dextrose Injection with 0.225% or 0.45% saline solution

NORMOSOL† – M in D5-W

5% Dextrose Injection with 0.15% potassium chloride solution

Mannitol 2.5%, 5% and 10%

PRIMAXIN should not be mixed with or physically added to other antibiotics. However, PRIMAXIN may be administered concomitantly with other antibiotics, such as aminoglycosides.

HOW SUPPLIED

PRIMAXIN is supplied as a sterile powder mixture in vials and infusion bottles containing imipenem (anhydrous equivalent) and cilastatin sodium as follows:

No. 3514—250 mg imipenem equivalent and 250 mg cilastatin equivalent and 10 mg sodium bicarbonate as a buffer

NDC 0006-3514-74 in trays of 10 vials.

No. 3516—500 mg imipenem equivalent and 500 mg cilastatin equivalent and 20 mg sodium bicarbonate as a buffer

NDC 0006-3516-75 in trays of 10 vials.

No. 3515—250 mg imipenem equivalent and 250 mg cilastatin equivalent and 10 mg sodium bicarbonate as a buffer

NDC 0006-3515-74 in trays of 10 infusion bottles.

No. 3517—500 mg imipenem equivalent and 500 mg cilastatin equivalent and 20 mg sodium bicarbonate as a buffer

NDC 0006-3517-75 in trays of 10 infusion bottles.

MERCK SHARP & DOHME, Division of Merck & Co., INC. West Point, Pa. 19486

A.H.F.S. Category: 8:12.28

Issued November 1985   DC 7362400

---

†Registered trademark of Abbott Laboratories, Inc.